Beyond Assessment of Quality of Life in Schizophrenia

A. George Awad • Lakshmi N.P. Voruganti
Editors

Beyond Assessment of Quality of Life in Schizophrenia

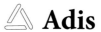

Editors
A. George Awad
Department of Psychiatry
University of Toronto and Humber
River Hospital
Toronto, Ontario
Canada

Lakshmi N.P. Voruganti
Department of Psychiatry
Oakville-Trafalgar Memorial Hospital
Oakville, Ontario
Canada

ISBN 978-3-319-30059-7   ISBN 978-3-319-30061-0   (eBook)
DOI 10.1007/978-3-319-30061-0

Library of Congress Control Number: 2016941540

Printed on acid-free paper

This Adis imprint is published by Springer Nature
The registered company is Springer International Publishing AG Switzerland

Foreword

A serious, systematic interest in assessing quality of life experiences of persons with schizophrenia appeared in the professional literature nearly four decades ago. As in other areas of health outcome assessment, there was a stirring sense at that time that simply measuring parameters of illness did not adequately capture the impacts of illness and treatment on the lives of patients. More broadly, this illness-focused approach did not adequately reflect the potential value of promoting and improving health. How do illness and treatment affect our ability to engage in all that life offers and our sense of well-being? These were heady questions, embedded in a broader sense of social activism, at a time when persons with schizophrenia lacked a voice about their care.

The context of this dawn of quality of life assessment provides context for this book. When quality of life assessment appeared on the scene, outcomes research in schizophrenia, as in most other disorders, stressed symptom reduction, symptom recurrence, and hospitalization. Strauss and Carpenter had only a few years earlier published their seminal work on the multiple dimensions of outcome in schizophrenia, showing that the course of symptoms, social functioning, and work impairment follow relatively independent trajectories. At the same time, leading policy voices raised critical social policy questions about how our changing systems of care were affecting persons with schizophrenia. Was deinstitutionalization a good thing? Were people with schizophrenia better off in the community? Quality of life assessment seemed a way to incorporate these health-related and humanistic concerns into the routine evaluation of treatments and social policies.

This early work on quality of life assessment in schizophrenia witnessed a proliferation of scales and primarily descriptive studies of quality of life experiences. At that time the focus was on a fairly broad notion of quality of life, capturing life experiences in many domains beyond health, such as housing, income, safety, interpersonal relationships, and neighborhoods. The advent of the newer generation of antipsychotic medications in the 1980s raised the hope these newer therapeutic agents with new modes of action and fewer (at least) different side effects would afford individuals with a better quality of life. We witnessed an intensified focus on quality of life outcomes in clinical trials. However, this hope did not pan out by and large. How could it be that these newer agents did not improve patient functioning and sense of well-being? This disappointment led to a much more critical consideration of the reliability and validity of self-reported quality of life, including how cognitive impairment inherent to schizophrenia may affect perception and judgment as well as how humans adapt psychologically to even the worst of circumstances to "make the best of things." Still, it appeared that at least from the perspective of patients, these new treatments were disappointing. Also, while quality of life assessment could document the adversity under which many persons with schizophrenia live, it was becoming clear that many of the vicissitudes of life – poverty, unemployment, substandard housing, violence, and social isolation – cannot be addressed directly by health care. Researchers realized that assessing the value of health care must be more focused. Hence the notion of "health-related quality of life" arose.

Despite all of these bumps in the road, assessment of quality of life has remained an important notion in health-care assessment. Why is this? This volume documents the many aspects of the history and current state of affairs of quality of life assessment. We see that it continues to evolve, both in how it is conceptualized and how it is measured. It seems embedded in our current notions of "patient-centered care" and "value-based treatment." It also certainly remains relevant today to considering the social circumstances of persons with schizophrenia living in our communities. One hopes that as our scientific understanding of the disorders that we now call schizophrenia grows and as new treatments emerge, we will truly be able to effectively incorporate quality of life into "value-based" assessments of "patient-centered" care. Finally we must retain the social values that led to interest in the quality of life of persons living with schizophrenia in the first place.

Baltimore, MD, USA   Anthony F. Lehman
October 2015

Preface

Quality of life has emerged over the past few decades as an attractive and important concept that reflects a new image of health, viewed from a biopsychosocial perspective. The concept has been applied as an important attribute in patient care, in clinical outcome studies, and in health economic analysis.

In psychiatry and the mental health field, quality of life, particularly in schizophrenia, evolved as the result of increased concerns about the plight of the chronically mentally ill who were discharged into the community as a result of deinstitutionalization in the 1960s. The pioneering efforts of Professor Antony F. Lehman, who has kindly and graciously contributed a foreword to this book, is credited for the significant growth of research interest in quality of life in schizophrenia. Such heightened interest has led to the extensive development of measuring tools and clearly documented the poor state of quality of life among persons suffering from schizophrenia. As publications multiplied, the majority of them have concerned themselves with measurement and documentation of the state of quality of life, and only a few publications have gone beyond assessments into how quality of life can impact clinical care, become an important component in pharmaco and health economics, as well as impacting resource utilization and health policy decision-making. Such gaps, in spite of the initial enthusiasm, have gradually undermined the usefulness of such construct and led to noticeable erosion in clinical and research interest. As we believe that the construct of quality of life in schizophrenia continues to be important and relevant, the idea of this book became clearer. We believe that the construct of quality of life in schizophrenia needs to be revisited for the purpose of refining it conceptually, bridging the gaps and going beyond measurement to its significant applications in impacting clinical care and health economics. We have been fortunate to be able to sign in contributions from a number of leading experts in the field who share with us in the importance of quality of life assessment in schizophrenia going beyond assessments, and for that we are most grateful.

The topics covered in this book are constructed under four major parts. The first part deals with basic and conceptual issues, which includes a synopsis of psychopathology of schizophrenia issues, issues that slowed progress in the development of quality of life in schizophrenia, social cognition and its relevance to quality of life, cultural adaptation, and the role of culture in assessments of health-related quality of life in schizophrenia.

The second part includes a critical review of quality of life measures currently in use, modern approaches in scaling and the development of measuring tools, the electronic technology and its role in future advances in assessments of outcomes, quality of life assessments in the development and clinical trials of antipsychotics from the pharmaceutical industry perspective, and assessment of burden of care and quality of life of caregivers in schizophrenia.

The third part deals with important issues beyond assessment and includes a model for integration of quality of life assessments in care plans, quality of life as an outcome and mediator of other outcomes, use of quality of life measurement in cost-effectiveness and how to impact public health policy and resource allocation. A case study from India as a developing country illustrates the interplay of clinical, cultural, economic, and resources issues.

The final part provides an outline of future challenges in an effort to reinvigorate the construct of quality of life in schizophrenia.

Developing a book with multiple contributors, as in any extensive project, requires a high level of coordination and editorial management, which, in our case, has been efficiently provided by Ms. Pamela Walsh, for whom we acknowledge her assistance. We hope that this book can prove of value to clinicians, researchers, health- and pharmaco-economists, as well as health policy decision-makers. We hope this book is perceived in terms, not as conclusions, but as the beginning of an important conversation that needs to take place among all stakeholders, in an effort to invigorate such an important and relevant construct, not only for the benefit of the individual, but for the society as a whole.

Toronto, Canada   A. George Awad
Oakville, Canada   Lakshmi N.P. Voruganti

Contents

Contributors

Susana Al-Halabí, PhD Centro de Investigación Biomédica en Red de Salud Mental, CIBERSAM, Oviedo, Spain

Pascal Auquier, MD, PhD Research Unit, Public Health, Chronic Diseases and Quality of Life, Aix – Marseille University, EA3279, Marseille, France

A. George Awad Department of Psychiatry, The Institute of Medical Science, University of Toronto, Toronto, ON, Canada

Vicent Balanzá-Martinez, MD, PhD Teaching Unit of Psychiatry, Department of Medicine, School of Medicine, La Fe University and Polytechnic Hospital, University of Valencia, CIBERSAM, Valencia, Spain

María Teresa Bascarán, MD, PhD Centro de Investigación Biomédica en Red de Salud Mental, CIBERSAM, Oviedo, Spain

Karine Baumstarck, MD, PhD Research Unit, Public Health, Chronic Diseases and Quality of Life, Aix – Marseille University, EA3279, Marseille, France

Per Bech, MD, PhD Psychiatric Research Unit, CCMH, Mental Health Centre North Zealand, Hillerød, Denmark

Jakob B. Bjorner Patient Insights, Lincoln, RI, USA

Department of Public Health, University of Copenhagen, Copenhagen, Denmark

National Research Centre for the Working Environment, Copenhagen, Denmark

Julio Bobes, MD, PhD Department of Psychiatry, University of Oviedo, Oviedo, Spain

Centro de Investigación Biomédica en Red de Salud Mental, CIBERSAM, Oviedo, Spain

María Teresa Bobes-Bascaran, PhD Centro de Investigación Biomédica en Red de Salud Mental, CIBERSAM, Valencia, Spain

Laurent Boyer, MD PhD Research Unit, Public Health, Chronic Diseases and Quality of Life, Aix–Marseille University, EA3279, Marseille, France

Sofia Brissos, MD Centro Hospitalar Psiquiátrico de Lisboa (Lisbon's Psychiatric Hospitalar Centre), Lisbon, Portugal

Raimund Buller, MD Clinical Development, Lundbeck, Issy-les-Moulineaux, France

Monika Bullinger, PhD Institute for Medical Psychology, Centre for Psychosocial Medicine, University Medical Centre Hamburg-Eppendorf, Hamburg, Germany

Jerome Carson School of Education and Psychology, University of Bolton, Bolton, UK

Santosh K. Chaturvedi, MD, FRCPsych Department of Mental Health Education, National Institute of Mental Health & Neurosciences, Bangalore, India

Department of Psychiatry, National Institute of Mental Health & Neurosciences, Bangalore, India

Leticia García-Álvarez, PhD Department of Psychiatry, University of Oviedo, Oviedo, Spain

Centro de Investigación Biomédica en Red de Salud Mental, CIBERSAM, Oviedo, Spain

María Paz García-Portilla, MD, PhD Department of Psychiatry, University of Oviedo, Oviedo, Spain

Centro de Investigación Biomédica en Red de Salud Mental, CIBERSAM, Oviedo, Spain

Domenico Giacco, MD, PhD Unit for Social and Community Psychiatry, WHO Collaborating Centre for Mental Health Services Development, Queen Mary University of London, East London NHS Foundation Trust, Newham Centre for Mental Health, London, UK

Lieuwe de Haan Psychotic Disorders, AMC Academic Psychiatric Centre, Amsterdam, The Netherlands

Early Psychosis, AMC Psychiatry, Amsterdam, AZ, The Netherlands

Frank Holloway, FRCPsych South London and Maudsley NHS Foundation Trust, Beckenham, UK

Maudsley Hospital, Denmark Hill, London, UK

Amir Kalali, MD Neuroscience Center of Excellence, Quintiles, San Diego, CA, USA

Anne Karow, MD Department of Psychiatry and Psychotherapy & Department of Child and Adolescent Psychiatry, Centre for Psychosocial Medicine, University Medical Centre Hamburg-Eppendorf, Hamburg, Germany

Richard Keefe, PhD Psychiatry & Behavioral Sciences and Psychology & Neuroscience, Duke University Medical Center, Durham, NC, USA

Martin Lambert, MD Department of Psychiatry and Psychotherapy & Department of Child and Adolescent Psychiatry, Centre for Psychosocial Medicine, University Medical Centre Hamburg-Eppendorf, Hamburg, Germany

Pilar A. Sáiz Martínez, MD, PhD Department of Psychiatry, University of Oviedo, Oviedo, Spain

Centro de Investigación Biomédica en Red de Salud Mental, CIBERSAM, Oviedo, Spain

Isabel Menendez-Miranda, MD PhD Mental Health Services of Asturias, Oviedo, Spain

Inez Myin-Germeys Department of Neuroscience, Centre for Contextual Psychiatry, KU Leuven, Belgium

Department of Psychiatry and Psychology, School of Mental Health and Neuroscience, Maastricht University, Maastricht, The Netherlands

Elizabeth Pappadopulos, PhD Pfizer Inc, New York, NY, USA

Abhishek Pathak, MD Department of Psychiatry, National Institute of Mental Health & Neurosciences, Bangalore, India

Guilherme Pereira, MD Centro Hospitalar Psiquiátrico de Lisboa (Lisbon's Psychiatric Hospitalar Centre), Lisbon, Portugal

M. Krishna Prasad, MD Department of Psychiatry, National Institute of Mental Health & Neurosciences, Bangalore, India

Stefan Priebe, DiplPsych, DrMedHabil, FRCPsych Unit for Social and Community Psychiatry, WHO Collaborating Centre for Mental Health Services Development, Queen Mary University of London, Newham Centre for Mental Health, London, UK

Christophe Sapin, MSc Global Analytics, Lundbeck A/S, Issy-les-Moulineaux, France

Mary V. Seeman Department of Psychiatry, The Institute of Medical Science, University of Toronto, Toronto, ON, Canada

Monika Vance Santium Mental Health, Vaughan, ON, Canada

Lakshmi N.P. Voruganti, MD, Msc, PhD Department of Psychiatry, Oakville-Trafalgar Memorial Hospital, Oakville, ON, Canada

Iris de Wit, MSc Early Psychosis, AMC Psychiatry, Amsterdam, AZ, The Netherlands

Department Early Psychosis, AMC, Academic Psychiatric Centre, Amsterdam, AZ, The Netherlands

Part I
Basic and Conceptual Issues

Chapter 1
Schizophrenia and Its Sequelae

Mary V. Seeman

The psychiatric disease category, schizophrenia, is defined by its symptoms – e.g., hallucinations (false perceptions), delusions (false beliefs), and disorganized speech and behavior, often accompanied by defects in attention, memory, reasoning, and judgment. The same symptoms are seen in other forms of psychotic illness, but when they endure over time, when emotional and linguistic expression is restricted or out of keeping with the situation, when there is difficulty in initiating goal-directed behavior, and when the person experiencing the symptoms becomes functionally disabled over time, the disorder is called schizophrenia. It is important to know that symptoms may come and go, sometimes disappear, sometimes peak, and that any two individuals diagnosed with schizophrenia may suffer from substantially different symptoms (American Psychiatric Association APA 2013). The degree of suffering and the degree of subsequent disability varies among individuals similarly diagnosed. Although schizophrenia used to be referred to as *dementia praecox*, the person with schizophrenia is not demented in the way the term is used today. When cognitively tested, he or she may do relatively poorly on objective tests of verbal fluency, short-term and working memory, and speed of processing new information, but vocabulary, grammar, and spatial skills will probably remain intact (Sheffield et al. 2014).

The diagnosis of schizophrenia is currently symptom-based, and symptoms are ascertained by standardized questionnaires. The most important diagnostic criterion, however, is functional decline, which means that persons with schizophrenia are seen by others, and see themselves, as disabled. Diagnostic divisions into historic subcategories such as paranoid, disorganized, catatonic forms of illness are no longer current. A dimensional approach to psychiatric diagnosis, based on the realization that underlying brain impairments cut across today's diagnostic categories, is currently being considered (Insel et al. 2010), but is not yet generally accepted.

M.V. Seeman
Department of Psychiatry, The Institute of Medical Science, University of Toronto, Toronto, ON, Canada
e-mail: mary.seeman@utoronto.ca

© Springer International Publishing Switzerland 2016   3
A.G. Awad, L.N.P. Voruganti (eds.), *Beyond Assessment of Quality of Life in Schizophrenia*, DOI 10.1007/978-3-319-30061-0_1

1.1 Epidemiology

Schizophrenia is diagnosed in every country in the world. Global prevalence is in the range of 1.4–4.6 per 1,000, and incidence rate is in the range of 0.16–0.42 per 1,000 people (Kirkbride et al. 2012). The disorder affects approximately 50 million people worldwide, and its global economic burden is calculated to be between 1.5 and 3 % of total health expenditures (Charrier et al. 2013). Men show a somewhat higher incidence than women, an earlier onset age, more negative symptoms, more neurologic deficits, a worse premorbid history, a worse course of illness until about age 50, and a poorer response to most treatments (Abel et al. 2010; Seeman 2012b). This implicates sex-specific factors in pathophysiology. Among first- and second-generation immigrants to Western countries, important ethnic differences have been found in incidence rates of the disorder (Kirkbride et al. 2012). Since rates in the respective countries of origin are unremarkable, the process of immigration and resettlement looms as a potential risk factor for some newcomers, but not for others.

1.2 Etiology

There is no single cause of schizophrenia. The disorder appears to result from multiple factors that take the form of genetic and epigenetic "hits," environmental and psychological traumas, and hormonal as well as immune changes that, together, alter the brain's chemistry and function. Approximately 80 % of the variation in whether one is or is not diagnosed with schizophrenia has been attributed to genetic factors (Sullivan et al. 2003). Current day thinking is that many common genetic alterations, each with a small effect, can raise the risk for schizophrenia. Among others, genetic regions involved in immune function have been strongly associated with schizophrenia in genome-wide association studies. In addition to multiple genes of small effect, there may be a few uncommon genetic alterations, still unspecified, that exert a larger influence (Doherty et al. 2012). Diagnostic specificity for risk genes is modest at best. The same genes that contribute to the risk for schizophrenia also appear to confer risk for other psychiatric disorders (Stefansson et al. 2009).

Susceptibility genes often do not act alone, but interact with environmental factors to increase risk. An example is the AKT1 gene that codes for a serine/threonine kinase and plays a role in regulating cell survival, insulin signaling, angiogenesis, and tumor formation. There appears to be an interaction between this gene and the use of cannabis on the risk of psychosis (Di Forti et al. 2012). In other words, cannabis smoking seems to be a risk for psychosis only in those with a specific genetic makeup. Other similar examples of gene-environment interactions have been reported (European Network of National Networks studying Gene-Environment Interactions in Schizophrenia EU-GEI 2014).

Inflammation may be important in the pathophysiology of schizophrenia (Bergink et al. 2014) as levels of cytokines are increased in this disorder (Song et al. 2013).

Because the risk for schizophrenia is raised for those born in winter and spring months, viral causation has been hypothesized. A high incidence among those living in crowded conditions – low socioeconomic conditions, urban residence, and cohabiting large families – also implies a role for infectious agents. It is known that a pregnant mother's exposure to viral infection raises the risk for schizophrenia in her child (Khandaker et al. 2013). A bi-directional association has also been proposed between psychosis and autoimmune disease, with both forms of illness increasing the risk of the other form (Benros et al. 2012). All these facts point to inflammation as a potential etiological factor in psychosis. Oxidative stress as a causative factor has also been proposed (Flatow et al. 2013). Cerebral anoxia is another hypothetical causative factor (Tejkalová et al. 2007). Studies have reported increased schizophrenia risks in association with obstetrical problems such as bleeding during pregnancy, prolonged labor, short gestation, and low birthweight (Suvisaari et al. 2013), all of which are capable of causing oxygen deprivation in the fetus and newborn.

From a psychological perspective, many environmental stressors such as early parental loss and neglect or abuse in childhood have been hypothesized as risk factors for schizophrenia, operating via biological stress pathways (Lodge and Grace 2011). No less than three-quarters of patients in early psychosis programs endorse childhood exposure to trauma (Barker et al. 2015, Duhig et al. 2015).

To make sense of the relatively high rates of schizophrenia in low socioeconomic classes and in immigrants, especially black immigrants to white societies, the social defeat hypothesis has been proposed in which long-term exposure to the experience of social defeat is thought to sensitize the mesolimbic dopamine system and, through such sensitization, increase the risk for schizophrenia (Selten et al. 2013).

Many other causative factors have been considered, but all are difficult to investigate because each potential factor interacts with so many others and may only be operative during specific time periods of heightened vulnerability. Specificity remains problematic because the outcome of the same risk factors can be schizophrenia, mood disorder, addictive disorder, or personality disorder.

1.3 Pathology

Neurochemically, schizophrenia is associated with brain dopamine system disruption. More than 20 animal models of schizophrenia show an excessive amount of the high-affinity state of the dopamine D2 receptor in postmortem brain. This causes biochemical and behavioral dopamine overactivity (Seeman 2011). Other neurotransmitters (GABA and glutamate) may also play a role in the expression of schizophrenia (Moghaddam and Javitt 2012).

Imaging techniques have shown structural alterations in the brain, such as enlargement of the third and lateral ventricles and modest reductions in whole-brain gray matter volume and in temporal, frontal, and limbic regions (Shepherd et al. 2012). There appears to be abnormal maturation of prefrontal networks in schizophrenia during late adolescence and early adulthood, perhaps a result of excessive pruning of synapses and dendritic spines during this period (Feinberg 1982). Myelination of nerve tracts is also abnormal (Matthews et al. 2012). Functional imaging studies have pointed to reduced activation of the dorsolateral prefrontal cortex during tasks of executive function (Minzenberg et al. 2009) and unusual limbic system activation during experimental tasks that use emotional stimuli (Gur et al. 2007).

Diffusion tensor imaging has shown white matter changes in frontal and temporal lobes, suggesting decreased connectivity among these regions (Yao et al. 2013) so much so that schizophrenia has been conceptualized as a disorder of disrupted connections between nerve cells and between brain circuits (Zhang et al. 2015).

1.4 Life Course

Although schizophrenia is considered a neurodevelopmental disorder (Lewis and Levitt 2002), with pathogenic factors already operative in fetal life, symptoms are not usually expressed until adolescence or early adulthood (Harrop and Trower 2001). Onset is later in women, who may not develop symptoms until their fourth or fifth decade (Abel et al. 2010; Seeman 2012b). Some subtle signs (memory problems, impairments in gross motor skills, attention problems, mixed handedness, eye tracking dysfunction, social deficits) may, in some cases, be apparent premorbidly in childhood (Niemi et al. 2005). The first 5–10 years after symptoms start are typically the most difficult and are a dangerous period with respect to potential suicide. The severity of illness tends to plateau after middle age, at least in men (Schultz et al. 1997). In women, the postmenopausal years may be particularly taxing (Abel et al. 2010; Seeman 2012b).

1.5 Sequelae of Schizophrenia

The experience of living with schizophrenia may result in severe depression and lead to suicide attempts in between 20 and 50 % of people. Approximately 10 % of schizophrenia patients die by suicide (Carlborg et al. 2010). Other potential sequelae of the disorder are anxiety (Braga et al. 2013); a decline in cognitive skills; a decline in educational and occupational functioning (Vargas et al. 2014); perceived discrimination at the hands of family, friends, employers, and strangers (Gerlinger et al. 2013); social isolation; and the usual consequences of low socioeconomic status – poor housing, poor nutrition, poor health, and few opportunities for improvement. Smoking and substance abuse are prevalent and can lead to a variety of physical ailments that contribute to high mortality rates in this population (Laursen et al. 2014). Most people with schizophrenia remain single, but approximately 50 % of women with schizophrenia give birth; they may not, however, retain custody of their children, and, whether reared at home or in foster care, their children show high rates of psychiatric disability (Seeman 2012a). In competitive societies, employment rates of people with schizophrenia are low (Greve and Nielsen 2013). Imprisonment rates are high (Ghoreishi et al. 2015); violence rates are high (van Dorn et al. 2012);

victimization rates are disproportionately high (Bengtsson-Tops and Ehliasson 2012). Regardless of symptoms and symptom control, the sequelae of schizophrenia undermine the quality of life available to individuals with this diagnosis.

1.6 Treatment

In analogy to other illnesses, early effective treatment of symptoms or shortening the duration of untreated psychosis leads to improved long-term outcome. Some advocate treatment (though not necessarily with antipsychotic medication) starting in the prodromal stage because approximately 35 % of those in the "ultrahigh-risk state" (Simon and Umbricht 2010) will go on to develop schizophrenia. Most of those who do not develop schizophrenia develop other kinds of psychopathology necessitating treatment (Lin et al. 2015).

Early intervention during the prodrome (Schmidt et al. 2015) usually focuses on psychoeducation for the patient and the family, the teaching of self-management skills, often in a group format; the treatment of depression, anxiety, obsessions, insomnia, anorexia, or other nonpsychotic symptoms; and the promotion of social support within the community. Motivational interviewing is used to enhance interest in self-help and in skills learning. Attention is paid to diet and exercise, and links are established with schools and vocational agencies.

Acute episodes of schizophrenia in the emergency department or inpatient ward are treated with antipsychotic drugs, sometimes by injection in order to calm the patient quickly. Antianxiety agents can be used as adjuncts. Usually, the patient is then switched to an oral drug, although depot drugs (monthly injections) can also be used for maintenance. The full benefit of a drug can take 6–8 weeks to be evident. Drugs are continued as long as symptoms persist and usually later. Doses can be considerably reduced but, once vulnerability to psychosis has emerged, stopping drugs altogether often precipitates a relapse. Drug choices and doses need to be regularly monitored for effectiveness against symptoms, for their effect on daily life, and for their potential adverse effects (Hasan et al. 2012).

Schizophrenia needs to be seen as a chronic illness. That does not mean that the patient cannot recover from most of the symptoms, or cannot enjoy life to the fullest, but it does mean that, after an acute episode, the patient continues to be vulnerable to relapse.

1.6.1 Psychosocial Maintenance Treatment

To guard against relapse and to promote an acceptable quality of life, effective medication management needs to be accompanied by psychosocial interventions (Dixon et al. 2010). Motivational interviewing encourages patients to change risky behavior (nonadherence to treatment, sedentary habits, social avoidance, dangerous sexual or aggressive behavior, unhealthy eating, smoking, beer drinking, and illegal drug use). The effect has been most studied with respect to adherence with antipsychotic treatment (Barkhof et al. 2013) and abstinence from substance abuse (Barrowclough et al. 2001), but can apply to any behavior that needs changing.

Assertive Community Treatment (ACT) is an evidence-based, multidisciplinary team approach to serving seriously mentally ill patients in the community. Mental health workers and peer support workers visit patients and provide practical help with health, income, housing, employment, schooling, family issues including parenting, and leisure time and occupation needs. ACT is a long-term approach aimed at preventing relapse and improving quality of life (Huguelet et al. 2012).

Cognitive remediation therapy (Wykes et al. 2007) targets cognitive deficits in attention, memory, and executive function. It is usually computer-based and can be fun for the patient to engage in, but gains acquired may not last. Cognitive behavioral therapy (CBT) aims to break cycles of repetitive thoughts and behaviors that maintain dysfunction. This therapy can be aimed at specific symptoms and has been more successful in ameliorating hallucinations and delusions (Wykes et al. 2008) than it has been in reducing negative symptoms (Elis et al. 2013). Gains must be periodically reinforced; otherwise they are lost. Acceptance and commitment therapy is based on mindfulness principles. The idea is to encourage people to observe their thoughts and feelings from a distance, to accept their symptoms as natural phenomena that do not need to be repudiated, resisted, or suppressed. Once symptoms and diagnoses are accepted and a normative meaning is attached to them, patients are guided toward meeting their individual recovery goals (Bach and Hayes 2002).

Vocational programs are aimed at preparing the patient for employment and helping to place the patient in either sheltered or full-time supported positions (Bond et al. 2008). Housing programs (Gilmer et al. 2014) provide appropriate housing for severely mentally ill people as a priority, before engagement in treatment. Parenting programs (Krumm et al. 2013) support parents with mental illness and model parenting skills. Social skills training is a behavioral method that targets social deficits in order to improve interpersonal interaction (Horan et al. 2011). Because improvements in social skills are reinforced in daily life, they may persist once taught (Rus-Calafell et al. 2014).

Family psychoeducation teaches family members about the nature of the illness and about the role of stress in exacerbating symptoms. Families are taught how to recognize early warning signs, how to intervene in a crisis, how to solve problems as they emerge, and how to cope with difficult situations. Family members are also taught how to temper their own critical or hostile remarks toward the patient and how to deal more effectively with their own personal difficulties (Lucksted et al. 2012).

1.6.2 Pharmacological Treatment

Drugs that reverse neurochemical abnormalities are the cornerstone of the treatment of schizophrenia. All current drugs interfere with dopamine transmission by blocking the dopamine D2 receptor (Seeman 2006), which reduces psychotic symptoms but leaves negative symptoms essentially untouched. The general efficacy of all the antipsychotic drugs is similar (Leucht et al. 2013), but their side effects differ and individuals may, for unknown reasons, respond better to one drug than to another. Patients who are resistant to many drugs will often respond to clozapine, used in North America as a drug of last resort (McEvoy et al. 2006). Unfortunately this drug has many side effects, one of which, agranulocytosis, requires routine blood monitoring. Long-acting injectable antipsychotics (once a month depots) are helpful in the treatment of patients who find it difficult to regularly take oral medication, but depot drugs do not help to develop patients' abilities to self-manage their symptoms (Kreyenbuhl et al. 2011).

Antipsychotic drugs have many side effects that can create difficulties for patients and can further undermine their quality of life. Most side effects, but not all, are dose dependent, with low doses ensuring freedom from unwanted effects. The older antipsychotic drugs, as a group, tend to induce extrapyramidal effects of which the most serious is tardive dyskinesia, unsightly and uncomfortable motor movements that persist even when the drug is stopped. The newer drugs, as a group, induce weight gain, with subsequent risk for diabetes, cardiovascular problems, and metabolic syndrome. Antipsychotic drugs also may result in sexual difficulties, hormonal problems, and daytime sedation that interferes with daily function (Leucht et al. 2009). Men and women suffer from somewhat different adverse effects of antipsychotic drugs (Seeman 2009). Adjunctive drugs, diet plans, and exercise programs can help prevent or reduce these adverse effects.

Because of the current interest in the role of inflammation and oxidative stress in the pathophysiology of schizophrenia, anti-inflammatory and antioxidant agents are being tried as adjunctive treatments, with aspirin, estrogen, and N-acetylcysteine showing some positive effects (Sommer et al. 2014). There is relatively limited information on the effectiveness of the use of adjunctive pharmacological agents for negative or cognitive symptoms or for the treatment of concomitant substance abuse (Kreyenbuhl et al. 2011).

1.7 Conclusion

Schizophrenia is considered one of the most serious mental illnesses in terms of its adverse impact on quality of life, not only of the patient but also of the patient's family and of the patient's community. Many individuals with schizophrenia, however, are content with their lives. In one study, the level of happiness experienced by patients with schizophrenia correlated with psychological factors such as low perceived stress, a sense of resilience, of optimism, and of personal mastery, but, contrary to expectation, did not correlate with sociodemographic characteristics, duration of illness, severity of symptoms, physical function, medical comorbidity, or cognitive functioning (Palmer et al. 2014). Much remains to be understood about the factors that contribute to satisfaction with one's life.

Quality of life in the context of illness is a complex concept. It depends not only on the severity of symptoms and the degree to which they interfere with life's goals but, in addition, on a number of interacting social, economic, health, psychological, and treatment variables. Maintaining hope in a better future is an important ingredient of satisfaction with one's life (Kylmä et al. 2006), but, in schizophrenia, at least one study has shown that quality of life worsens with age (Cichocki et al. 2015). Ensuring that future studies come to different conclusions is the purpose of researching quality of life issues in schizophrenia.

References

Abel KM, Drake R, Goldstein JM. Sex differences in schizophrenia. Int Rev Psychiatry. 2010;2:417–28.

American Psychiatric Association (APA). Diagnostic and statistical manual of mental disorders. 5th ed. Arlington: American Psychiatric Publishing; 2013.

Bach P, Hayes SC. The use of acceptance and commitment therapy to prevent the rehospitalization of psychotic patients: a randomized controlled trial. J Consult Clin Psychol. 2002;70:1129–39.

Barker V, Gumley A, Schwannauer M, Lawrie SM. An integrated biopsychosocial model of childhood maltreatment and psychosis. Br J Psychiatry. 2015;206:177–80.

Barkhof E, Meijer CJ, de Sonneville LM, Linszen DH, de Haan L. The effect of motivational interviewing on medication adherence and hospitalization rates in nonadherent patients with multi-episode schizophrenia. Schizophr Bull. 2013;39:1242–51.

Barrowclough C, Haddock G, Tarrier N, Lewis SW, Moring J, O'Brien R, et al. Randomized controlled trial of motivational interviewing, cognitive behavior therapy, and family intervention for patients with comorbid schizophrenia and substance use disorders. Am J Psychiatry. 2001;158:1706–13.

Bengtsson-Tops A, Ehliasson K. Victimization in individuals suffering from psychosis: a swedish cross-sectional study. J Psychiatr Ment Health Nurs. 2012;19:23–30.

Benros ME, Mortensen PB, Eaton WW. Autoimmune diseases and infections as risk factors for schizophrenia. Ann N Y Acad Sci. 2012;1262:56–66.

Bergink V, Gibney SM, Drexhage HA. Autoimmunity, inflammation, and psychosis: a search for peripheral markers. Biol Psychiatry. 2014;75:324–31.

Bond GR, Drake RE, Becker DR. An update on randomized controlled trials of evidence-based supported employment. Psychiatr Rehabil J. 2008;31:280–90.

Braga RJ, Reynolds GP, Siris SG. Anxiety comorbidity in schizophrenia. Psychiatry Res. 2013;210:1–7.

Carlborg A, Winnerbäck K, Jönsson EG, Jokinen J, Nordström P. Suicide in schizophrenia. Expert Rev Neurother. 2010;10:1153–64.

Charrier N, Chevreul K, Durand-Zaleski I. The cost of schizophrenia: a literature review. Encéphale. 2013;39 Suppl 1:S49–56.

Cichocki Ł, Cechnicki A, Franczyk-Glita J, Błądziński P, Kalisz A, Wroński K. Quality of life in a 20-year follow-up study of people suffering from schizophrenia. Compr Psychiatry. 2015;56:133–40.

Di Forti M, Iyegbe C, Sallis H, Kolliakou A, Falcone MA, Paparelli A, et al. Confirmation that the AKT1 (rs2494732) genotype influences the risk of psychosis in cannabis users. Biol Psychiatry. 2012;72:811–6.

Dixon LB, Dickerson F, Bellack AS, Bennett M, Dickinson D, Goldberg RW, et al. The 2009 schizophrenia PORT psychosocial treatment recommendations and summary statements. Schizophr Bull. 2010;36:48–70.

Doherty JL, O'Donovan MC, Owen MJ. Recent genomic advances in schizophrenia. Clin Genet. 2012;81:103–9.

Duhig M, Patterson S, Connell M, Foley S, Capra C, Dark F, Gordon A, Singh S, Hides L, McGrath JJ, Scott J. The prevalence and correlates of childhood trauma in patients with early psychosis. Aust N Z J Psychiatry. 2015;49:651–9.

Elis O, Caponigro JM, Kring AM. Psychosocial treatments for future directions. Clin Psychol Rev. 2013;33:914–28.

European Network of National Networks studying Gene-Environment Interactions in Schizophrenia (EU-GEI). Identifying gene-environment interactions in schizophrenia: contemporary challenges for integrated, large-scale investigations. Schizophr Bull. 2014;40:729–36.

Feinberg I. Schizophrenia: caused by a fault in programmed synaptic elimination during adolescence? J Psychiatr Res. 1982;17:319–34.

Flatow J, Buckley P, Miller BJ. Meta-analysis of oxidative stress in schizophrenia. Biol Psychiatry. 2013;74:400–9.

Gerlinger G, Hauser M, Hert M, Lacluyse K, Wampers M, Correll CU. Personal stigma in schizophrenia spectrum disorders: a systematic review of prevalence rates, correlates, impact and interventions. World Psychiatry. 2013;12:155–64.

Ghoreishi A, Kabootvand S, Zangani E, Bazargan-Hejazi S, Ahmadi A, Khazaie H. Prevalence and attributes of criminality in patients with schizophrenia. J Inj Violence Res. 2015;7:7–12.

Gilmer TP, Stefancic A, Katz ML, Sklar M, Tsemberis S, Palinkas LA. Fidelity to the housing first model and effectiveness of permanent supported housing programs in California. Psychiatr Serv. 2014;65:1311–7.

Greve J, Nielsen LH. Useful beautiful minds-an analysis of the relationship between schizophrenia and employment. J Health Econ. 2013;32:1066–76.

Gur RE, Loughead J, Kohler CG, Elliott MA, Lesko K, Ruparel K, et al. Limbic activation associated with misidentification of fearful faces and flat affect in schizophrenia. Arch Gen Psychiatry. 2007;64:1356–66.

Harrop C, Trower P. Why does schizophrenia develop at late adolescence? Clin Psychol Rev. 2001;21:241–65.

Hasan A, Falkai P, Wobrock T, Lieberman J, Glenthoj B, Gattaz WF, et al. World Federation of Societies of Biological Psychiatry (WFSBP) Guidelines for Biological Treatment of Schizophrenia, part 1: update 2012 on the acute treatment of schizophrenia and the management of treatment resistance. World J Biol Psychiatry. 2012;13:318–78.

Horan WP, Kern RS, Tripp C, Hellemann G, Wynn JK, Bell M, et al. Efficacy and specificity of social cognitive skills training for outpatients with psychotic disorders. J Psychiatr Res. 2011;45:1113–22.

Huguelet P, Koellner V, Boulguy S, Nagalingum K, Amani S, Borras L, Perroud N. Effects of an assertive community program in patients with severe mental disorders and impact on their families. Psychiatry Clin Neurosci. 2012;66:328–36.

Insel T, Cuthbert B, Garvey M, Heinssen R, Pine DS, Quinn K, et al. Research domain criteria (RDoC): toward a new classification framework for research on mental disorders. Am J Psychiatry. 2010;167:748–51.

Khandaker GM, Zimbron J, Lewis G, Jones PB. Prenatal maternal infection, neurodevelopment and adult schizophrenia: a systematic review of population-based studies. Psychol Med. 2013;43:239–57.

Kirkbride JB, Errazuriz A, Croudace TJ, Morgan C, Jackson D, Boydell J, et al. Incidence of schizophrenia and other psychoses in England, 1950–2009: a systematic review and meta-analyses. PLoS One. 2012;7:e31660.

Kreyenbuhl J, Buchanan R, Kelly D, Noel J, Boggs D, Fischer B, et al. The 2009 schizophrenia patient outcomes research team (PORT) psychopharmacological treatment recommendations. Int Clin Psychopharmacol. 2011;26:e54–5.

Krumm S, Becker T, Wiegand-Grefe S. Mental health services for parents affected by mental illness. Curr Opin Psychiatry. 2013;26:362–8.

Kylmä J, Juvakka T, Nikkonen M, Korhonen T, Isohanni M. Hope and schizophrenia: an integrative review. J Psychiatr Ment Health Nurs. 2006;13:651–64.

Laursen TM, Nordentoft M, Mortensen PB. Excess early mortality in schizophrenia. Annu Rev Clin Psychol. 2014;10:425–48.

Leucht S, Corves C, Arbter D, Engel RR, Li C, Davis JM. Second-generation versus first-generation antipsychotic drugs for schizophrenia: a meta-analysis. Lancet. 2009;373:31–41.

Leucht S, Cipriani A, Spineli L, Mavridis D, Orey D, Richter F, et al. Comparative efficacy and tolerability of 15 antipsychotic drugs in schizophrenia: a multiple-treatments meta-analysis. Lancet. 2013;382:951–62.

Lewis DA, Levitt P. Schizophrenia as a disorder of neurodevelopment. Annu Rev Neurosci. 2002;25:409–32.

Lin A, Wood SJ, Nelson B, Beavan A, McGorry P, Yung AR. Outcomes of nontransitioned cases in a sample at ultra-high risk for psychosis. Am J Psychiatry. 2015;172:249–58.

Lodge DJ, Grace AA. Developmental pathology, dopamine, stress and schizophrenia. Int J Dev Neurosci. 2011;29:207–13.

Lucksted A, McFarlane W, Downing D, Dixon L. Recent developments in family psychoeducation as an evidence-based practice. J Marital Fam Ther. 2012;38:101–21.

Matthews PR, Eastwood SL, Harrison PJ. Reduced myelin basic protein and actin-related gene expression in visual cortex in schizophrenia. PLoS One. 2012;7, e38211.

McEvoy JP, Lieberman JA, Stroup TS, Davis SM, Meltzer HY, Rosenheck RA, et al. Effectiveness of clozapine versus olanzapine, quetiapine, and risperidone in patients with chronic schizophrenia who did not respond to prior atypical antipsychotic treatment. Am J Psychiatry. 2006;163:600–10.

Minzenberg MJ, Laird AR, Thelen S, Carter CS, Glahn DC. Meta-analysis of 41 functional neuroimaging studies of executive function in schizophrenia. Arch Gen Psychiatry. 2009;66:811–22.

Moghaddam B, Javitt D. From revolution to evolution: the glutamate hypothesis of schizophrenia and its implication for treatment. Neuropsychopharmacology. 2012;37:4–15.

Niemi LT, Suvisaari JM, Haukka JK, Lönnqvist JK. Childhood predictors of future psychiatric morbidity in offspring of mothers with psychotic disorder results from the Helsinki High-Risk Study. Br J Psychiatry. 2005;186:108–14.

Palmer BW, Sirkin MA, Depp CA, Glorioso DK, Jeste DV. Wellness within illness: happiness in schizophrenia. Schizophr Res. 2014;159:151–6.

Rus-Calafell M, Gutiérrez-Maldonado J, Ribas-Sabaté J. A virtual reality integrated program for improving social skills in patients with schizophrenia: a pilot study. J Behav Ther Exp Psychiatry. 2014;45:81–9.

Schmidt SJ, Schultze-Lutter F, Schimmelmann BG, Maric NP, Salokangas RK, Riecher-Rössler A, et al. EPA guidance on the early intervention in clinical high risk states of psychoses. Eur Psychiatry. 2015;30:388–404.

Schultz SK, Miller DD, Oliver SE, Arndt S, Flaum M, Andreasen NC. The life course of schizophrenia: age and symptom dimensions. Schizophr Res. 1997;23:15–23.

Seeman P. Targeting the dopamine D2 receptor in schizophrenia. Expert Opin Ther Targets. 2006;10:515–31.

Seeman MV. Secondary effects of antipsychotics: women at greater risk than men. Schizophr Bull. 2009;35:937–48.

Seeman P. All roads to schizophrenia lead to dopamine supersensitivity and elevated dopamine D2High receptors. CNS Neurosci Ther. 2011;17:118–32.

Seeman MV. Intervention to prevent child custody loss in mothers with schizophrenia. Schizophr Res Treatment. 2012a;2012:796763.

Seeman MV. Women and psychosis. Womens Health. 2012b;8:215–24.

Selten JP, van der Ven E, Rutten BP, Cantor-Graae E. The social defeat hypothesis of schizophrenia: an update. Schizophr Bull. 2013;39:1180–6.

Sheffield JM, Gold JM, Strauss ME, Carter CS, MacDonald III AW, Ragland JD, et al. Common and specific cognitive deficits in schizophrenia: relationships to function. Cogn Affect Behav Neurosci. 2014;14:161–74.

Shepherd AM, Laurens KR, Matheson SL, Carr VJ, Green MJ. Systematic meta-review and quality assessment of the structural brain alterations in schizophrenia. Neurosci Biobehav Rev. 2012;36:1342–56.

Simon AE, Umbricht D. High remission rates from an initial ultra-high risk state for psychosis. Schizophr Res. 2010;116:168–72.

Sommer IE, van Westrhenen R, Begemann MJ, de Witte LD, Leucht S, Kahn RS. Efficacy of anti-inflammatory agents to improve symptoms in patients with schizophrenia: an update. Schizophr Bull. 2014;40:181–91.

Song X, Fan X, Song X, Zhang J, Zhang W, Li X, et al. Elevated levels of adiponectin and other cytokines in drug naïve, first episode schizophrenia patients with normal weight. Schizophr Res. 2013;150:269–73.

Stefansson H, Ophoff RA, Steinberg S, Andreassen OA, Cichon S, Rujescu D, et al. Common variants conferring risk of schizophrenia. Nature. 2009;460:744–7.

Sullivan PF, Kendler KS, Neale MC. Schizophrenia as a complex trait: evidence from a meta-analysis of twin studies. Arch Gen Psychiatry. 2003;60:1187–92.

Suvisaari JM, Taxell-Lassas V, Pankakoski M, Haukka JK, Lönnqvist JK, Häkkinen LT. Obstetric complications as risk factors for schizophrenia spectrum psychoses in offspring of mothers with psychotic disorder. Schizophr Bull. 2013;39:1056–66.

Tejkalová H, Kaiser M, Klaschka J, Stastny F. Does neonatal brain ischemia induce schizophrenia-like behavior in young adult rats? Physiol Res. 2007;56:815–23.

Van Dorn R, Volavka J, Johnson N. Mental disorder and violence: is there a relationship beyond substance use? Soc Psychiatry Psychiatr Epidemiol. 2012;47:487–503.

Vargas G, Strassnig M, Sabbag S, Gould F, Durand D, Stone L, et al. The course of vocational functioning in patients with schizophrenia: Re-examining social drift. Schizophr Res Cogn. 2014;1:e41–6.

Wykes T, Reeder C, Landau S, Everitt B, Knapp M, Patel A, Romeo R. Cognitive remediation therapy in schizophrenia randomised controlled trial. Br J Psychiatry. 2007;190:421–7.

Wykes T, Steel C, Everitt B, Tarrier N. Cognitive behavior therapy for schizophrenia: effect sizes, clinical models, and methodological rigor. Schizophr Bull. 2008;34:523–37.

Yao L, Lui S, Liao Y, Du M, Hu N, Thomas JA, Gong Q. White matter deficits in first episode schizophrenia: an activation likelihood estimation meta-analysis. Prog Neuropsychopharmacol Biol Psychiatry. 2013;45:100–6.

Zhang R, Wei Q, Kang Z, Zalesky A, Li M, Xu Y, et al. Disrupted brain anatomical connectivity in medication-naïve patients with first-episode schizophrenia. Brain Struct Funct. 2015;220:1145–59.

Chapter 2
Issues That Slowed Progress in Assessments of Health-Related Quality of Life in Schizophrenia

A. George Awad and Lakshmi N.P. Voruganti

2.1 Quality of Life in Schizophrenia: A Historical Note

Though the early origins of the concept of quality of life is unknown, the term "quality of life" made its first modern appearance after the Second World War. The post-war economic prosperity and the enhanced standard of living in Western societies brought in various expectations, such as satisfaction, happiness and well-being. Such vague notions at that time were picked up by social scientists who pursued population-based quality of life research that led to the collection of extensive social indicators data (Campbell et al. 1976). In 1964, US president Johnson introduced the concept of quality of life into the political arena in his address on the great society that followed the influential publication by the economist John Kenneth Galbraith's book, *The Affluent Society* (Galbraith 1958). Once the term "quality of life" got popularized in the societal and political arena, it stimulated a good deal of research interest in many scientific disciplines, including medicine. Applying the broad concept of quality of life in medical research quickly led to the realization that such a broad concept includes a good deal of "non-health" issues that complicate its use as an outcome in health research, particularly in psychiatry and mental health research.

In 1947, the World Health Organization (WHO) broadened the definition of health to include mental health, in addition to physical health (World Health Organization WHO 1947). Psychological and social issues, such as satisfaction and feelings of

A.G. Awad (✉)
Department of Psychiatry, The Institute of Medical Science, University of Toronto,
Toronto, ON, Canada
e-mail: gawad@hrh.ca

Lakshmi N.P. Voruganti, MD, MSc, PhD
Department of Psychiatry, Oakville-Trafalgar Memorial Hospital,
3001 Hospital Gate, Oakville, ON L6M 0L8, Canada
e-mail: doctor@voruganti.net

© Springer International Publishing Switzerland 2016
A.G. Awad, L.N.P. Voruganti (eds.), *Beyond Assessment of Quality of Life in Schizophrenia*, DOI 10.1007/978-3-319-30061-0_2

well-being, got recognized as important attributes in the definition of the state of health. Narrowing the concept of quality of life into health-related issues has enabled researchers to develop more appropriate scales for measurements applicable for use in clinical services. The new construct of "health-related quality of life" was quickly embraced by a number of medical specialties, such as oncology and cardiovascular and chronic pulmonary diseases. Soon after, health-related quality of life came to represent the new face of modern medicine emphasizing not only prolongation of life but also a better quality of life. In psychiatry and the mental health field, such development seemed to be slow at the beginning, lagging behind other medical fields. However, the deinstitutionalization movement in the early 1960s that led to the precipitous discharge of chronic psychiatric patients from mental hospitals to a community not prepared to receive them, pushed quality of life issues to the forefront (Bacharach 1976; Lehman et al. 1982, 1986; Lehman 1983). The concerns about the plight of chronic psychiatric patients in the community particularly their poor housing and deteriorated social conditions in a community not prepared to welcome them stimulated a good deal of research interests among psychiatrists and social scientists. In the 1970s and early 1980s, a number of prominent contributors have been successful in documenting the poor quality of life of discharged chronic psychiatric patients in the community (Bacharach 1976; Lehman 1983). Such early pioneering efforts stimulated a good deal of research interest, in terms of development of measurement scales that allowed for documenting quality of life among psychiatric populations. Applying the concept of quality of life to the population suffering from schizophrenia identified a number of significant barriers that slowed its development, which include a number of challenges related to the concept of quality of life itself and its definition, challenges related to the illness and the impact of its psychopathology and also as the impact of its management, particularly the side effects of antipsychotic medications, which has emerged as the cornerstone in management of the schizophrenia disorder (Awad et al. 1995; Awad and Voruganti 2007).

2.2   Lack of Agreement on a Definition of Health-Related Quality of Life in Schizophrenia

Early in the development of quality of life as a general concept, it was referred to as "a vague and ethereal entity, something that many people talk about but which nobody clearly knows what to do about" (Campbell et al. 1976; Campbell 1981). Though the introduction of health-related quality of life may have narrowed the concept by limiting its boundaries to health-related issues in an effort to avoid the many non-health-related elements related to life situation, yet the definition continued to be somewhat vague and open to different interpretations. An earlier study that included a critical appraisal of health-related quality of life literature in 75 published papers revealed a lack of quality of life definition in 85 % of published reports (Gill & Feinstein 1995). No published paper distinguished overall quality of life from health-related quality of life, and in only 17 % of the reviewed reports, self-appraisal of quality of life was included. Clearly, the lack of agreement on a definition has led to multiplicity of definitions, depending on the theoretical orientation of the researcher as expressed in the choice of the particular measurement scale. Such multiplicity of definitions without having common metrics to compare measurement data has undermined for a number of years the utility of such important construct. Defining health-related quality of life in recent years as representing the functional effects of an illness and its therapy upon a patient as perceived by the patient has allowed for improved measurement approaches, but did not resolve the conflict between the subjective nature of quality of life as narrowly defined and the subsequent broadening of the definition to include objective measures, that relates more to "standards of living" (Skantz et al. 1992; Awad and Voruganti 2012). Considering the various stages of the schizophrenia disorder from acute to chronic and the remissions in between, as well as the multiplicity of theoretical orientations, pointed to the reality that there may be no single definition that can appropriately cover such diverse clinical stages of the illness. Diversity of definitions has also led a number of researchers to distinguish between subjective quality of life preserving the original concept and objective quality of life which include socioeconomic sufficiency, housing, employment and social functioning (Skantz et al. 1992). An alternative, as suggested early by Skantz et al. (1992) and as later supported by us (Awad and Voruganti 2012), is to group such objective measures as "quality of living" in distinction to the subjective nature of quality of life, as originally conceptualized. The challenge then, as we indicated in an earlier publication, is how to reconcile both dimensions, maintaining the subjective nature of quality of life with the quest for objectivity (Voruganti et al. 1998). We believe the field should accept the reality that there may not be a forthcoming agreement on a single definition and has to move beyond the quest for a uniformed approach to definition. It is incumbent, then, on researchers to define health-related quality of life as applied in their own studies. It also makes it important for journal editors to require such information for publishing health-related quality of life reports.

2.3   Lack of Conceptual Integrative Models

In a recent update about measurement of health-related quality of life in persons with schizophrenia (Awad and Voruganti 2012), we noted that the field requires a good deal of theoretical and conceptual thinking in order to enhance the scientific foundation and further better understanding that can allow for more appropriate scale development which can lead ultimately to accurate interpretation of data.

Historically, as the concept of quality of life in schizophrenia became prominent, as the result of increasing concerns about the chronically mentally ill and their quality of life in the community, it is not surprising then that the initial conceptualization of quality of life in the 1960s was mostly focused on such issues as personal safety, poverty and lack of adequate community psychosocial support (Lehman et al. 1982, 1986). One of the early conceptual models advanced by Calman defined quality of life as the gap between the patient's expectation and achievements (Calman 1984). According to such conceptual model, quality of life is expressed in terms of satisfaction, fulfilment, growth and setting self-goals. The model, despite seemingly promising and able of circumventing the absence of a gold standard against which quality of life can be measured, has not been vigorously pursued. Similarly, the conceptual model proposed by Ware (1996), which was based on an earlier proposal by Wood and Williams (1987), equates the concept of reintegration into normal living "to quality of life". Such a model would broaden the concept of quality of life from an individual personal perspective to a wider social and societal context. Though the model is creative, in terms of the multiplicity of layers of concern that revolve around the centre, which is the individual patient, unfortunately the model was not adequately tested.

As it is recognized that schizophrenia is a multidimensional disorder that affects multiple domains of mental functioning, such as affect, thinking and cognition, its treatments also require diverse approaches including pharmacological, psychosocial and rehabilitative interventions (see Chap. 1, by M. Seeman). Accordingly, measurement of quality of life with persons with schizophrenia requires integrative conceptual models to capture the various components of the disorder as well as the impact of its treatment, including the many side effects of antipsychotic medications (Awad et al. 1997). In an attempt to capture the impact of the illness and its treatment, we proposed an integrative model for quality of life in medicated persons with schizophrenia. According to this clinically intuitive model, quality of life is defined as the outcome of the dynamic interactions between three major determinants: psychotic symptoms and their severity, medications and their side effects as well as psychosocial performance, all arranged in a circular model emphasizing the impact of each factor on other factors (Awad et al. 1997). The model also includes a number of second-order modulators of quality of life that include personality characteristics, premorbid adjustments, values and attitudes towards health/illness and medications. A subsequent study has confirmed the validity of such a conceptual construct and has also provided a basis for its use in testing new antipsychotics in clinical trials (Voruganti et al. 2007; Voruganti et al. 1998). A study designed to correlate subjective quality of life and clinical indices on 63 stable patients with the confirmed diagnosis of schizophrenia on medications revealed a positive correlation between subjective self-rated quality of life and the positive subscale of PANSS (positive and negative symptom scale) (0.34, $p < 0.001$), negative PANSS subscale (0.42, $p < 0.001$), general psychopathology (0.55, $p < 0.001$) and total PANSS score (0.61, $p < 0.0001$) (Voruganti et al. 1998). Correlating medication side effects, akathisia emerged to have the strongest negative correlation with quality of life (0.41, $p < 0.0001$), which is consistent with observations from clinical practice. Negative subjective tolerability to antipsychotics as measured by the Drug Attitude Inventory (DAI) showed significant negative correlation with self-rated quality of life (-0.28, $p < 0.05$). On the other hand, there was no significant correlation with antipsychotic medication dosage.

A subsequent model, the distress/protection vulnerability model of quality of life impairment, was proposed by Ritsner in 2000 (Ritsner 2007). According to this model, subjective quality of life is defined as the outcome of the interaction of an array of distress and protection factors. Dimensions such as physical health, subjective feelings, leisure activities, social relationships, general activities and pharmacotherapy can be classified as protective, but their impairment can also be a source of distress.

Another model, the mediational model, was proposed by Zissi et al. (1998), based on linking subjective quality of life with objective constructs such as improvement in lifestyle, autonomy and positive self-concepts. According to this model improvement of lifestyle, greater autonomy and positive concepts correlate with improved quality of life. In developing this model, the absence of a direct relationship between objective indicators and subjective quality of life was noted. The lack of such correlation continues to be an unresolved issue since it was earlier reported by the Gothenberg group (Skantz et al. 1992; Skantz 1998). We believe that at the present time, there seems to be more acceptance based on research findings as well as clinical experiences, that both subjective and objective constructs are different and though are possibly overlapping are likely to be impacted upon by different factors (Awad and Voruganti 2012; Fitzgerald et al. 2001; Hayhurst et al. 2014). This, in turn, raises the challenge of how to reconcile subjective constructs with the quest for objectivity (Voruganti et al. 1998).

A more recent model of subjective quality of life for outpatients with schizophrenia and other psychosis was advanced by Eklund and Backstrom (2005). The authors hypothesized that objective life circumstances, self-variables, psychopathology, activity level, satisfaction with daily activities and satisfaction with medical care would be determinants of quality of life. In their conclusion, the authors identified a self-variable that showed the strongest association with quality of life with two aspects that should be feasible to influence mental health care, daily activity and medical care, both contributed to the subjects' self-rated quality of life.

We believe as Najman and Levine (1981) concluded that "relying solely on objective indicators is not informative and may have little to contribute to clear understanding of the quality of life personal experience". On the other hand, relying only on subjective appraisal of quality of life, an illness like schizophrenia, can pose limitations related to the impact of the illness itself on the ability of the person for accurate self-appraisal. Even though we do believe that the majority of persons with stable schizophrenia are capable of accurately assessing their inner feelings and their level of satisfaction, we strongly believe that both subjective self-appraisal and objective "quality of living" indicators need to be included in any conceptualization, but without any assumption that they are closely related. It is worth nothing that there seems to be some confusion among researchers defining what is meant by "objective" measures. A large number of reports equates "objective" with the rater- or clinician-conducted appraisal. Others define objective as denoting functional or socioeconomic aspects. Such confusion requires resolution and an agreement on a standard nomenclature. We believe that "objective" measures need to be reserved for assessment of functional and socioeconomic issues and appraisal by a rater or a clinician to be expressed as "observer's rating" or "clinician's rating".

2.4   Reliability of Patients' Self-Reports

Clinicians have frequently viewed with some scepticism patients' self-assessment of treatment outcomes and whether they are capable of accurately self-appraising their inner feelings and level of satisfaction. It is true that patients with schizophrenia frequently experience disturbed thinking, altered feelings and impaired communication; however, it has been adequately documented that the majority of stable patients with schizophrenia are capable of providing consistent and accurate appraisal of their inner feelings and their level of satisfaction. As early as 1982, Glazer et al. reported high agreement between the reports of patients and their significant others demonstrating the reliability of patients with schizophrenia to report their social adjustment. We conducted probably the most extensive study, exploring the reliability of persons with schizophrenia self-reports (Awad et al. 1997; Voruganti et al. 1998). Using a global measure of quality of life (Gurin's Global Scale, Gurin et al. 1960) compared to another multidimensional scale (Modified Sickness Impact Profile M-SIP, Bergner 1978), as well as measures for clinical indices that included Personal and Social Performance scale (PSP) (Stuart and Wykes 1987), Global Assessment of Functioning scale (GAF) (Luborsky and Bachrach 1974), Drug Attitude Inventory (DAI) (Hogan et al. 1983; Awad 1993) and neurocognitive assessment (COGLAB, Spaulding et al. 1981), we demonstrated the reliability and consistency of patients' self-reports over a 4-week period. In order to determine the influence of illness severity and treatment-related factors on the reliability of patient self-reports, the patient sample was divided into three groups, according to the severity of their illness. Repeated measures analysis of variance (ANOVA) failed to detect any group by week interaction for the severity of symptoms, side effects, neurocognitive deficits, antipsychotic drug doses or attitudes. The lack of such interaction indicated that M-SIP scores remained fairly consistent for all the subgroups across time. In other words, the subgroup of patients with a higher level of symptoms was as reliable in their self-reports as the subgroup of patients with a lower level of symptoms. Our study clearly demonstrated that clinically stable patients with schizophrenia are capable of evaluating and reporting their quality of life with a high degree of reliability, regardless of illness severity and/or treatment-related factors. Similarly, self-reported quality of life ratings were fairly accurate when compared to clinicians' assessment (Voruganti et al. 1998). A high degree of concordance between self-reports and clinicians' rated evaluations was achieved by adopting a situation-specific multidimensional measurement approach. Our conclusions were supported by other researchers (Russo et al. 1998; Khatri et al. 2001; Becchi et al. 2004). More recently, Reininghaus et al. (2012) reported the validity of subjective quality of life measures in psychotic patients with severe psychopathology and cognitive deficits employing an item response model analysis. Similarly, self-reported quality of life measure was reported as reliable and valid in outpatients suffering from schizophrenia with executive impairment (Baumstarck et al. 2013). Unfortunately, in spite of the extensive literature documenting the reliability of stable patients' self-reports, the issue still lingers and seems not completely settled. It is somewhat paradoxical that clinicians base their diagnostic formulations on what patients tell us about their unique and personal experiences, such as delusions or hallucinatory experiences, which are difficult to verify; however, patients' self-reports about their inner feelings as well as their level of satisfaction are frequently taken with some doubt. In the face of extensive evidence to the opposite, one has to concede that the only exception to this conclusion relates to the small group of chronic severely deteriorated patients with severe communication problems, which makes it impossible to achieve reliable self-reports.

2.5   Lack of Standardized Quality of Life Measures

The past two decades have seen the development of a large number of quality of life scales in schizophrenia that frequently lacked appropriate psychometrics (see Chap. 5 by Bobes-Bascaran et al., Chap. 7 by Bjorner and Bech). Many of the scales lack a theoretical or conceptual foundation and rely in large part on the developer's own conceptual theoretical orientation. Many of the scales are not appropriate for the life of a person with schizophrenia, in terms of being too long and taxing the already compromised cognitive abilities of the person, or are too short to convey meaningful information. Many scales suffer from the common limitations of many other scales, in terms of floor and ceiling effects. Many scales in use are not capable of capturing quality of life at different stages of the illness and also not being sensitive enough to pick up the relatively small changes in quality of life that are anticipated over time. The absence of common standardized metrics makes it difficult to compare data across studies. Over the past two decades, there has been good progress in the application of modern measurement theories, such as item response theory (IRT), item banks and computer adaptive testing in scale development (Adelen and Reeve 2007). Such developments have the potential to eliminate many of the shortcomings of currently available scales, and importantly, it provides common metrics for comparative effectiveness. Though the new approach in scale development has made inroads in other medical specialties, it has been slow in its development in psychiatric disorders in general, but even more so in schizophrenia.

2.6   The Perception of Lack of Impact of Quality of Life Assessments on Clinical Management

Over the past two decades, there has been substantial growth in the number of published quality of life reports in schizophrenia. A recent update review that covered publications between 2000 and 2010 revealed that the vast majority of published studies dealt with aspects of measurement of quality of life in schizophrenia (Awad and Voruganti 2012). Very few studies have gone beyond quality of life assessments to important applications, such as integration in care plans or impacting health economics, or health policy decision-making. Such a significant gap has likely contributed to the perceived erosion in the utility of the concept of quality of life in schizophrenia. Though the concept seemed promising initially as the new ideal of modern medicine and psychiatry, the expectations that quality of life assessments can lead to improvement in clinical management did only partially materialize, at best. Paradoxically, as the concept of quality of life has become popular, it is in danger of fading away (Awad and Voruganti 2012). The emerging perception of lack of usefulness of quality of life assessments has undermined its utility, yet it highlighted important gaps that require further research interests and also has motivated us to develop this book by going beyond assessments of quality of life into specific clinical and health economic applications.

2.7   Summary and Conclusions

The deinstitutionalization movement in the 1960s seems to have accelerated interest in the construct of quality of life, as a result of the deteriorated living situations of the precipitously discharged psychiatric patients from mental hospitals to a community which was not prepared for them. In subsequent years, as measurement tools were developed and the number of quality of life-related publications increased, a number of factors seem to have impeded further development. Prominent among such factors have been the lack of agreement on the definition of quality of life in schizophrenia, which has resulted in a multiplicity of definitions and a broad range of theoretical and conceptual understandings. There is a lack of appropriate conceptual models that can prove helpful in understanding the theoretical underpinning of the concept of quality of life, as well as impacting on the development of more appropriate scales that can capture the impact of the illness and its treatment. Though the reliability of patients with schizophrenia to provide consistent self-appraisal of their satisfaction and inner feelings has been adequately documented, there is still lingering doubt about such ability among the majority of stable patients with schizophrenia. Many of the measurement tools in use at the present time seem to suffer from a good deal of deficiencies and make it impossible to identify comparative effectiveness among studies, in the absence of common metrics. Some of the erosion in interest in recent years seems to do with a growing perception that the concept of quality of life and its measurement in schizophrenia is not very useful, as a result of lack of integrative approaches in clinical care, as well as the limited impact on pharmacoeconomics, policy decision-making and resource allocations.

We do believe that the construct of quality of life in schizophrenia continues to be important and valid, and needs to be almost reinvented, in order to maximize its usefulness and deal with the conflicts within the construct itself and the gaps in its application.

References

Adelen MO, Reeve BP. Applying item response theory (IRT) modeling to questionnaire development, evaluation and refinement. Qual Life Res. 2007;16:5–18.

Awad AG. Subjective response to neuroleptics in schizophrenia. Schizophr Bull. 1993;19: 609–18.

Awad AG, Voruganti LN. Antipsychotics, schizophrenia and the issue of quality of life. In: Ritsner M, Awad AG, editors. Quality of life impairment in schizophrenia, mood and anxiety disorders. Dordrecht: Springer; 2007. p. 307–19.

Awad AG, Voruganti LN. Measurement of quality of life in patients with schizophrenia – an update. Pharmacoeconomics. 2012;30:183–95.

Awad AG, Voruganti LN, Heslegrave RJ. The aim of antipsychotic medications: what are they and are they being achieved? CNS Drugs. 1995;19:609–18.

Awad AG, Voruganti LN, Heslegrave RS. Preliminary validation of a conceptual model to assess quality of life in schizophrenia. Qual Life Res. 1997;6:21–6.

Bacharach LL. Deinstitutionalization: an analytic review and sociological perspective. Rockville: National Institute of Health; 1976.

Baumstarck K, Boyer L, Boucekine M. Self-reported quality of life measure is reliable and valid in adult patients suffering from schizophrenia with executive impairment. Schizophr Res. 2013;147:58–67.

Becchi A, Rucci P, Placentino A, Veri G, de Girolamo G. Quality of life in patients with schizophrenia – comparison of self-reports and proxy assessments. Soc Psychiatry Psychiatr Epidemiol. 2004;30:397–401.

Bergner M. The sickness impact profile: development and brief summary of its purpose, uses and administration. Seattle/Washington: University of Washington; 1978.

Calman KC. Quality of life in cancer patients: an hypothesis. J Med Ethics. 1984;10:124–7.

Campbell A. The sense of well-being in america. New York: McGraw-Hill; 1981.

Campbell A, Converse PE, Rogers WC. Subjective measures of well-being. Am Psychol. 1976;31:117–24.

Eklund M, Backstrom M. A model of subjective quality of life for outpatients with schizophrenia and other psychoses. Qual Life Res. 2005;14:1157–68.

Fitzgerald PB, Williams CL, Cortiling N, Filig SL, Brewer K, Adams A, deCastella AR, Rolfe T, Davey P, Kulkarni J. Subject and observer-rated quality of life in schizophrenia. Acta Psychiatr Scand. 2001;103:387–92.

Galbraith JK. The affluent society. Boston: Houghton & Mifflin; 1958.

Gill TM, Feinstein AR. Critical appraisal of the quality of quality-of-life measurements. JAMA. 1995;272:619–26.

Glazer W, Sholomskas D, Williams D, Weissman M. Chronic schizophrenia in the community: are they able to report their social adjustment? Am J Orthopsychiatry. 1982;52:166–71.

Gurin G, Verhof J, Feld S. Americans view their mental health. New York: Russel Sage Foundation; 1960.

Hayhurst KP, Massie S, Dunn G, Lewis S, Drake RJ. Validity of subjective versus objective quality of life in people with schizophrenia. BMC Psychiatry. 2014;14:365–9.

Hogan TP, Awad AG, Eastwood RA. A self-rated scale predictive of drug compliance in schizophrenia: reliability and discriminative abilities. Psychol Med. 1983;13:177–83.

Khatri N, Romney D, Pelletier G. Validity of self-reports about quality of life among patients with schizophrenia. Psychiatr Serv. 2001;52:534–5.

Lehman A. The well-being of chronic mental patients: assessing their quality of life. Arch Gen Psychiatry. 1983;40:369–73.

Lehman A, Ward N, Linn L. Chronic mental patients: the quality of life issue. Am J Psychiatry. 1982;139:1271–6.

Lehman A, Possidente S, Hawker F. The quality of life of chronic patients in state hospitals and in community residences. Hosp Community Psychiatry. 1986;37:901–7.

Luborsky L, Bachrach H. Factors influencing clinicians' judgments of mental health: eighteen experiences with the health-sickness rating scale. Arch Gen Psychiatry. 1974;31:292–9.

Najman JM, Levine S. Evaluating the impact of medical care and technologies on the quality of life: a review and critique. Soc Sci Med. 1981;15:107–15.

Reininghaus U, McCabe R, Burns T, Croudace T, Priebe S. The validity of subjective quality of life measures in psychotic patients with severe psychopathology and cognitive deficits: an item response model analysis. Qual Life Res. 2012;2012:237–46.

Ritsner M. The distress/protection vulnerability model of quality of life impairment syndrome. In: Ritsner M, Awad AG, editors. Quality of life impairment in schizophrenia, mood and anxiety disorders. Dodrecht: Springer; 2007. p. 3–20.

Russo J, Trufillo CA, Wengerson D. The MOS-36 item short form health survey: reliability, validity and preliminary findings in schizophrenic outpatients. Med Care. 1998;36:752–6.

Skantz K. Subjective quality of life and standard of living: a 10-year follow-up of outpatients with schizophrenia. Acta Psychiatr Scand. 1998;98:390–8.

Skantz K, Malm U, Denker SJ. Comparison of quality of life with standard of living in schizophrenic outpatients. Br J Psychiatry. 1992;161:797–801.

Spaulding W, Hargrave S, Crincan W, Martin T. A microcomputer based laboratory for psychopathology research in rural settings. Behav Res Meth Instrum. 1981;13:616–23.

Stuart E, Wykes T. Assessment schedules for chronic psychiatric patients. Psychol Med. 1987;17:485–93.

Voruganti LN, Heselgrave R, Awad AG, Seeman M. Quality of life measurement in schizophrenia: reconciling the question of subjectivity with question of reliability. Psychol Med. 1998;28: 165–72.

Voruganti LN, Awad AG, Parker G, Forrest C, Usmani Y, Fernando MLD, Senthislal S. Cognition, functioning and quality of life in schizophrenia treatment: results of one year randomized controlled trial of olanzapine and quetiapine. Schizophr Res. 2007;96:146–55.

Ware Jr JE. The SF-36 health survey in quality of life and pharmacoeconomics clinical trials. In: Spilker B, editor. Quality of life and pharmacoeconomics in clinical trials. Philadelphia: Lippincott-raven; 1996. p. 337–45.

Wood S, William JI. Reintegration to normal living as a proxy to quality of life. J Chronic Dis. 1987;40:497–509.

World Health Organization (WHO). The constitution of the World Health Organization. WHO Chron. 1947;1:29–43.

Zissi A, Barry MU, Cochrane RA. A mediational model of quality of life for individuals with severe mental health problems. Psychol Med. 1998;28:1221–30.

Chapter 3
Quality of Life, Cognition, and Social Cognition in Schizophrenia

Sofia Brissos, Guilherme Pereira, and Vicent Balanzá-Martinez

3.1 Introduction

Nowadays, the main objective in treating patients with schizophrenia (SZ) is not only to attain and maintain symptomatic remission, in order to reach recovery, but also to avoid relapses and reach a level of personal and social functioning, as well as of quality of life (QoL), as near as possible to that of the general population (Hasan et al. 2013). In that sense, psychosocial functioning and QoL are increasingly recognized as important treatment outcomes in SZ (Juckel and Morosini 2008; Remington et al. 2010; Figueira and Brissos 2011).

But while contemporary pharmacologic strategies are effective at managing certain SZ symptoms, mainly positive ones, they have had little impact on the poor outcome associated with this disorder (DSM-IV 2000). Thus, understanding determinants of outcome in SZ, and, namely, of QoL, has become a central goal of study.

Symptoms are known to negatively impact subjective QoL (Norman et al. 2000; Hofer et al. 2004; Ruggeri et al. 2005), and depressive mood may be the most important determinant of subjective QoL (Dickerson et al. 1998; Fitzgerald et al. 2001; Reine et al. 2003; Harvey et al. 2007; Aki et al. 2008; Margariti et al. 2015). However, symptoms alone seem to explain only a modest proportion of variance in QoL (Tolman and Kurtz 2012), and symptom reduction alone often does not result in meaningful improvements in QoL (Narvaez et al. 2008; Priebe et al. 2011). This is probably due to the fact that other problems interfering with QoL persist even

S. Brissos, MD (✉) • G. Pereira, MD
Department of Psychiatry, Centro Hospitalar Psiquiátrico de Lisboa
(Lisbon's Psychiatric Hospitalar Centre), Lisbon, Portugal
e-mail: brissos.sofia@gmail.com

V. Balanzá-Martinez, MD, PhD
Teaching Unit of Psychiatry, Department of Medicine, School of Medicine, La Fe University and Polytechnic Hospital, University of Valencia, CIBERSAM, Valencia, Spain

© Springer International Publishing Switzerland 2016
A.G. Awad, L.N.P. Voruganti (eds.), *Beyond Assessment of Quality of Life in Schizophrenia*, DOI 10.1007/978-3-319-30061-0_3

when patients are stable or in remission, such as lack of social contacts, unemployment, stigmatization, and difficulties in social functioning (Narvaez et al. 2008).

Cognitive deficits are a core feature of SZ and may be the prime driver of the significant disabilities in occupational, social, and economic functioning in patients with SZ (Keefe and Harvey 2012). A wealth of studies conducted over the last two decades has supported a link between cognitive skills and functional outcomes for SZ patients (e.g., Green 1996; Green et al. 2000, 2004), and longitudinal studies have suggested that cognitive deficits play a particularly important role in the ability of patients to benefit from integrated programs of behavioral rehabilitation (Woonings et al. 2003; Brekke et al. 2007, 2009; Kurtz et al. 2008). Therefore, it would seem intuitive to think that cognitive deficits would negatively impact on variables such as personal and social functioning, which could in turn affect QoL. However, despite some studies have found such an association, others have not.

Whether social cognition and neurocognition are distinct domains in SZ remains controversial (Sergi et al. 2007; Van Hooren et al. 2008). Although probably related, they have been generally viewed as distinct constructs (Sergi et al. 2007; Schmidt et al. 2011), given that only a small proportion of the variance in social cognition (i.e., about 10 %) is shared with (or can be explained by) variation in neurocognition (Sergi et al. 2007; Van Hooren et al. 2008; Ventura et al. 2013; Mehta et al. 2014).

Understanding the role of neurocognition and social cognition in SZ patients' QoL is important because antipsychotic treatment does not seem to have a large effect on QoL (Kilian and Angermeyer 2005), and interventions that focus on symptoms or functioning alone may fail to improve subjective QoL to the same level (Karow et al. 2014). Therefore, knowledge of the determinants of QoL is of key importance in tailoring effective interventions to improve the lives of people with this disorder (Tolman and Kurtz 2012). Despite this fact, an understanding of determinants of QoL in SZ remains elusive, especially regarding neurocognition and social cognition.

In the present chapter, we present recent data concerning the eventual association between neurocognition, social cognition, and QoL in SZ patients and possible implications for planning and implementing treatment strategies.

3.2   Quality of Life in Schizophrenia

Although there is no unanimous definition of QoL, the WHO considers it a broadranging concept which takes into account the individual's perception of his or her position in life, within the cultural context and value system where he or she lives in and in relation to his or her goals, expectations, parameters, and social relations (The WHOQOL Group 1995).

QoL usually involves objective and subjective indicators across parallel life domains (Lehman 1988). Objective measures of QoL include indicators of health and living conditions, sociodemographic items, and role functioning and are usually assessed by a third person, namely, through clinician ratings; subjective QoL refers to client satisfaction in general and within different life domains (Harvey et al. 2007; Tolman and Kurtz 2012) and is usually based on self-report/ an appreciation of the patient himself or herself.

QoL can also be divided into two main categories: (1) one representing the outward (extrinsic) features of QoL, which include instrumental, interpersonal, and daily activities, and (2) another, representing the inward (intrinsic) features of QoL that relate to the subjective feeling of well-being (Tas et al. 2013). Social cognitive skills such as mental state reasoning may be key predictors of the inward aspects of QoL, whereas neurocognitive faculties and negative symptoms may be more related with outward features (Tas et al. 2013).

Although it is traditionally assumed that SZ patients' self-report is unrealistic (Yamauchi et al. 2008), QoL can be accurately and consistently rated by patients (Voruganti et al. 1998; Lambert et al. 2003; Becchi et al. 2004), especially in the non-acute phase, and self-report measures of QoL may be more valid than clinician-reported QoL evaluations. On the other hand, the phase of illness is also significant for QoL research, especially the exacerbation phase, where, besides the patient's perception, research should include a more objective aspect of QoL – the family's, the doctor's, and other healthcare professionals' perceptions (Lehman 1996). Moreover, depending on the severity of cognitive impairment and the stage of illness, SZ patients may be less aware of the severity of their disorder and its impact on their functioning; as cognition and insight improve, there may be a paradoxical decline in perceived self-reported QoL (Chue 2006). Nevertheless, subjective QoL, while related to objective measures, may be influenced by illness features quite differently than those for objective QoL (Kurtz et al. 2012).

Therefore, despite importance expressed by consumers, subjective QoL as an outcome domain has been a relatively neglected area of research relative to objective indices of QoL in SZ (Kurtz et al. 2013). This is of utmost importance, since in patients with SZ, scores on objectively and subjectively rated measures of QoL can differ markedly; overall, patients with depressive symptoms will value their QoL lower, and those with low insight will value their QoL higher (Boyer et al. 2012; Hayhurst et al. 2014). SZ patients' QoL also depends on the cultural background, some studies showing a better prognosis in less developed and poorer communities in comparison to urban societies (Chisholm and Bhugra 1997). Finally, although QoL represents a direct consequence of mental health, better QoL itself can improve the level of mental functioning (Jakovljević et al. 2010).

3.3 Measures of Quality of Life in Schizophrenia Patients

No single instrument captures all key concepts of importance to patients with SZ, and the appropriateness of a patient-reported outcomes' instrument should be considered in light of its development history, face and content validity, psychometric properties, and purpose for use. Many of the instruments used to assess patient functioning were developed in a general or non-SZ patient population (e.g., the Medical Outcomes Study Short Form [SF-36], Sickness Impact Profile [SIP], and

Social Adjustment Scale [SAS] I and II). Consequently, relevant concepts may not have been adequately measured (Kitchen et al. 2012; Papaioannou et al. 2011).

The combination out of standardized generic and disease-specific QoL instruments may be a useful alternative. In fact, while generic QoL assessment might be a valuable tool in the comparison of different populations of patients, disease-specific QoL assessment might be more useful to detect specific treatment effects (Heinrichs et al. 1984).

Scales to assess objective QoL may also have some biases, e.g., the Quality of Life Scale (QLS), although disease specific, was originally designed to assess deficit symptoms (Heinrichs et al. 1984); therefore, scores on the QLS show very high correlations with negative symptoms and may be contaminated (Norman et al. 2000). Regarding subjective QoL, the WHOQOL-BREF is one of the most used instruments (Karow et al. 2014), has undergone rigorous international development, and is sensitive to the health-related QoL status of those with long-term mental illness (Herrman et al. 2002).

Although controversy persists as to which instrument should best be used for measuring QoL in SZ, there seems to be not one "best" scale for all research questions; therefore, the best-fitting scale has to be selected depending on each study design or study sample.

For a more in-depth reading about scales to evaluate QoL in SZ, we suggest the reader to go over Chap. 4 of the present book.

3.4   Cognitive Deficits in Schizophrenia

Cognitive deficits are a core feature of SZ, being present during childhood and early adolescence, thus predating the typical/modal age of onset of psychosis (Keefe 2013). Furthermore, antipsychotic treatment seems to have little impact on cognition (Keefe 2013), and conventional antipsychotics may even exacerbate already impaired cognitive functioning (Burton 2006; Moncrieff et al. 2009). Whether these cognitive deficits are static or changeable across the patient's life span is still under debate.

The importance of cognitive deficits in SZ is that they impact negatively on the ability to perform everyday living skills, not only as measured in assessment settings (Patterson et al. 2001; Evans et al. 2003) but also in real-world community functioning (Green 1996; Percudani et al. 2004; Hofer et al. 2005; Rosenheck et al. 2006; Nuechterlein et al. 2011), being the prime driver of the significant disabilities in occupational, social, and economic functioning in patients with SZ (Keefe and Harvey 2012).

Neurocognitive tests often assess more than one neurocognitive domain, and many tests do not fit neatly into a single domain. Thus, descriptions of the profile of cognitive deficits in SZ have varied across literature reviews. However, research suggests that the profile of cognitive deficits and level of performance in patients with SZ include almost no aspect of cognition that is similar to those in healthy control subjects (Brissos et al. 2011a). This profile includes many of the most important aspects of human cognition: attention, memory, reasoning, and processing speed.

Given the apparent impact of cognitive deficits in so many aspects of SZ patients' life, it would seem logical that these might also have an impact on patients' QoL; this has been the subject of recent research, which will be presented ahead.

3.5 Social Cognition in Schizophrenia

Social cognition is defined as the mental operations involved in understanding, perceiving, and interacting with other humans (Fiske and Taylor 1991; Gallotti and Frith 2013). Despite the agreement about the value of this construct, until recently, there were some divergences regarding terms, definitions, and measurement approaches. Meanwhile, five relevant domains have been identified: theory of mind, social perception, social knowledge, attributional bias, and emotion processing (Green et al. 2008).

Theory of mind, also known as mental state attribution, mentalizing, mind reading, or perspective taking, encompasses the capacity to infer intentions, dispositions, and beliefs of others. The resemblance between impairment in social functioning in SZ and autism partially explains why this construct has been applied to SZ. Assessment of this domain relies on tests adopted from psychological tasks developed to test children's capacity to infer mental states of others (Brüne 2005). Tasks like interpretation of complex emotions from pictures of the eye region of multiple faces (e.g., Eyes Task, Baron-Cohen et al. 2001), picture sequencing tasks (e.g., Langdon et al. 1997), and tests of comprehension of hints behind indirect speech, metaphor, and irony (e.g., Hinting Task, Corcoran et al. 1995, and Faux Pas Test, Stone et al. 1998) have been used in this area.

Social perception, in turn, accounts for the capacity to appraise social roles, societal rules, relationships, and social context through identifying and using social cues. Its assessment comprises tasks wherein individuals are asked to make judgments about complex or ambiguous social situations or interactions, hinging upon nonverbal, paraverbal, and verbal social cues (e.g., Profile of Nonverbal Sensitivity (PONS), Rosenthal et al. 1979, and Social Cue Recognition Test (SCRT), Corrigan 1997).

Social knowledge concerns acquaintance with social roles, rules, and goals that underlie social situations and interactions (Subotnik et al. 2006). This domain overlaps with social perception, inasmuch as the former demands the latter.

Attributional bias accounts for the individual style of bringing forth causal explanations for particular positive or negative life events. Attributions are categorized as internal (cause due to oneself) or external. External attributions are either sorted as personal (causes attributed to another person) or situational (causes attributed to situational factors). Personalizing bias, i.e., the proneness to attribute good outcomes to oneself's skills and poor outcomes to others, instead of situational factors, is associated with paranoid ideation throughout schizophrenic patients and controls (Langdon et al. 2010; Bentall et al. 2001). Measurement of this domain includes questionnaires like the Internal, Personal, and Situational Attributions Questionnaire (IPSAQ) (Kinderman and Bentall 1997) and the Ambiguous Intentions Hostility Questionnaire (AIHQ) (Combs et al. 2007) or methods by which attributions are inferred from the natural speech of the subjects, such as the Leeds Attributional Coding System (LACS) (Munton et al. 1999).

Lastly, *emotion processing* is a broad concept that mainly refers to perception and utilization of emotions. Despite the impairment of emotions' expression observed in SZ patients, there is growing evidence that their subjective emotional experience may not be reduced and intense negative emotions could be experienced (Kret and Ploeger 2015). According to the influential Four-Branch Model of Emotional Intelligence, four components are considered (perceiving, facilitating, understanding, and managing emotions) and can be assessed in the Mayer–Salovey–Caruso Emotional Intelligence Test (Mayer et al. 2001).

There is a wealth of evidence showing that SZ patients have social cognitive deficits that are a stable feature of the disorder (e.g., Penn et al. 1997) and that are closely linked to a variety of outcome domains (see Couture et al. (2006) for a review). In fact, a growing number of experts have suggested that in SZ, functional outcomes (both cross-sectional and longitudinal) can be better understood by specific aspects of social cognition, for example, the ability to accurately make attributions about another's intentions, or theory of mind (ToM), and the ability to decode facial affect (see 2006 NIMH Workshop on Social Cognition in Schizophrenia, Green et al. 2008). These, in turn, would have an impact on patients' objective and/or subjective QoL.

Finally, although social cognition has traditionally been viewed as a separate construct from basic neurocognitive function, with independent and distinct upward causal effects on functional outcome, and the need for distinct remediation approaches (Hoe et al. 2012), recent studies suggest that a one-factor model (considering these two dimensions of cognition) fits data better than when considered as different constructs (Lin et al. 2013), especially when regarding an association with QoL. This is probably why more recent studies have included measures of both social and basic neurocognition, to evaluate the effect of each of them and of both on patients' QoL, as can be seen in the following sections.

3.6 Neurocognition and Quality of Life in Schizophrenia

Over the last two decades, an inverse relationship between domains of neurocognition and subjective QoL has been reported; one potential explanation for this is that patients with stronger cognitive abilities may have greater insight into their illness and functional disability, enabling negative social comparison and thus lower subjective QoL (Kurtz et al. 2012). In fact, insight has been found to associate inversely with subjective QoL in SZ patients (Boyer et al. 2012), even though the effects of awareness of the consequences of illness on QoL may (also) be largely mediated by depressive symptoms (Margariti et al. 2015), and not better insight itself.

As can be seen in Table 3.1, the majority of studies found that neurocognitive performance was positively correlated with measures of objective QoL; however, a different picture emerges when measures of subjective QoL are used (Table 3.2). This had already been pointed by Kurtz and Tolman (2011) in their review, where they used a quantitative analysis as well as homogeneity and moderator variable analyses.

Overall and looking at studies published from 2000 onward (see Tables 3.1 and 3.2), there seem to be positive relationships between measures of crystallized verbal ability, working memory, verbal list learning, processing speed, and measures of executive function and objective QoL, but as Tolman and Kurtz (2012) stated, these seem to be in the small to medium effect size range. This suggests that there are likely many other individual and social determinants of *objective QoL* in addition to elementary neurocognition. Indeed, learning potential (Green et al. 2000), negative symptoms (Bowie et al. 2008), and social cognition (namely, affect recognition) may moderate the relationship between neurocognitive deficits and objective QoL (Addington et al. 2006). In fact, although cognitive dysfunction in attention and processing speed domain may be most strongly associated with lowered objective QoL in SZ (Ueoka et al. 2011), the majority of studies on neurocognition and functional outcome suggest that measures of attention are more strongly associated with performance-based measures of skill acquisition and social problem solving than measures of objective community functioning that overlap with measures of objective QoL (Green 1996; Tolman and Kurtz et al. 2012).

Another cognitive function highly associated with functional outcome in SZ has been memory; memory has strong correlations to community functioning, social problem solving, as well as psychosocial skill acquisition (Green et al. 2000) and has been shown to be predictive of most QoL subscales including those measuring aspects of community functioning such as subjective measures of satisfaction with health and daily activities and objective measures of money spent on self. Verbal memory problems are prevalent in SZ and have been proposed as the most likely aspect of cognition to mediate functional outcome and QoL in SZ (Heinrichs and Zakzanis 1998; Green et al. 2000). However, change in verbal memory function over time rather than absolute performance levels may (also) mediate patients' perceptions of QoL (Sota and Heinrichs 2004).

Regarding objective QoL, four studies since Tolman and Kurtz's review (2012) reported positive associations (Ueoka et al. 2011; Kurtz et al. 2012; Tas et al. 2013; Corbera et al. 2013), whereas Lin et al. (2013), using a mediation model, found that the link between neurocognition and QoL was mediated by clinical symptoms, mainly negative ones. On the other hand, poorer social cognitive and neurocognitive skills may have a detrimental effect on perceived self-competency, and this may consequently reduce QoL scores in stable patients (Lysaker et al. 2005; Tas et al. 2013). In other words, it may be that patients with less severe negative symptoms and impaired social cognitive abilities may make inaccurate judgments about their own competency; this would consequently have a negative impact on their own perception of QoL, i.e., the Intrapsychic Foundation domain of QoL (Tas et al. 2013).

Table 3.1 Studies of neurocognition, social cognition, and objective quality of life

Study	Sample characteristics	Neurocognitive measures	Social cognition measures	QoL measures	Main findings
Nahum et al. (2014)	17 SZ patients and 17 matched HC		Penn Facial Memory Test; PROID; MSCEIT's perceiving emotions and managing emotions branches	QLS	Post-training performance on the SocialVille tasks were similar to initial performance of HC. Patients also showed improvements on social cognition, social functioning, and motivation. No improvements were recorded for emotion recognition indices on the MSCEIT or on QoL
Tas et al. (2013)	28 stable SZ patients	WMS-III; WCST; TMT-A and B; CPT; RAVLT; Benton Judgment of Line Orientation test	FEIT; FEDT; RMET; Hinting Task; UOT; IPSAQ	QLS	Executive functioning and social cognition had some power in predicting QoL. Mental state reasoning was specifically found to be most strongly related with the Intrapsychic Foundation subdomain of QoL, whereas neurocognition and symptom severity were associated with other subdomains of QoL. Social cognition did not show a potential mediating effect among all predictors and QoL subdomains
Lin et al. (2013)	302 clinically stable SZ individuals from inpatient and day-care units	Category Fluency, TMT-A; WAIS-III Digit Symbol Coding; CPT; WMS-III backward digit span and nonverbal spatial span, word listing, visual, maze	MSCEIT V2.0. Social cognition assessed by the "managing emotions" branch	QLS	Using a mediation model, the link between cognitive function and QoL was mediated by clinical symptoms, mainly negative symptoms
Corbera et al. (2013)	44 stable SZ and SZA outpatients and 24 HC	MCCB	SAT-MC; BLERT; the Hinting Task; BORRTI Egocentricity and Alienation scales; IRI	QLS	Basic social cognition correlated with the QLS in both samples together, but no differences were found between groups in this relationship. Interpersonal discomfort showed a strong negative correlation with social competence on the SSPA and QLS in HC but not in patients

Bell et al. (2013)	First phase: 77 stable SZ and SZA outpatients Second phase: 63 stable SZ and SZA outpatients		Social Attribution Task-Multiple Choice version; Bell-Lysaker Emotion Recognition Task; Hinting Task; BORRTI; MCCB Social Cognition Index (composed of scores from the MSCEIT, Emotion Management Task, and Social Management Task)	QLS	The group with high social cognition stood out with significantly better QLS total scores than patients with low social cognition or patients with high negative symptoms
Kurtz et al. (2012)	44 stable SZ and SZA outpatients	WAIS-III Vocabulary, and the Digit Symbol and Symbol Search subtests; PCPT; CVLT-II; PCET	PEAT	QLS	Verbal memory and facial affect recognition were linked to improvements in objective QoL Facial affect recognition partially mediated the relationship between verbal memory and improvements in objective QoL
Tas et al. (2012)	19 clinically stable SZ patients received F-SCIT 26 clinically stable SZ patients received SS	TMT-B; WMS-R	FEIT; FEDT; Hinting Task; UOT; IPSAQ	QLS	Patients who received F-SCIT significantly improved in QoL, social functioning, and social cognition, whereas the SS group worsened in nearly all outcome variables
Ueoka et al. (2011)	61 stabilized SZ outpatients	BACS: List Learning, Digit Sequencing Task, Token Motor Task, Category Instances and COWA, Symbol Coding, and Tower of London		QLS	The BACS composite score, attention and speed of information processing score, and verbal memory score showed significant and positive correlations with QLS

(continued)

Table 3.1 (continued)

Study	Sample characteristics	Neurocognitive measures	Social cognition measures	QoL measures	Main findings
Lipkovich et al. (2009)	414 SZ and SZA outpatients	WAIS Letter–Number Sequencing, RAVLT (with 10 min Crawford alternative)		QLS	At baseline, multiple QLS domains significantly related to processing speed, working memory, and verbal memory
Savilla et al. (2008)	57 SZ outpatients	BACS: List Learning, Digit Sequencing Task, Token Motor Task, Category Instances and COWA, Symbol Coding, and Tower of London		QLS	Poorer cognition associated with poorer QoL
Narvaez et al. (2008)	88 SZ+SZA outpatients	WAIS Digit Span, Digit Symbol, Letter–Number Sequencing subtests; WMS-LMI, LMII; WCST-PE, CAT		Objective section of QoL interview	Severity of depressive symptoms predicted subjective QoL. Severity of negative symptoms predicted objective QoL. List learning and WCST measures were positively associated with objective QoL
Fiszdon et al. (2008)	151 SZ and SZA outpatients	WAIS Digit Span and Digit Symbol subtests; WMS-LMI; HVLT-immediate		QLS	None of the neurocognitive variables were significantly associated with QLS total
Matsui et al. (2008)	53 SZ outpatient and 31 HC	Subtests of the Rule Shift Cards Test, Temporal Judgment Test, Zoo Map Test, Ball Search Test, Japanese Sentence Memory Test, JVLT, Digit Span, and the Script Test		QLS	QLS score was significantly predicted by the script and sentence memory tests

Study	Sample	Cognitive measures	Social cognition measures	QoL measure	Results
Addington and Addington (2008)	50 first-episode patients (88% SZ), 53 multi-episode SZ patients, and 55 HC	WAIS Digit Symbol, Letter–Number Sequencing; CPT; WMS-LMI, LMII; RAVLT-immediate, delayed; WCST-CAT, PE		QLS	Cognition predicted QLS scores at time 1 and time 2 for FE, ME, and NPC groups
Kohler et al. (2007)	11 stable SZ and SZA patients received donepezil 11 stable SZ and SZA patients received placebo	Standardized computerized neurocognitive assessment, including tests of abstraction, attention, verbal and spatial memory, and spatial abilities	Tests for emotion discrimination and differentiation	QLS	No treatment effects were found on any cognitive functions or clinical symptoms in placebo or donepezil groups
Lysaker and Davis (2004)	65 SZ and SZA outpatients	WAIS Vocabulary subtest; HVLT-delayed, WCST-PE		QLS	All neurocognitive measures were correlated with at least one domain of the QLS
Dickinson and Coursey (2002)	40 SZ and SZA outpatients	WAIS Vocabulary, Digit Span, Letter–Number Sequencing, and Digit Symbol subtests		LOF	Neurocognitive measures (except for Digit Span) were positively associated with LOF

BACS Brief Assessment of Cognition in Schizophrenia, *BLERT* Bell-Lysaker Emotion Recognition Task, *BORRT* Bell Object Relations and Reality Testing Inventory, *COWA* Controlled Oral Word Association Test, *CPT* Continuous Performance Test, *CVLT* California Verbal Learning Test, *FE* first episode of psychosis, *FEDT* Facial Emotion Discrimination Task, *FEIT* Facial Emotion Identification Task, *F-SCIT* family-assisted social cognition and interaction training, *HC* healthy controls, *HVLT* Hopkins Verbal Learning Test, *IPSAQ* Internal, Personal, and Situational Attributions Questionnaire, *IRI* Interpersonal Reactivity Index, *JVLT* Japanese Verbal Learning Test, *LMI* Logical Memory Immediate Recall, *LMII* Logical Memory Delayed Recall, *LOF* Strauss–Carpenter Level of Functioning Scale, *MCCB* MATRICS Consensus Cognitive Battery, *ME* multi-episode schizophrenia, *MSCEIT* Mayer–Salovey–Caruso Emotional Intelligence Test, *NPC* nonpsychiatric controls, *PCET* Penn Conditional Exclusion Test, *PCPT* Penn Continuous Performance Test, *PEAT* Penn Emotion Acuity Test, *PROID* Prosody Identification Test, *QLS* Heinrichs–Carpenter Quality of Life Scale, *QoL* quality of life, *RAVLT* Rey Auditory Verbal Learning Test, *RMET* Reading the Mind in the Eyes Test (Revised), *SAT-MC* Social Attribution Test-Multiple Choice, *SIP* Sickness Impact Profile, *SS* social stimulation, *SSPA* Social Skills Performance Assessment, *SZ* schizophrenia, *SZA* schizoaffective disorder, *TMT* Trail Making Test, *UOT* Unexpected Outcomes Test, *WAIS* Wechsler Adult Intelligence Scale, *WCST* Wisconsin Card Sorting Test (*CAT* categories, *PEs* perseverative errors), *WMS* Wechsler Memory Scale

Table 3.2 Studies of neurocognition, social cognition, and subjective quality of life

Study	Sample characteristics	Neurocognitive measures	Social cognition measures	QoL measures	Main findings
Caqueo-Urizar et al. (2015)	253 SZ patients	GEOPTE Scale of Social Cognition for Psychosis (items 1–7 for neurocognitive functions)	GEOPTE Scale of Social Cognition for Psychosis (items 8–15 for social cognitive function)	SQL-18	Patient perceptions of their social cognitive function (but not neurocognitive functioning) were strongly associated with QoL
Hasson-Ohayon et al. (2014)	39 SZ patients and 60 HC		FEIT; Faux Pas Task; IPII; MAS-A to assess metacognition	Wisconsin QLI-MH social domain	A diagnosis of SZ and metacognitive capacity, but not social cognition, predicted social QoL. Self-reflectivity had a negative relationship to social QoL, while understanding of others' minds had a positive relation to social QoL
Gigaux et al. (2013)	10 SZ outpatients and 10 HC	RWD task; TMT; Stroop Color Test; HSC; Go/No-Go Test		SQL-18	No relationship between QoL and cognitive inhibition was found
Boyer et al. (2012)	113 outpatients with stable SZ	WMS-III verbal learning and memory from logical memory subtests, visual learning and memory from the visual reproduction subtests; D2 attention task; TMT-A, B; verbal fluency (letter fluency)		SQL-18	Elementary neuropsychological measures were not statistically associated with QoL

Maat et al. (2012)	1120 patients with non-affective psychosis, 1057 of their siblings, 919 of their parents, and 590 unrelated HC	BFRT; WAIS-III	DFART; Hinting Task	WHOQOL-BREF	Total PANSS score was a moderator of the influence of the Hinting Task on QoL; in patients with a relatively low PANSS score, Hinting Task was not associated with QoL, while in patients with a mean or relatively high PANSS score, a better performance on the Hinting Task was associated with a poor QoL. This illness-related association is further emphasized by the finding that in siblings and HC, QoL is not related to social cognition but to neurocognition Social cognition, rather than neurocognition, is associated with QoL in SZ, and theory of mind is a more important domain of social cognition than emotion perception in relation to QoL of SZ patients
Kurtz et al. (2012)	44 stable SZ and SZA outpatients	WAIS-III Vocabulary, and the Digit Symbol and Symbol Search subtests; PCPT; CVLT-II; PCET	PEAT	SWL	Verbal memory and crystallized verbal skill were linked to improvements in SWL

(continued)

Table 3.2 (continued)

Study	Sample characteristics	Neurocognitive measures	Social cognition measures	QoL measures	Main findings
Woon et al. (2010)	83 SZ outpatients and 47 HC	BACS: List Learning, Digit Sequencing Task, Token Motor Task, Category Instances and COWA, Symbol Coding, and Tower of London and with the WRAT		WHOQOL-BREF	Poorer neurocognitive function especially in working and verbal memory, as well as lower level of psychosocial functioning, was correlated with poorer subjective QoL
Chino et al. (2009)	36 SZ outpatients	RAVLT-immediate; letter fluency test		WHOQOL-BREF	Neurocognitive test results were not correlated with subjective QoL
Brissos et al. (2008)	23 SZ remitted patients, 30 euthymic bipolar I patients, and 23 HC	WAIS Digit Span subtest; WMS-LMI, LMII; Symbol Digit Modalities Test; TMT-A, B; COWAT-letter fluency		WHOQOL-BREF	No correlations between any of the domains of the WHOQOL-BREF and any neurocognitive variables
Narvaez et al. (2008)	88 SZ and SZA outpatients	WAIS Digit Span, Digit Symbol, Letter–Number Sequencing subtests; letter fluency; WMS-LMI, LMII, TMT-A, B; WCST-PE, CAT		Subjective section of QOLI	Better neuropsychological functioning independently predicted worse subjective QoL

Study	Sample	Cognitive tests	Other measures	QoL measure	Findings
Williams et al. (2008)	56 FES outpatients and 112 HC	"IntegNeuro" battery tests (verbal interference, switching of attention, choice reaction time, verbal learning and recall, digit span, span of visual memory, sustained attention, tapping, letter fluency, semantic fluency, maze)	BRIEF; Neuroticism from the NEO-FFI	WHOQOL-BREF	Working memory capacity, verbal memory, sustained attention/vigilance, and negativity strongly predicted poorer social functioning in FES, along with poorer QoL in psychological, social, and health satisfaction facets
Hofer et al. (2005)	60 SZ outpatients	MWT-B, WCST, CVLT-immediate, TAP, BVRT, COWA		WHOQOL-BREF	No significant relationship found between neurocognitive variables and subjective QoL
Prouteau et al. (2005)	55 SZ spectrum disorder patients in a rehabilitation program	CANTAB		A measure of subjective QoL	Worse baseline sustained attention predicted better self-rated QoL
Alptekin et al. (2005)	38 SZ clinically stable SZ outpatients and 31 HC	WAIS Digit Span; COWAT-letter fluency		WHOQOL-BREF	The social domain scores of the WHOQOL were positively correlated with digit span and COWAT
Wegener et al. (2005)	51 SZ, SZA, schizophreniform, drug-induced psychosis, and BD patients	WAIS, Rey Complex Figure, RAVLT, CPT, Delis–Kaplan Executive Function System		WHOQOL-BREF	When psychiatric symptoms were considered, neurocognitive variables no longer predicted QoL
Herman (2004)	46 SZ + substance abuse inpatients and 43 SZ inpatients	WAIS Vocabulary, Digit Span, Digit Symbol subtests; COWAT-letter fluency; WMS-LMI, LMII, TMT-A, B		WHOQOL-BREF	Subjective QoL was only positively correlated with COWAT

(continued)

Table 3.2 (continued)

Study	Sample characteristics	Neurocognitive measures	Social cognition measures	QoL measures	Main findings
Sota and Heinrichs (2004)	55 neuroleptic-naïve SZ patients (assessed at index and 3 years later)	Vocabulary and Block Design subtests of the WAIS-R, CVLT, WCST, Purdue Pegboard		SIP	Cognitive measures predicted subjective QoL 3 years later
Voruganti et al. (2007)	86 SZ patients evaluated at baseline, 3, 6, 9, and 12 months after randomization to quetiapine or olanzapine	SSTICS (a computer-assisted cognitive test battery – COGLAB)		SIP	Quetiapine improved self-rated cognitive dysfunction and performance on selected neurocognitive tasks, but benefits of drug therapy were not reflected as significant gains in QoL
Fujii et al. (2004)	30 SZ, SZA, BD, and psychosis NOS	WAIS/WAIS-R IQ scale and Digit Span, Halstead categories, WMS Memory Quotient, Finger Tapping		BQLI	Neurocognitive variables predicted both objective and subjective QoL scores

BACS Brief Assessment of Cognition in Schizophrenia, *BD* Bipolar Disorder, *BFRT* Benton Facial Recognition Test, *BQLI* Brief Quality of Life Inventory, *BRIEF* Brain Resource Inventory of Emotional Intelligence Factor, *BVRT* Benton Visual Retention Test, *CANTAB* Cambridge Neuropsychological Test Automated Battery, *COWA* Controlled Oral Word Association Test, *COWAT* Controlled Word Association Test, *CPT* Continuous Performance Test, *CVLT* California Verbal Learning Test, *DFART* Degraded Facial Affect Recognition Task, *FEIT* Facial Emotion Identification Task, *FES* first-episode schizophrenia, *FFI* Five-Factor Inventory, *HC* healthy controls, *HSC* Hayling Sentence Completion Test, *IPII* Indiana Psychiatric Illness Interview, *LMI* Logical Memory Immediate Recall, *LMII* Logical Memory Delayed Recall, *MAS-A* Metacognition Assessment Scale-Abbreviated, *MWT-B* Mehrfachwahl–Wortschatz-Test B, *NOS* not otherwise specified, *PCPT* Penn Continuous Performance Test, *PEAT* Penn Emotion Acuity Test, *QLI-MH* Quality of Life Index for Mental Health, *QoL* quality of life, *QOLI* Lehman Quality of Life Interview, *RAVLT* Rey Auditory Verbal Learning Test, *RWD* reading with distraction, *SIP* Sickness Impact Profile, *SSTICS* subjective scale to investigate cognition in schizophrenia, *SWL* Satisfaction with Life Scale, *SZ* schizophrenia, *SZA* schizoaffective disorder, *TAP* Test of Attentional Performance, *TMT* Trail Making Test, *WAIS* Wechsler Adult Intelligence Scale, *WCST* Wisconsin Card Sorting Test (*CAT* categories, *PEs* perseverative errors), *WHOQOL-BREF* World Health Organization Quality of Life Scale (short form), *WMS* Wechsler Memory Scale, *WRAT* Wide Range Achievement Test

Concerning *subjective QoL* findings, the associations are overall nonsignificant, especially in measures of attention, working memory, verbal memory, and executive function. Furthermore, in the study by Prouteau et al. (2005), worse baseline sustained attention predicted better self-reported QoL. Measures of crystallized verbal ability and processing speed were both negatively correlated with subjective QoL, and verbal fluency seems to be the only measure found to be positively correlated with subjective QoL. Nevertheless, intellectual, executive, and motor skills have been shown to be valid joint predictors of subjective QoL in SZ patients 3 years after initial assessment (Sota and Heinrichs 2004). Since the review by Tolman and Kurtz (2012), two studies found significant associations between cognition and subjective QoL (Kurtz et al. 2012; Woon et al. 2010), whereas the other four found no associations (Caqueo-Urízar et al. 2015; Gigaux et al. 2013; Boyer et al. 2012; Maat et al. 2012).

One potential explanation for the inverse relationship between domains of neurocognition and subjective QoL is that individuals with stronger cognitive abilities may have greater insight into their illness and functional disability, enabling negative social comparison and thus lower life satisfaction (Narvaez et al. 2008; Karow and Pajonk 2006; Brekke et al. 2001).

Finally, cognition may play a common role in influencing SZ patients' ability to benefit from psychosocial and cognitive rehabilitation interventions, as measured by objective milestones of psychosocial success (attaining competitive employment, increasing the number and quality of social interactions) and the subjective experience of success in these same life domains (Kurtz et al. 2012).

Regarding intervention studies, Tas et al. (2012) reported that patients who received family-assisted social cognition and interaction training (F-SCIT) significantly improved in QoL, social functioning, and social cognition, whereas the social stimulation group worsened in nearly all outcome variables.

While the very different relationships between neurocognition and objective vs. subjective QoL might appear paradoxical, a wealth of research has revealed that objective QoL instruments that measure social and vocational status do not correlate with subjective QoL instruments that measure satisfaction with these same life domains (Lehman 1988; Savilla et al. 2008). This dissociation in constructs supports the notion that objective QoL and subjective QoL could have different sets of predictors in SZ patients. This has implications for the choice of scales used in studies.

3.7 Social Cognition and QoL in Schizophrenia

In recent years, social cognition has arisen as a significant predictor of social functioning in SZ (Couture et al. 2011), possibly by acting as a mediator factor (Ventura et al. 2009). Evidence also suggests that QoL and functional outcome in patients with SZ are related (Brekke et al. 2001). This fact raised the possibility that social cognition could be a factor influencing QoL in SZ patients. Until recently, few studies have explored this issue; we identified seven studies regarding social cognition and objective QoL and five concerning social cognition and subjective QoL (see Tables 3.1 and 3.2).

Regarding *objective QoL*, Kurtz et al. (2012) in a longitudinal study found that facial affect recognition partially mediated the relationship between verbal memory and improvements in objective QoL, suggesting that social cognitive skills could mediate the relationship between elemental aspects of cognition and observer-rated community functioning. In line with the aforementioned study, in the study by Bell et al. (2013), the group with high social cognition stood out with significantly better QLS total scores as compared to patients with low social cognition or to patients with high negative symptoms. Thus, it appears that better community functioning, as measured by the QLS, requires both the absence of prominent negative symptoms and better social cognition.

On the other hand, using structural equation modeling, a more powerful method than multiple regression to analyze a set of interactive factors simultaneously (Hoyle 1995; Lin et al. 2013) tested the mediation effect of clinical symptoms on the relationship between basic neurocognition and social cognition and functional outcome, in a large sample of patients with chronically stable SZ. Clinical symptoms, mainly negative ones, were found to mediate the relationship between neuro-/social cognitions and functional outcome, namely, QoL (Lin et al. 2013). They hypothesize that negative symptoms impair neuro- and social cognition possibly through lowered motivation to attend the tasks, negatively impacting on functioning, or negative symptoms decrease the motivation to participate in social activities, directly influencing functional outcome (Lin et al. 2013). These data support the importance of symptomatic remission to achieve a better social functioning (Brissos et al. 2011b).

However, some studies on objective QoL found no effect of social cognition in mediating predictors of QoL subdomains (Tas et al. 2013). Since the negative symptoms on the PANSS include items that directly reflect social contact, this may inflate the relationships between QoL and psychopathology, and this strong relationship may consequently obscure the mediation effect of social cognition (Tas et al. 2013).

Regarding *subjective QoL*, Maat et al. (2012) were the first to explore the specific role of social cognition in subjective QoL in SZ; they found that although better functional outcome correlated with a higher social cognition, subjective QoL did not and advanced the possibility that those patients with severe psychotic symptoms overall, but relatively preserved social cognition, may have good insight into their situation and therefore may actively withdraw from community life, which would reflect in a lower subjective QoL.

On the other hand, poorer social cognitive and neurocognitive skills may have a detrimental effect on perceived self-competency, and this may consequently reduce QoL scores in clinically stable SZ patients (Tas et al. 2013; Lysaker et al. 2005). In other words, it may be that stable SZ patients with less severe negative symptoms and impaired social cognitive abilities may make inaccurate judgments about their own competency; this would consequently have a negative impact on their own perception of their QoL, i.e., the Intrapsychic Foundation domain of QoL (Tas et al. 2013).

Finally, Hasson-Ohayon et al. (2014) have gone further and explored the distinction between social cognition and metacognition (i.e., the ability of thinking about thinking) and their associations with QoL's social domain in SZ; their results are consistent with the possibility that social cognition and metacognition constitute separate capacities and that the social domain of QoL was related to metacognition but not social cognition.

In sum, while some studies confirm the importance of social cognition in SZ patients' objective and subjective QoL, others have found no such association (Nahum et al. 2014; Tas et al. 2013; Hasson-Ohayon et al. 2014), raising the need for further investigation in this area. This is important to plan and implement treatment strategies, since the improvement on social cognition, social functioning, and motivation after social cognitive training may not reflect in improvements in QoL (Nahum et al. 2014).

3.8 Limitations of Studies

Despite the effort placed in recent research regarding basic neurocognition and social cognition and QoL in SZ patients, several methodological limitations have to be taken into account when interpreting the results.

The samples evaluated in most studies were relatively small and did not have control groups to evaluate potential differences between patients and healthy individuals. Longitudinal studies are also scarce.

Regarding symptoms, and especially depressive symptoms, known to be important predictors and/or mediators of the potential effect of neurocognition and social cognition on QoL, there is a low use of scales besides the PANSS, and not all studies use it; the use of scales to specifically assess insight and depressive symptoms in SZ patients might prove useful in the future, since depressive symptoms may mediate the effect between cognition and QoL, directly or through their interaction with illness awareness (Margariti et al. 2015).

Other variables such as cultural influences, (un)employment status, familiar relations, as well as illness duration, negative and positive symptom scores, or medication type and dosage have all been insufficiently taken into consideration in moderator analyses and may influence either neuro- or social cognition, as well as objective and/or subjective QoL.

As Tolman and Kurtz (2012) noted, several moderator analyses revealed that the type of QoL measure within the subjective QoL domains influenced the relationship of elementary neurocognition and QoL, suggesting that there is considerable between-measure variability in the assessment of the construct of subjective QoL. Moreover, cross-sectional predictors of objective and subjective satisfaction with life may be different from longitudinal predictors of treatment response (Kurtz et al. 2013).

Regarding neurocognitive evaluation, one of the critical issues associated with sophisticated cognitive neuroscience tests is whether these will manifest the substantial and consistent correlations seen between standard neuropsychological tests and indices of everyday functioning. One of the reasons that these standard tests may be so strongly correlated with everyday functioning is because they are so global and nonspecific (Keefe and Harvey 2012). It is possible that these sophisticated tests will be highly sensitive to focal brain functioning and only modestly sensitive to disability, especially that associated with SZ. This is of utmost importance, since the ultimate goal of treatment of cognitive dysfunction, as currently conceptualized, is to translate into meaningful functional outcomes (e.g., daily functioning, QoL) and reduce disability (Harvey and Keefe 2015). If task performance is uncorrelated with disability, then it seems implausible to think that improving performance would reduce disability (Keefe and Harvey 2012).

On the other hand, statistical significant differences in neurocognitive performance between groups, or changes before and after interventions, may not translate into clinical real-world benefits and, namely, in QoL. Therefore, translating research findings into real-world clinical practice is an even bigger challenge.

Regarding testing itself, some elementary neurocognitive domains have not been well represented in terms of numbers of measures (e.g., attention, nonverbal memory) in some studies, and current findings will be strengthened with the addition of other neurocognitive measures designed to measure similar constructs. The same is true for studies of social cognition.

3.9 Summary and Future Directions

QoL is a valid and useful outcome criterion, since subjective and patient-centered outcomes are more and more important in SZ research; as such, it should be consistently applied in clinical trials (Karow et al. 2014) and probably more often in clinical practice. However, the lack of consensus on QoL scales hampers research on its predictive validity. Future research needs to find a consensus on the concept and measures of QoL and to test whether QoL predicts better outcomes with respect to remission and recovery under consideration of different treatment approaches in patients with SZ (Karow et al. 2014). Moreover, studies taking into account staging systems for SZ are not known to us and would probably be useful in planning treatment strategies.

Given the above evidence, it seems intuitive that enhancement of neurocognition and social cognition in SZ patients might have benefits in terms of personal and social functioning, vocational outcome, and QoL.

Cognitive remediation on neurocognition has been shown to improve not only neurocognitive performance but also SZ patients' self-reported QoL (Garrido et al. 2013); on the other hand, negative results have also been reported (Wykes et al. 2007; Voruganti et al. 2007). In fact, antipsychotics such as quetiapine have been shown to improve self-rated cognitive dysfunction and subjects' performance on selected neurocognitive tasks; the accrued benefits of drug therapy, however, were not reflected as significant gains in daily functioning and QoL (Voruganti et al. 2007).

On the other hand, this may prove to be true for objective QoL only, since overall, results indicate that neurocognition is largely unrelated and, for some neurocognitive domains, even negatively related to subjective QoL; therefore, there is a need for clinical researchers to craft new interventions alongside those targeting cognition in order to ensure that integrated treatment interventions attend to individuals' subjective life satisfaction in addition to improving objective QoL.

If social cognition has an influence on QoL, then social cognition training could indirectly improve QoL. In fact, social cognition has been shown to be improved by psychosocial interventions and social cognitive training (Horan et al. 2008; Roberts et al. 2010; Kurtz 2011), and remediation training that specifically targets social cognition has been shown to significantly improve patients' self-reports of all subdomains of QoL (Tas et al. 2012). Interventions such as family-assisted social cognition and interaction training (F-SCIT), developed by Roberts and Penn (Roberts and Penn 2009), could constitute an approach to improve social cognition and QoL for SZ patients.

On the other hand, since neurocognition and social cognition are better viewed as a single construct, tests of both dimensions should always be included when studying this area. In fact, the MATRICS has proposed that social cognition and neurocognition should constitute an integral whole when measuring cognitive function in SZ.

Finally, clinical symptoms may mediate the cognition–functional outcome relationship, namely, QoL (Lin et al. 2013). Treating symptoms with antipsychotics, although keeping an eye for side effects that may impair QoL, or using approaches such as cognitive rehabilitation to reach clinical remission might be able to improve the functioning and QoL of patients with SZ (Lin et al. 2013).

In sum, it is evident that the interdependent relationship between symptomatology, neurocognition, social cognition, and QoL in SZ may be deterministic, and therefore it seems crucial to take a more holistic and integrative approach to understanding QoL when trying to see the bigger picture in this complex and severe disorder (Tas et al. 2013).

References

Addington J, Addington D. Social and cognitive functioning in psychosis. Schizophr Res. 2008;99(1):176–81.

Addington J, Saeedi H, Addington D. Influence of social perception and social knowledge on cognitive and social functioning in early psychosis. Br J Psychiatry. 2006;189(4):373–8.

Aki H, Tomotake M, Kaneda Y, Iga J-I, Kinouchi S, Shibuya-Tayoshi S, Tayoshi S-Y, Motoki I, Moriguchi K, Sumitani S. Subjective and objective quality of life, levels of life skills, and their clinical determinants in outpatients with schizophrenia. Psychiatry Res. 2008;158(1):19–25.

Alptekin K, Akvardar Y, Akdede BB, Dumlu K, Işık D, Pirinçci F, Yahssin S, Kitiş A. Is quality of life associated with cognitive impairment in schizophrenia? Prog Neuro-Psychopharmacol Biol Psychiatry. 2005;29(2):239–44.

American Psychiatric Association. Diagnostic and statistical manual-text revision. 4th ed., text rev. Washington, DC: Author; 2000.

Baron-Cohen S, Wheelwright S, Hill J, Raste Y, Plumb I. The "Reading the Mind in the Eyes" test revised version: a study with normal adults, and adults with Asperger syndrome or high-functioning autism. J Child Psychol Psychiatry. 2001;42(2):241–51.

Becchi A, Rucci P, Placentino A, Neri G, de Girolamo G. Quality of life in patients with schizo-phrenia—comparison of self-report and proxy assessments. Soc Psychiatry Psychiatr Epidemiol. 2004;39(5):397–401.

Bell MD, Corbera S, Johannesen JK, Fiszdon JM, Wexler BE. Social cognitive impairments and negative symptoms in schizophrenia: are there subtypes with distinct functional correlates? Schizophr Bull. 2013;39(1):186–96.

Bentall RP, Corcoran R, Howard R, Blackwood N, Kinderman P. Persecutory delusions: a review and theoretical integration. Clin Psychol Rev. 2001;21(8):1143–92.

Bowie CR, Leung WW, Reichenberg A, McClure MM, Patterson TL, Heaton RK, Harvey PD. Predicting schizophrenia patients' real-world behavior with specific neuropsychological and functional capacity measures. Biol Psychiatry. 2008;63(5):505–11.

Boyer L, Aghababian V, Richieri R, Loundou A, Padovani R, Simeoni M, Auquier P, Lancon C. Insight into illness, neurocognition and quality of life in schizophrenia. Prog Neuro-Psychopharmacol Biol Psychiatry. 2012;36(2):271–6.

Brekke JS, Kohrt B, Green MF. Neuropsychological functioning as a moderator of the relationship between psychosocial functioning and the subjective experience of self and life in schizophre-nia. Schizophr Bull. 2001;27(4):697.

Brekke JS, Hoe M, Long J, Green MF. How neurocognition and social cognition influence func-tional change during community-based psychosocial rehabilitation for individuals with schizo-phrenia. Schizophr Bull. 2007;33(5):1247–56.

Brekke J, Hoe M, Green M. Neurocognitive change, functional change and service intensity during community-based psychosocial rehabilitation for schizophrenia. Psychol Med. 2009;39(10):1637–47.

Brissos S, Dias VV, Soeiro-de-Souza MG, Balanzá-Martínez V, Kapczinski F. The impact of a history of psychotic symptoms on cognitive function in euthymic bipolar patients: a compari-son with schizophrenic patients and healthy controls. Rev Bras Psiquiatr. 2011a;33(4):353–61.

Brissos S, Dias VV, Balanzá-Martinez V, Carita AI, Figueira ML. Symptomatic remission in schizophrenia patients: relationship with social functioning, quality of life, and neurocognitive performance. Schizophr Res. 2011b;129(2):133–6.

Brissos S, Dias VV, Carita AI, Martinez-Arán A. Quality of life in bipolar type I disorder and schizophrenia in remission: clinical and neurocognitive correlates. Psychiatry Res. 2008;160(1):55–62.

Brüne M. Emotion recognition, 'theory of mind,' and social behavior in schizophrenia. Psychiatry Res. 2005;133(2):135–47.

Burton S. Symptom domains of schizophrenia: the role of atypical antipsychotic agents. J Psychopharmacol. 2006;20(6 suppl):6–19.

Caqueo-Urízar A, Boyer L, Baumstarck K, Gilman SE. Subjective perceptions of cognitive deficits and their influences on quality of life among patients with schizophrenia. Qual Life Res. 2015;24(11):2753–60.

Chino B, Nemoto T, Fujii C, Mizuno M. Subjective assessments of the quality of life, well-being and self-efficacy in patients with schizophrenia. Psychiatry Clin Neurosci. 2009;63(4):521–28.

Chisholm D, Bhugra D. Sociocultural and economic aspects of quality of life measurement. Eur Psychiatry. 1997;12(4):210–5.

Chue P. The relationship between patient satisfaction and treatment outcomes in schizophrenia. J Psychopharmacol. 2006;20(6 Suppl):38–56.

Combs DR, Penn DL, Wicher M, Waldheter E. The Ambiguous Intentions Hostility Questionnaire (AIHQ): a new measure for evaluating hostile social-cognitive biases in paranoia. Cogn Neuropsychiatry. 2007;12(2):128–43.

Corbera S, Wexler BE, Ikezawa S, Bell MD. Factor structure of social cognition in schizophrenia: is empathy preserved? Schizophr Res Treatment. 2013;2013:409205.

Corcoran R, Mercer G, Frith CD. Schizophrenia, symptomatology and social inference: investigat-ing "theory of mind" in people with schizophrenia. Schizophr Res. 1995;17(1):5–13.

Corrigan PW. The social perceptual deficits of schizophrenia. Psychiatry. 1997;60(4):309–26.

Couture SM, Penn DL, Roberts DL. The functional significance of social cognition in schizophrenia: a review. Schizophr Bull. 2006;32 Suppl 1:S44–63.

Couture SM, Granholm EL, Fish SC. A path model investigation of neurocognition, theory of mind, social competence, negative symptoms and real-world functioning in schizophrenia. Schizophr Res. 2011;125(2):152–60.

Dickinson D, Coursey RD. Independence and overlap among neurocognitive correlates of community functioning in schizophrenia. Schizophr Res. 2002;56(1):161–70.

Dickerson F, Ringel N, Parente F. Subjective quality of life in out-patients with schizophrenia: clinical and utilization correlates. Acta Psychiatr Scand. 1998;98(2):124–7.

Evans JD, Heaton RK, Paulsen JS, Palmer BW, Patterson T, Jeste DV. The relationship of neuropsychological abilities to specific domains of functional capacity in older schizophrenia patients. Biol Psychiatry. 2003;53(5):422–30.

Figueira ML, Brissos S. Measuring psychosocial outcomes in schizophrenia patients. Curr Opin Psychiatry. 2011;24(2):91–9.

Fiske ST, Taylor SE. Social cognition. 2nd ed. New York: McGraw-Hill; 1991. p. 16–5.

Fiszdon JM, Choi J, Goulet J, Bell MD. Temporal relationship between change in cognition and change in functioning in schizophrenia. Schizophr Res. 2008;105(1):105–13.

Fitzgerald PB, Williams C, Corteling N, Filia S, Brewer K, Adams A, De Castella A, Rolfe T, Davey P, Kulkarni J. Subject and observer-rated quality of life in schizophrenia. Acta Psychiatr Scand. 2001;103(5):387–92.

Fujii DE, Wylie AM, Nathan JH. Neurocognition and long-term prediction of quality of life in outpatients with severe and persistent mental illness. Schizophrenia Res. 2004; 69(1):67–73.

Gallotti M, Frith CD. Social cognition in the we-mode. Trends Cogn Sci. 2013;17(4):160–5.

Garrido G, Barrios M, Penadés R, Enríquez M, Garolera M, Aragay N, Pajares M, Vallès V, Delgado L, Alberni J. Computer-assisted cognitive remediation therapy: cognition, self-esteem and quality of life in schizophrenia. Schizophr Res. 2013;150(2):563–9.

Gigaux J, Le Gall D, Jollant F, Lhuillier J, Richard-Devantoy S. Cognitive inhibition and quality of life in schizophrenia: a pilot study. Schizophr Res. 2013;143(2):297–300.

Green MF. What are the functional consequences of neurocognitive deficits in schizophrenia? Am J Psychiatry. 1996;153(3):321.

Green MF, Kern RS, Braff DL, Mintz J. Neurocognitive deficits and functional outcome in schizophrenia: are we measuring the "right stuff"? Schizophr Bull. 2000;26(1):119.

Green MF, Kern RS, Heaton RK. Longitudinal studies of cognition and functional outcome in schizophrenia: implications for MATRICS. Schizophr Res. 2004;72(1):41–51.

Green MF, Penn DL, Bentall R, Carpenter WT, Gaebel W, Gur RC, Kring AM, Park S, Silverstein SM, Heinssen R. Social cognition in schizophrenia: an NIMH workshop on definitions, assessment, and research opportunities. Schizophr Bull. 2008;34(6):1211–20.

Harvey PD, Keefe RS. Methods for delivering and evaluating the efficacy of cognitive enhancement. In: Cognitive Enhancement. Springer International Publishing; 2015. p. 5–25.

Harvey PD, Velligan DI, Bellack AS. Performance-based measures of functional skills: usefulness in clinical treatment studies. Schizophr Bull. 2007;33(5):1138–48.

Hasan A, Falkai P, Wobrock T, Lieberman J, Glenthoj B, Gattaz WF, Thibaut F, Möller H-J. World Federation of Societies of Biological Psychiatry (WFSBP) guidelines for biological treatment of schizophrenia, part 2: update 2012 on the long-term treatment of schizophrenia and management of antipsychotic-induced side effects. World J Biol Psychiatry. 2013;14(1):2–44.

Hasson-Ohayon I, Avidan-Msika M, Mashiach-Eizenberg M, Kravetz S, Rozencwaig S, Shalev H, Lysaker PH. Metacognitive and social cognition approaches to understanding the impact of schizophrenia on social quality of life. Schizophr Res. 2014;161(2):386–91.

Hayhurst KP, Massie JA, Dunn G, Lewis SW, Drake RJ. Validity of subjective versus objective quality of life assessment in people with schizophrenia. BMC Psychiatry. 2014;14(1):365.

Heinrichs RW, Zakzanis KK. Neurocognitive deficit in schizophrenia: a quantitative review of the evidence. Neuropsychology. 1998;12(3):426.

Heinrichs DW, Hanlon TE, Carpenter WT. The Quality of Life Scale: an instrument for rating the schizophrenic deficit syndrome. Schizophr Bull. 1984;10(3):388.

Herrman H, Hawthorne G, Thomas R. Quality of life assessment in people living with psychosis. Soc Psychiatry Psychiatr Epidemiol. 2002;37(11):510–8.

Herman M. Neurocognitive functioning and quality of life among dually diagnosed and non-substance abusing schizophrenia inpatients. Int J Ment Health Nurs. 2004;13(4):282–91.

Hoe M, Nakagami E, Green M, Brekke J. The causal relationships between neurocognition, social cognition and functional outcome over time in schizophrenia: a latent difference score approach. Psychol Med. 2012;42(11):2287–99.

Hofer A, Kemmler G, Eder U, Edlinger M, Hummer M, Fleischhacker WW. Quality of life in schizophrenia: the impact of psychopathology, attitude toward medication, and side effects. J Clin Psychiatry. 2004;65(7):932–9.

Hofer A, Baumgartner S, Bodner T, Edlinger M, Hummer M, Kemmler G, Rettenbacher MA, Fleischhacker WW. Patient outcomes in schizophrenia II: the impact of cognition. Eur Psychiatry. 2005;20(5):395–402.

Horan WP, Kern RS, Green MF, Penn DL. Social cognition training for individuals with schizophrenia: emerging evidence. Am J Psychiatr Rehabil. 2008;11(3):205–52.

Hoyle RH. Structural equation modeling: concepts, issues, and applications. Thousand Oaks: Sage Publications; 1995.

Jakovljević M, Tomić Z, Maslov B, Skoko I. New image of psychiatry, mass media impact and public relations. Psychiatr Danub. 2010;22(2):145–8.

Juckel G, Morosini PL. The new approach: psychosocial functioning as a necessary outcome criterion for therapeutic success in schizophrenia. Curr Opin Psychiatry. 2008;21(6):630–9.

Karow A, Pajonk FG. Insight and quality of life in schizophrenia: recent findings and treatment implications. Curr Opin Psychiatry. 2006;19(6):637–41.

Karow A, Wittmann L, Schöttle D, Schäfer I, Lambert M. The assessment of quality of life in clinical practice in patients with schizophrenia. Dialogues Clin Neurosci. 2014;16(2):185.

Keefe R. The longitudinal course of cognitive impairment in schizophrenia: an examination of data from premorbid through posttreatment phases of illness. J Clin Psychiatry. 2013; 75:8–13.

Keefe RS, Harvey PD. Cognitive impairment in schizophrenia. In: Novel antischizophrenia treatments. Springer Berlin Heidelberg; 2012. p. 11–37.

Kilian R, Angermeyer MC. The effects of antipsychotic treatment on quality of life of schizophrenic patients under naturalistic treatment conditions: an application of random effect regression models and propensity scores in an observational prospective trial. Qual Life Res. 2005;14(5):1275–89.

Kinderman P, Bentall RP. Causal attributions in paranoia and depression: internal, personal, and situational attributions for negative events. J Abnorm Psychol. 1997;106(2):341.

Kitchen H, Rofail D, Heron L, Sacco P. Cognitive impairment associated with schizophrenia: a review of the humanistic burden. Adv Ther. 2012;29(2):148–62.

Kohler CG, Martin E A, Kujawski E, Bilker W, Gur RE, Gur RC. No effect of donepezil on neurocognition and social cognition in young persons with stable schizophrenia. Cogn Neuropsychiatry. 2007;12(5):412–21.

Kret ME, Ploeger A. Emotion processing deficits: a liability spectrum providing insight into comorbidity of mental disorders. Neurosci Biobehav Rev. 2015;52:153–71.

Kurtz MM. Neurocognition as a predictor of response to evidence-based psychosocial interventions in schizophrenia: what is the state of the evidence? Clin Psychol Rev. 2011;31(4): 663–72.

Kurtz MM, Tolman A. Neurocognition, insight into illness and subjective quality-of-life in schizophrenia: what is their relationship? Schizophr Res. 2011;127(1):157–62.

Kurtz MM, Wexler BE, Fujimoto M, Shagan DS, Seltzer JC. Symptoms versus neurocognition as predictors of change in life skills in schizophrenia after outpatient rehabilitation. Schizophr Res. 2008;102(1):303–11.

Kurtz MM, Bronfeld M, Rose J. Cognitive and social cognitive predictors of change in objective versus subjective quality-of-life in rehabilitation for schizophrenia. Psychiatry Res. 2012;200(2):102–7.

Kurtz MM, Olfson RH, Rose J. Self-efficacy and functional status in schizophrenia: relationship to insight, cognition and negative symptoms. Schizophr Res. 2013;145(1):69–74.

Lambert M, Schimmelmann BG, Karow A, Naber D. Subjective well-being and initial dysphoric reaction under antipsychotic drugs-concepts, measurement and clinical relevance. Pharmacopsychiatry. 2003;36:S181–90.

Langdon R, Michie PT, Ward PB, McConaghy N, Catts SV, Coltheart M. Defective self and/or other mentalising in schizophrenia: a cognitive neuropsychological approach. Cogn Neuropsychiatry. 1997;2(3):167–93.

Langdon R, Ward PB, Coltheart M. Reasoning anomalies associated with delusions in schizophrenia. Schizophr Bull. 2010;36(2):321–30.

Lehman AF. Measures of quality of life among persons with severe and persistent mental disorders. Soc Psychiatry Psychiatr Epidemiol. 1996;31(2):78–88.

Lehman AF. A quality of life interview for the chronically mentally ill. Eval Program Plann. 1988;11(1):51–62.

Lin C-H, Huang C-L, Chang Y-C, Chen P-W, Lin C-Y, Tsai GE, Lane H-Y. Clinical symptoms, mainly negative symptoms, mediate the influence of neurocognition and social cognition on functional outcome of schizophrenia. Schizophr Res. 2013;146(1):231–7.

Lipkovich IA, Deberdt W, Csernansky JG, Sabbe B, Keefe RS, Kollack-Walker S. Relationships among neurocognition, symptoms and functioning in patients with schizophrenia: a path-analytic approach for associations at baseline and following 24 weeks of antipsychotic drug therapy. BMC psychiatry. 2009;9(1):1.

Lysaker PH, Carcione A, Dimaggio G, Johannesen J, Nicolò G, Procacci M, Semerari A. Metacognition amidst narratives of self and illness in schizophrenia: associations with neurocognition, symptoms, insight and quality of life. Acta Psychiatr Scand. 2005;112(1):64–71.

Lysaker PH, Davis LW. Social function in schizophrenia and schizoaffective disorder: associations with personality, symptoms and neurocognition. Health Qual Life Outcomes. 2004;2(1):1.

Maat A, Fett A-K, Derks E, Investigators G. Social cognition and quality of life in schizophrenia. Schizophr Res. 2012;137(1):212–8.

Margariti M, Ploumpidis D, Economou M, Christodoulou GN, Papadimitriou GN. Quality of life in schizophrenia spectrum disorders: associations with insight and psychopathology. Psychiatry Res. 2015;225(3):695–701.

Matsui M, Sumiyoshi T, Arai H, Higuchi Y, Kurachi M. Cognitive functioning related to quality of life in schizophrenia. Prog Neuro-Psychopharmacol Biol Psychiatry. 2008;32(1):280–7.

Mayer JD, Salovey P, Caruso DR, Sitarenios G. Emotional intelligence as a standard intelligence. Emotion (Washington, DC). 2001;1(3):232–42.

Mehta UM, Bhagyavathi HD, Thirthalli J, Kumar KJ, Gangadhar BN. Neurocognitive predictors of social cognition in remitted schizophrenia. Psychiatry Res. 2014;219(2):268–74. doi:10.1016/j.psychres.2014.05.055.

Moncrieff J, Cohen D, Mason J. The subjective experience of taking antipsychotic medication: a content analysis of internet data. Acta Psychiatr Scand. 2009;120(2):102–11.

Munton AG, Silvester J, Stratton P. Attributions in action: a practical approach to coding qualitative data. John Wiley & Sons Inc.; 1999.

Nahum M, Fisher M, Loewy R, Poelke G, Ventura J, Nuechterlein KH, Hooker CI, Green MF, Merzenich MM, Vinogradov S. A novel, online social cognitive training program for young adults with schizophrenia: a pilot study. Schizophr Res Cogn. 2014;1(1):e11–9.

Narvaez JM, Twamley EW, McKibbin CL, Heaton RK, Patterson TL. Subjective and objective quality of life in schizophrenia. Schizophr Res. 2008;98(1):201–8.

Norman RM, Malla AK, McLean T, Voruganti LP, Cortese L, McIntosh E, Cheng S, Rickwood A. The relationship of symptoms and level of functioning in schizophrenia to general wellbeing and the Quality of Life Scale. Acta Psychiatr Scand. 2000;102(4):303–9.

Nuechterlein KH, Subotnik KL, Green MF, Ventura J, Asarnow RF, Gitlin MJ, Yee CM, Gretchen-Doorly D, Mintz J. Neurocognitive predictors of work outcome in recent-onset schizophrenia. Schizophr Bull. 2011;37 Suppl 2:S33–40.

Papaioannou D, Brazier J, Parry G. How valid and responsive are generic health status measures, such as EQ-5D and SF-36, in schizophrenia? A systematic review. Value Health. 2011;14(6):907–20.

Patterson TL, Goldman S, McKibbin CL, Hughs T, Jeste DV. UCSD Performance-Based Skills Assessment: development of a new measure of everyday functioning for severely mentally ill adults. Schizophr Bull. 2001;27(2):235–45.

Penn DL, Corrigan PW, Bentall RP, Racenstein J, Newman L. Social cognition in schizophrenia. Psychol Bull. 1997;121(1):114.

Percudani M, Barbui C, Tansella M. Effect of second-generation antipsychotics on employment and productivity in individuals with schizophrenia. Pharmacoeconomics. 2004;22(11): 701–18.

Priebe S, Katsakou C, Yeeles K, Amos T, Morriss R, Wang D, Wykes T. Predictors of clinical and social outcomes following involuntary hospital admission: a prospective observational study. Eur Arch Psychiatry Clin Neurosci. 2011;261(5):377–86.

Prouteau A, Verdoux H, Briand C, Lesage A, Lalonde P, Nicole L, Reinharz D, Stip E. Cognitive predictors of psychosocial functioning outcome in schizophrenia: a follow-up study of subjects participating in a rehabilitation program. Schizophr Res. 2005;77(2):343–53.

Reine G, Lancon C, Di Tucci S, Sapin C, Auquier P. Depression and subjective quality of life in chronic phase schizophrenic patients. Acta Psychiatr Scand. 2003;108(4):297–303.

Remington G, Foussias G, Agid O. Progress in defining optimal treatment outcome in schizophrenia. CNS Drugs. 2010;24(1):9–20.

Roberts DL, Penn DL. Social cognition and interaction training (SCIT) for outpatients with schizophrenia: a preliminary study. Psychiatry Res. 2009;166(2):141–7.

Roberts DL, Penn DL, Labate D, Margolis SA, Sterne A. Transportability and feasibility of Social Cognition And Interaction Training (SCIT) in community settings. Behav Cogn Psychother. 2010;38(01):35–47.

Rosenheck R, Leslie D, Keefe R, McEvoy J, Swartz M, Perkins D, Stroup S, Hsiao JK, Lieberman J. Barriers to employment for people with schizophrenia. Am J Psychiatry. 2006;163(3): 411–7.

Rosenthal R, Hall J, Archer D, DiMatteo M, Rogers P. The PONS test manual. New York: Irvington; 1979.

Ruggeri M, Nose M, Bonetto C, Cristofalo D, Lasalvia A, Salvi G, Stefani B, Malchiodi F, Tansella M. Changes and predictors of change in objective and subjective quality of life Multiwave follow-up study in community psychiatric practice. Br J Psychiatry. 2005;187(2):121–30.

Savilla K, Kettler L, Galletly C. Relationships between cognitive deficits, symptoms and quality of life in schizophrenia. Aust N Z J Psychiatry. 2008;42(6):496–504.

Schmidt SJ, Mueller DR, Roder V. Social cognition as a mediator variable between neurocognition and functional outcome in schizophrenia: empirical review and new results by structural equation modeling. Schizophr Bull. 2011;37 Suppl 2:S41–54.

Sergi MJ, Rassovsky Y, Widmark C, Reist C, Erhart S, Braff DL, Marder SR, Green MF. Social cognition in schizophrenia: relationships with neurocognition and negative symptoms. Schizophr Res. 2007;90(1):316–24.

Sota TL, Heinrichs RW. Demographic, clinical, and neurocognitive predictors of quality of life in schizophrenia patients receiving conventional neuroleptics. Compr Psychiatry. 2004;45(5):415–21.

Stone VE, Baron-Cohen S, Knight RT. Frontal lobe contributions to theory of mind. J Cogn Neurosci. 1998;10(5):640–56.

Subotnik KL, Nuechterlein KH, Green MF, Horan WP, Nienow TM, Ventura J, Nguyen AT. Neurocognitive and social cognitive correlates of formal thought disorder in schizophrenia patients. Schizophr Res. 2006;85(1):84–95.

Tas C, Danaci AE, Cubukcuoglu Z, Brüne M. Impact of family involvement on social cognition training in clinically stable outpatients with schizophrenia—a randomized pilot study. Psychiatry Res. 2012;195(1):32–8.

Tas C, Brown E, Cubukcuoglu Z, Aydemir O, Danaci AE, Brüne M. Towards an integrative approach to understanding quality of life in schizophrenia: the role of neurocognition, social cognition, and psychopathology. Compr Psychiatry. 2013;54(3):262–8.

The WHOQOL Group. The World Health Organization quality of life assessment (WHOQOL): position paper from the World Health Organization. Soc Sci Med. 1995;41(10):1403–9.

Tolman AW, Kurtz MM. Neurocognitive predictors of objective and subjective quality of life in individuals with schizophrenia: a meta-analytic investigation. Schizophr Bull. 2012; 38(2):304–15.

Ueoka Y, Tomotake M, Tanaka T, Kaneda Y, Taniguchi K, Nakataki M, Numata S, Tayoshi S, Yamauchi K, Sumitani S. Quality of life and cognitive dysfunction in people with schizophrenia. Progr Neuro-Psychopharmacol Biol Psychiatry. 2011;35(1):53–9.

Van Hooren S, Versmissen D, Janssen I, Myin-Germeys I, à Campo J, Mengelers R, Van Os J, Krabbendam L. Social cognition and neurocognition as independent domains in psychosis. Schizophr Res. 2008;103(1):257–65.

Ventura J, Hellemann GS, Thames AD, Koellner V, Nuechterlein KH. Symptoms as mediators of the relationship between neurocognition and functional outcome in schizophrenia: a meta-analysis. Schizophr Res. 2009;113(2):189–99.

Ventura J, Wood RC, Jimenez AM, Hellemann GS. Neurocognition and symptoms identify links between facial recognition and emotion processing in schizophrenia: meta-analytic findings. Schizophr Res. 2013;151(1):78–84.

Voruganti L, Heslegrave R, Awad A, Seeman M. Quality of life measurement in schizophrenia: reconciling the quest for subjectivity with the question of reliability. Psychol Med. 1998; 28(01):165–72.

Voruganti L, Awad A, Parker G, Forrest C, Usmani Y, Fernando M, Senthilal S. Cognition, functioning and quality of life in schizophrenia treatment: results of a one-year randomized controlled trial of olanzapine and quetiapine. Schizophr Res. 2007;96(1):146–55.

Wegener S, Redoblado-Hodge MA, Wegener S, Redoblado-Hodge MA, Lucas S, Fitzgerald D, Harris A, Brennan J. Relative contributions of psychiatric symptoms and neuropsychological functioning to quality of life in first-episode psychosis. Aust N Z J Psychiatry. 2005; 39(6):487–92.

Williams LM, Whitford TJ, Flynn G, Wong W, Liddell BJ, Silverstein S, Gordon E. General and social cognition in first episode schizophrenia: identification of separable factors and prediction of functional outcome using the IntegNeuro test battery. Schizophr Res. 2008;99(1):182–191.

Woon P, Chia MY, Chan WY, Sim K. Neurocognitive, clinical and functional correlates of subjective quality of life in Asian outpatients with schizophrenia. Prog Neuro-Psychopharmacol Biol Psychiatry. 2010;34(3):463–8.

Woonings FM, Appelo MT, Kluiter H, Slooff CJ, van den Bosch RJ. Learning (potential) and social functioning in schizophrenia. Schizophr Res. 2003;59(2):287–96.

Wykes T, Reeder C, Landau S, Everitt B, Knapp M, Patel A, Romeo R. Cognitive remediation therapy in schizophrenia. Br J Psychiatry. 2007;190(5):421–7.

Yamauchi K, Aki H, Tomotake M, Iga JI, Numata S, Motoki I, Izaki Y, Tayoshi S, Kinouchi S, Sumitani S. Predictors of subjective and objective quality of life in outpatients with schizophrenia. Psychiatry Clin Neurosci. 2008;62(4):404–11.

Chapter 4
Conceptual Issues in Cultural Adaptation and the Role of Culture in Assessment of Health-Related Quality of Life in Schizophrenia

Monika Vance, Elizabeth Pappadopulos, Richard Keefe, and Amir Kalali

4.1 Introduction

Before we begin a discussion about the role of culture in evaluating health-related quality of life in schizophrenia, let's clarify some terms used in connection with measurement of psychiatric states and samples of behavior across clinical disciplines and related industries. For conceptual consistency of the discussion in this chapter, it's important to understand how terminology from other scientific disciplines is used across healthcare and pharmaceutical industries that describes, or simply refers to, psychometric measurement and the tools that are used for such purpose.

The most basic fact is that an instrument used to systematically and empirically measure sample function or behavior is a *psychological test*. Psychological tests are scientifically constructed instruments that are used to objectively measure states and/or traits within a specifically defined conceptual framework (e.g., attitudes, aptitudes, competencies, cognition, mood, physical function, and so on). Such

M. Vance (✉)
Santium Mental Health, 13-3120 Rutherford Road, Suite 339,
Vaughan, ON L4K 0B2, Canada
e-mail: mvance@santium.com

E. Pappadopulos, PhD
Pfizer Inc, 235 East 42nd Street, New York, NY 10017, USA
e-mail: elizabeth.pappadopulos@pfizer.com

R. Keefe, PhD
Psychiatry & Behavioral Sciences and Psychology & Neuroscience, Duke University
Medical Center, Durham, NC, USA
e-mail: richard.keefe@duke.edu

A. Kalali, MD
Neuroscience Center of Excellence, Quintiles,
10188 Telesis Court, San Diego, CA 92121, USA
e-mail: Amir.Kalali@quintiles.com

© Springer International Publishing Switzerland 2016
A.G. Awad, L.N.P. Voruganti (eds.), *Beyond Assessment of Quality of Life in Schizophrenia*, DOI 10.1007/978-3-319-30061-0_4

conceptual frameworks can be generalized to quality of life or become slightly more targeted to health-related quality of life, or be highly specific, such as measuring types and severity of hallucinations in schizophrenia.

Psychological tests were originally created to aid in making decisions about people in the contexts of educational competencies and occupational fit and were later adopted for clinical differentiation between "normal" and "abnormal" behavior and functioning. For lack of better alternatives, at least for now, well-designed psychological tests remain to be particularly useful for evaluating interrelationships of cognitive, affective, and behavioral traits (Urbina 2014). This transition in application ultimately progressed into scientific research and experimentation with therapeutic treatments.

In the context of this chapter, we will treat health-related quality of life tests the same as any psychological test used for clinical assessment purposes, because at its core, a quality of life test is still a psychometric instrument despite its typically generalized construct in relation to psychopathologies of mental disorders. Because it is a psychometric instrument, the same amount of rigor in evaluation, selection, and adaptation should be applied to it as to any of the other and more complex clinically focused psychological tests.

4.2   Test Adoption: Culture, Purpose, and Fit

Most commercially available psychological tests were developed in the course of routine clinical practice within busy clinics and psychiatric institutions and assigned by their developers to test publishers for marketing, global distribution, and copyright management. Many more remain hidden in thousands of international scientific journals, doctoral dissertations, obscure databases owned by academic institutions and professional associations, and an array of compendia of measures commonly used within a specific psychiatric specialty. Most of these instruments were developed in the 1970s with intent to improve empirical data in clinical research, quality of longitudinal care for a certain groups of patients, and later also for justification of importance and effectiveness of treatment programs for managed care reimbursement purposes. Successes with methods of treatment monitoring and outcome reporting from these initiatives have been, and continue to be, publicized in journals and sometimes also through marketing efforts by test publishers and their international affiliates. This leads to clinicians practicing in other settings, or in other countries, or treating different types of patient groups (i.e., immigrants who do not yet speak the language), to adopt such instruments in their local settings. While having access to new instruments is generally viewed as an advancement in mental health treatment methods, adopting an instrument for use within a new culture, with groups of people speaking different languages and harboring different behavioral norms, can become exceptionally challenging and sometimes impossible. If the instrument is used in the context for which it was not designed, a perceived and well-intentioned "advancement in mental health care" can actually result in unintended harm to patients and potentially to their caregivers as well.

4.3 Considerations in Cross-Cultural Assessment of Mental Health States

4.3.1 The Role of Emic and Etic Perspectives in Assessment and Testing

Psychological testing is a scientifically standardized method of measuring mental capabilities and behavioral styles of specific groups of people, confirmed by validity and reliability that collectively represent psychometric accuracy. It is therefore important for both researchers and clinicians to think about how meaningful the information generated by a psychological test will be when he or she takes into consideration the differences and similarities between a cultural group for which an instrument was developed and the innate traits of the cultural group to which the instrument will be applied. Although there are distinctly different opinions in the fields of anthropology and linguistics about how cross-cultural data should be collected and interpreted, there does appear to be a consensus on two key approaches: (1) etic perspective and (2) emic perspective. Marvin Harris, an influential anthropologist and a prolific writer, applied the work of linguist Kenneth Pike to cultural anthropology and defined the terms *etic* and *emic* (Harris 1976) in parallel to Pike's linguistic context (Pike 1967). He defined *etics* as "domains or operations whose validity does not depend upon the demonstrations of conscious or unconscious significance or reality in the minds of natives" and *emics* as "domains and operations whose validity depends upon distinctions that are real or meaningful (but not necessarily conscious) to the natives themselves."

For clinicians and researchers alike, understanding cross-cultural data and its interpretability is critical for modeling successful outcomes of their treatment plans and research studies. In clinical practice, interpretability of information that clinicians elicit from their patients is largely subjective and inconsistent in quality. In medicine, practicing clinicians tend to have a strong aversion to structured interviewing and completing of questionnaires of any kind. Patients have become an important part of the data collection process, as they have vested interest in improving their quality of life, or at least maintaining it, and can provide a more comprehensive report on functioning, pain intensity, changes in quality of life, and important symptoms. In clinical psychology and in neuropsychology, structured data collection is accepted and part of routine assessment. In any case, however, information gathering and quality of data entered into patient registries are based on the depth of a clinicians' understanding of cultural differences and similarities between the patient and the environment in which the patient lives and/or is being treated. Better information provides deeper insight into patients' illness and promises more effective treatment. This is challenging, because sharing of pertinent information can be uncomfortable for the patients and caregivers and for some ethnic groups even culturally inappropriate. Trust and rapport between patient and clinician have been found to be an integral success factor in adherence to treatment in any culture. Therefore, for effective longitudinal treatment of mental illness, it is important for the clinician and the patient to develop a relationship of mutual respect. For example, when they choose to seek medical treatment, individuals from displaced ethnic groups tend to seek out physicians of the same ethnicity. A physician with the same cultural background provides a sense of familiarity of "home," because he or she is likely to speak their own language, understand their customs, willingly bare their bodies, and submit to certain types of invasive procedures and of his or her manner of communication. A much less conscious aspect of such a preference is that the physician will likely be familiar with common culture-bound ways in reporting symptoms, should be able to adapt Western idioms in relation to a specific condition to something conceptually equivalent in the patient's country and culture, will know how to ask culturally appropriate questions to elicit information that is needed for medical assessment, will be willing to collaborate with traditional healers if it's part of the patient's culture, and considers emic social stigmas when sharing information with patients and their caregivers. This connection to their origins and homeland lowers possible skepticism toward culturally unfamiliar modes of treatment and makes patients feel more comfortable, perhaps more secure, and more likely to comply with the clinician's direction.

In contrast, in the absence of access to a clinician with the same ethnic background, the risk of misdiagnosis is greater along with greater difficulty in eliciting clinically important information. For example, during psychotic episodes, thinking becomes increasingly disorganized, and patients who are usually bilingual tend to revert to their mother language. In such a state, they may be unable to communicate in the clinician's language to answer clinically important questions. In some cases, family members or other sources who are not medically trained are used to translate patients' feedback. As interpreters, they may not have adequate language skills to relay conceptually accurate information, and as kin to patients, they are likely to have strong emotional attachment that may result in decreased objectivity and unconscious omission of information that would be otherwise clinically relevant and important for accurate diagnosis and efficient treatment.

In clinical research, interpretability of collected data is far more stringent in methodology, it is etic in nature and assumes that more similarities exist rather than differences across cultural groups. In an effort to collect comparable and interpretable data, researchers and Western clinicians alike prefer to view psychopathology in a universal manner. Considering the variance in data collection practices between clinical practice and research, is psychopathology universal enough to assume that cross-cultural equivalence exists and collected data is truly comparable and interpretable?

4.3.2   Measuring Quality of Life in Schizophrenia Across Cultural Boundaries

Due to the heterogeneous nature of populations in most countries today, the social construct for quality of life, much like the patterning of symptom presentation, varies across even small subgroups within a single culture. The concept of quality of life is largely subjective, culturally dependent, multidimensional and intended to encompass all positive and negative aspects of a person's life within the context of their known and accepted norms. As discussed earlier, cultural values, sociocentricity, social notions, customs, spiritual beliefs, and rational mental health status influence the construct. So far, there is no consensus on what truly constitutes *quality of life* in any population group, and results from existing research conclude that concepts and ideas that exist in one culture cannot be expected to be present or meaningful in another culture (Brislin 1980; Hui and Triandis 1985; Sperber 1994; Triandis et al. 1972). Therefore, the perception of general quality of life is highly subjective to the cultural and socioeconomic norm that a patient lives within and expects or to which he or she is accustomed.

Health-related quality of life is usually a construct that is connected to a slightly more defined and objective rating of the patient's functional improvement and general health status and tends to be also associated with the patient's acceptance of that status, level of satisfaction with provided treatment and care, and allocation of reimbursement resources for outcome-based success in treatment effects. In North America, health-related quality of life in schizophrenia has a series of key dimensions measuring both subjective and objective well-being. They include functional status (i.e., skills and abilities: psychological, social, adaptive, motor, etc.), physical health status, perceived well-being, sustenance, and occupation/employment.

The choice of tests used for evaluating health-related quality of life in schizophrenia depends on the purpose of testing and inferred outcomes of treatment. The Global Assessment Scale (GAS), developed in 1976 by Endicott et al, is one of the most commonly used tests in North America to assess overall functional status and clinical condition in schizophrenia research (Endicott et al. 1976). Investigations in psychopharmacology and symptomatology for schizophrenia is centered on psychotic symptoms, namely, because they are behaviorally visible and socially disruptive. In 1984, Heinrichs et al. argued that fluctuations in psychotic symptoms occur against the abstract canvas of the patients' sociocentric environment with functional impairments in deficit symptomatology, characterized by most enduring and crippling continuity of premorbid, early morbid, and postpsychotic functional defects. Kraepelin (1971) described these defects as follows:

> ...a weakening of those emotional activities which permanently form the mainstrings of volition. In connection with this, mental activity and instinct for occupation become mute. The result ... is emotional dullness, failure of mental activities, loss of mastery over volition, of endeavor, and of ability for independent action. The essence of personality is thereby destroyed... (Kraepelin E., 1971, p. 741)

With the general aim to help schizophrenics control psychotic symptoms and to return to general public community, Heinrichs et al. developed a quality of life test with focus on methodical assessment of schizophrenic patients' deficit state (i.e., intrapsychic, instrumental, and interpersonal functioning), readiness to function adequately enough to regain independence, managing social and occupational adjustment, and individual well-being. Since patients' sociocentric environment varies across both emic and etic cultural parameters, the presence and absence of certain types of functional deficits can only be hypothetical from a clinical standpoint, and the innate cause of an observed or a reported behavior can and should be evaluated with sound clinical judgment and common sense by a clinician who is well experienced with treating and caring for schizophrenic patients.

The Heinrichs-Carpenter Quality of Life Scale (QLS) was developed to serve as a method for standardizing and quantifying these clinical judgments. Negative symptoms and functional deficit symptoms are interrelated, but do not uniformly correlate in scope, and hence functional deficit symptoms are not well represented in tests that measure negative symptom severities. In clinical research and in drug development, focusing on negative symptoms is appropriate due to the tightly controlled environment of clinical trial studies. However, in psychiatric practice, once a patient is medicated, focus on sustainable role performance and internal state becomes more valuable. The QLS is a 21-item observer-rated semi-structured interview and was designed to evaluate four dimensions that collectively represent the deficit syndrome construct in schizophrenia:

1. Intrapsychic foundations (i.e., sense of purpose, motivation, curiosity, empathy, ability to experience pleasure, and emotional interaction)
2. Interpersonal relations (i.e., capacity for intimacy, active vs. passive participation, avoidance, and withdrawal tendencies)
3. Instrumental role (i.e., parent, housekeeper, worker, student; level of accomplishment, degree of employment vs. talents and opportunities, and satisfaction derived from role)
4. Common objects and activities (i.e., degree of participation in day-to-day life, social and community activities, and possession of objects related to these activities and interests)

The QLS is currently one of the most widely used quality of life tests in schizophrenia. In addition to being developed as a standardized outcome criterion for clinical judgment, its purpose, sensitivity to detect change, and applicability in various clinical settings and its unique negative symptom-related focus on deficit symptoms in schizophrenia make its construct, when impacted, to be a considerable factor in clinical decision-making for treatment interventions and monitoring course of illness (Heinrichs et al. 1984).

With drastic changes in both American and Canadian healthcare systems, many mental health treatment centers and institutions shut down their doors. Inpatients who were thought to pose low risk in harming themselves, or someone else, were released and referred to live in various types of housing projects, with variable quality in community support services. Many previously institutionalized patients, including schizophrenics, ended up living on the street due to shortages in accommodation availabilities or in individual attempts to avoid being harmed by other cohabitants, having their few belongings stolen or damaged, and seeking or consenting to shelter only in extreme life-preserving situations. Additionally, adequate psychological and psychiatric treatment being relatively inaccessible to individuals with low incomes compounded the challenge of managing quality of life for individuals living with severe mental illness and who continue to decompensate with minimal or no social and medical support. Over time, with changes intending improvement in mental health-related healthcare systems and breadth of services, a pathoplastic phenomenon characterized by an ethically induced psychosocial change may play a part in evolving the construct of health-related quality of life in schizophrenia within North America and across international boundaries.

Measuring health-related quality of life for public policy decisions tends to focus on either generic or disease-specific assessment of cost utility versus overall benefit to patient for community-oriented purchasing of interventions and development of supporting programs. The empirical measurement is generalized, often down to a single item, and although patient input may have its purpose and value in this type of assessment, the analysis of information collected usually does not focus on patients' preferences for treatment, outcome, and/or satisfaction with care. The health-related economic perspective is that a patient's health state may change over time, and hence their preferences and benefit expectations will also, which could in turn make economic utility values longitudinally unstable and unreliable. Research conducted in valued states of existence cites *health* to be the most valued state (Revicki and Kaplan 1993; Rokeach 1973). Life expectation, including morbidity-free life expectancy, has increased dramatically since in the last century. Most countries around the world are now measuring health expectancy in various ways (Bone 1992; Robine 1992) and assessing whether the years we've gained in life are spent in good health or in poor health. Quality of life has become a term that is used interchangeably with health status. Since public health priorities, access to medical care, and quality of care and availability of support programs across international healthcare systems vary, the conceptual framework of health-related quality of life also varies across ethnic groups. The World Health Organization attempted to define the conceptual framework of health-related quality of life as a "state of complete physical, mental and social well-being, autonomy, and not merely the absence of disease or infirmity" (WHO 1947). In 1987, Ware et al. expanded on the construct, arguing that since the role of healthcare is to optimize health status, health-related dimensions of quality of life need to be defined. Ware proposed five intrinsic attributes of health-related quality of life: physical health, mental health, social functioning, role functioning, and general well-being (Bowling 1999).

Measuring health-related quality of life in schizophrenia follows the same set of principles. However, schizophrenic patients require a much higher level of care than individuals who cope with depression, anxiety, diabetes, or other illnesses that do not include psychosis and delirium in the psychopathological profile. Since the symptom patterning in schizophrenia is variable across cultures, a generalized approach targeting specific key factors that affect schizophrenics' quality of life is warranted. For the purpose of some kind of uniformity for comparative purposes across cultures, measuring treatment outcome in psychosis is a commonly used construct that has proven to be meaningful in outcomes research studies.

In 1996, van Os (van Os et al 1996) proposed six interrelated dimensions of course and outcome in psychosis:

1. Negative symptoms/disability
2. Illness severity/course
3. Time living independently

4. Unemployment
5. Prison/vagrancy
6. Depression/self-harm

The six dimensions can be measured with a battery of tests in combination of patient-reported experiences and structured clinical interviews. The tests used to measure any one of the desired dimensions should meet the following criteria:

- Fit the population group for which the tests were developed.
- Are intended for the use in the same type of setting (i.e., inpatient vs. outpatient programs).
- Have culturally relevant constructs of any combination of the above domains.
- Correlate to other well-validated measures using the same conceptual framework.
- Demonstrate strong correlation with culture-bound symptom severity.
- Are administered in the patient's preferred language or dialect.
- Demonstrate to be sensitive to change over the intended test-retest time frame.
- Are sensitive to treatment effect.
- Correlate with global clinical ratings.

Some tests have been fully adapted, with local norms and clinical samples, in the target cultures. In clinical research, particularly, it is worth the time and effort to think about the appropriateness of the construct and to search for and identify instruments that are already available. Some health-related quality of life tests were developed in European countries and then translated into English for the use in North America. In practice, the further apart two cultures are, the more difficult and cumbersome the translation and adaptation become; therefore, generalized construct, especially when translation and adaptation is needed, would be a better alternative to tests constructed in alignment with localized criteria for psychopathology. In naturalistic studies of health-related quality of life across cultures, it is also common to use various quality of life instruments with the same or comparable construct but different quantity of item content. In the next section, we will review some important considerations for translation and cultural adaptation of psychological tests.

4.3.3   Translating Item Content

Psychological tests come from the discipline of psychology, which has its own governing bodies within areas of application (i.e., education and clinical practice). These governing organizations produce standards and practices for translation and cultural adaptation of educational and psychological tests for their clinical psychology and psychometrics community in a unified effort to minimize scoring error. The pharmaceutical industry and the field of pharmaco-economic outcomes and research produced its own version of standards for translating a psychological test for their psychiatric research community, perhaps without being aware of what the field of psychology had already done.

4.4   Summary and Conclusions

In the context of an overall multicultural canvas, observation and understanding of cultural similarities and differences are critical for adaptation and for clinically meaningful interpretability of information collected with psychological tests, regardless of the tests' intended utilities and purposes. This includes at least working knowledge and understanding of emic norms for behaviors and communication styles, external cultural influences on emic societies, and culture-bound patterns in symptom presentation. Although the psychopathological profile of schizophrenia is consistent across cultures, the patterns in which symptoms present themselves across ethnic groups and individuals vary a great deal. Negative symptoms are easier to detect even with communication barriers; however, it is important that clinicians communicate well with patients and their caregivers to ensure that culturally bound behaviors, spiritual beliefs, somatic symptoms, reporting styles, immigration history and reasons, acculturation progress, caregiver support network, and details of challenges in functioning are collectively considered. Such considerations will help with ensuring that clinically important information is elicited for diagnostic and treatment monitoring purposes, for maximizing adherence to treatment, and that patients are assessed individually and in harmony with their unique histories. To make this possible, clinicians need to speak their patients' primary language and be familiar with their patients' social culture, medical care philosophy, and medical use of possible euphemisms for stigmatized disorders. When that is not practical, they should use a reliable interpreter who is familiar with such cultural nuances and to ensure that information provided by patients and their families are not being misinterpreted when judged from an etic standpoint, ultimately resulting in possible differential diagnoses, delayed treatment, and further symptomatic decompensation.

Quality of life is highly subjective and culturally specific, particularly for schizophrenia and other dissociative disorders with psychosis in the psychopathological profiles. Cross-culturally adapted quality of life tests will therefore be more meaningful if they measure a generalized construct consisting of key cross-cultural dimensions that represent domains responsible for observable disruption to an accepted norm. In order to do so, the tests must be adapted linguistically, contextually, and sometimes also in item content and level of difficulty. Linguist translators are generally not adequately qualified to accomplish such adaptations without high risk of negatively impacting content validity and hence the psychometric integrity of the test. Research in linguistics, anthropology, and psychology has provided guidance in linguistic and functional requirements for adapting psychological tests, methods for linguistic adaptation, and complete cultural standardization, along with an array of case studies describing challenges and successes in cross-cultural adaptation projects. These methods should be adopted by the life sciences industry since they have been proven to work. Due to the variability in considerations discussed in this chapter as they relate to adaptation of psychological tests, linguistic and cross-cultural adaptation projects should not be assigned to translation companies that do not have internal resources consisting of experts in psychometrics and test development and a reliable network of truly bilingual clinicians with disorder-specific emic clinical experience. These projects can become complicated during resolution of items that are difficult or impossible to translate and particularly when items require replacement or complete removal. For such projects, efficient teams comprised of psychometrists and emic clinicians with experience in development and cultural adaptation of psychological tests become invaluable resources, especially when item content needs to change and the test must be revalidated.

References

Bone MR. International efforts to measure health expectancy. J Epidemiol Community Health. 1992;46(6):555–8. http://doi.org/10.1136/jech.46.6.555.

Bowling A. Health-related quality of life: a discussion of the concept, its use and measurement background: the "quality of life." In: Presented to the adapting to change core course. 1999.

Brislin RW. Translation and content analysis of oral and written material. In: Triandis HC, Berry JW, editors. Handbook of cross-cultural psychology, vol. 2. Boston: Allyn & Bacon; 1980.

Endicott J, Spitzer RL, Fleiss JL, Cohen J. The global assessment scale. A procedure for measuring overall severity of psychiatric disturbance. Arch Gen Psychiatry. 1976;33(6):766–71. http://doi.org/10.1001/archpsyc.1976.01770060086012.

Harris M. History and Significance of the EMIC/ETIC Distinction. Ann Rev Anthropol. 1976. http://doi.org/10.1146/annurev.an.05.100176.001553.

Heinrichs DW, Hanlon TE, Carpenter WT. The Quality of Life Scale: an instrument for rating the schizophrenic deficit syndrome. Schizophr Bull. 1984;10(3):388–98. http://doi.org/10.1093/schbul/10.3.388.

Hui CH, Triandis HC. Measurement in cross-cultural psychology: a review and comparison of strategies. J Cross-Cultur Psychol. 1985;16(2):131–52. http://doi.org/10.1177/0022002185016002001.

Kraepelin E. Dementia praecox and paraphrenia. Huntington: Krieger; 1971.

Pike KL. Language in relation to a unified theory of the structure of human behavior. The Hague: Mouton; 1967.

Revicki DA, Kaplan RM. Relationship between psychometric and utility-based approaches to the measurement of health-related quality of life. Q Life Res Int J Q Life Aspects Treat Care Rehabil. 1993;2(6):477–87. http://doi.org/10.1007/BF00422222.

Robine JM. Health expectancy: first workshop of the international healthy life expectancy network REVES. H.M. Stationery Office. 1992.

Rokeach M. Rokeach values survey. The nature of human values. New York: The Free Press; 1973.

Sperber D. The modularity of thought and the epidemiology of representations. In: Mapping the mind: domain specificity in cognition and culture. 1994. p. 39–67.

Triandis HC, Malpass RS, Davidson AR. Psychology and culture. In: Mussen PH, editor. Annual review of psychology. 1972. p. 355–78.

Urbina S. Essentials of psychological testing PDF.pdf. In: Kaufman N, Kaufman A, editors. 2nd ed. Hoboken: Wiley & Sons Inc.; 2014.

Van Os J, Fahy TA, Jones P, Harvey I, Sham P, Lewis S, Bebbington P, Toone B, Williams M, Murray R. Psychopathological syndromes in the functional psychoses: associations with course and outcome. Psychol Med. 1996;26(1):161–76. http://doi.org/10.1017/S0033291700033808.

World Health Organization (WHO). The constitution of the World Health Organization. WHO Chron. 1947;1:29–43.

Part II
Methodological Issues

Chapter 5
A Review of Quality-of-Life Assessment Measures in Schizophrenia: Limitations and Future Developments

María Teresa Bobes-Bascarán, María Paz García-Portilla, Pilar A. Sáiz Martínez, Leticia García-Alvarez, Isabel Menéndez-Miranda, Susana Al-Halabí, María Teresa Bascarán, and Julio Bobes

5.1 Introduction

The assessment of quality of life (QoL) in patients with schizophrenia is an area of growing concern since it is considered an essential distal outcome for clinical trials and patient management (Auquier et al. 2003; Awad and Voruganti 2012) according to the patient-reported outcome (PRO) movement in medicine (see Fig. 5.1). Its evaluation is founded on the notion that every patient has a right to self-determination in health-care decisions and his/her subjective perspective should be considered in both diagnosis and care planning processes (Awad and Voruganti 2012; Badia et al. 1999; Bilker et al. 2003).

The evaluation of QoL in patients with mental disorders is replete with its own difficulties and nuances, and the specific assessment of this construct in patients with schizophrenia involves even greater challenges, as we will review in this chapter. Even though the construct has gone through many years of refinement, there is no

M.T. Bobes-Bascarán, PhD
Centro de Investigación Biomédica en Red de Salud Mental, CIBERSAM,
Valencia, Spain

M.P. García-Portilla, MD, PhD • P.A.S. Martínez, MD, PhD
L. García-Alvarez, PhD • J. Bobes, MD, PhD (✉)
Centro de Investigación Biomédica en Red de Salud Mental, CIBERSAM,
Oviedo, Spain

Department of Psychiatry, University of Oviedo, Oviedo, Spain
e-mail: bobes@uniovi.es

I. Menéndez-Miranda, MD PhD
Mental Health Services of Asturias, Oviedo, Spain

S. Al-Halabí, PhD • M.T. Bascarán, MD, PhD
Centro de Investigación Biomédica en Red de Salud Mental, CIBERSAM,
Oviedo, Spain

© Springer International Publishing Switzerland 2016
A.G. Awad, L.N.P. Voruganti (eds.), *Beyond Assessment of Quality of Life in Schizophrenia*, DOI 10.1007/978-3-319-30061-0_5

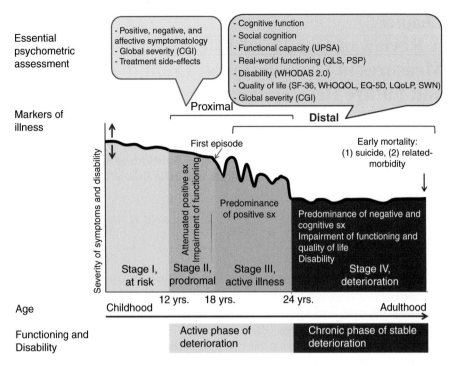

Fig. 5.1 Proximal and distal outcomes in schizophrenia (Modified from Lieberman et al. (2001); Insel 2010)

gold standard tool available at present. The most accepted fallback is to administer the tool most appropriate to each specific design, study sample (Bobes 2001), and the aim of the quality-of-life measurement (Bobes et al. 2005) – health economic analysis versus patient concerns.

A recent review of QoL scales used in studies investigating patients with schizophrenia over the past 5 years found 35 different generic and specific QoL scales currently used in this field (Bobes 2001). Surprisingly, 60 % of the scales (*n* = 432 studies) were used only once or twice. The generic QoL scales most often used in these studies were (a) the WHOQOL-BREF (abbreviated version of the WHOQOL-100) (Bobes et al. 2007), (b) the Short-Form 36 or Short-Form 12 (SF-36/SF-12) (Brooks 1996), and (c) the EuroQOL (EQ-5D) (Browne et al. 1996). The most widely used schizophrenia-specific QoL scales were (a) the Heinrichs-Carpenter Quality of Life Scale (QLS) (Bullinger and Quitmann 2014); (b) the Quality of Life, Enjoyment, and Satisfaction Questionnaire (Q-LRS-Q-18) (Calman 1984; Cella et al. 2010); and (c) the Subjective Well-Being Under Neuroleptics Scale (SWN) (Endicott et al. 1993).

We will now describe the most relevant, currently used instruments to assess QoL in schizophrenia, grouped into those that evaluate general aspects and those that survey-specific domains potentially affected in schizophrenia.

5.2 Types of Measures for Assessing Health-Related Quality of Life in Schizophrenia

5.2.1 Generic Quality-of-Life Instruments

5.2.1.1 The Short-Form Health Survey (SF-36, SF-12) (Brooks 1996; Evenson and Vieweg 1998; Fervaha et al. 2014)

The Medical Outcome Study (MOS) 36-Item Short-Form Health Survey (SF-36) is a well-established, widely used, generic quality-of-life instrument. It was not designed specifically to assess patients with schizophrenia, but its validity in this population has since been well established afterward (Fervaha and Remington 2013).

It consists of 36 items grouped into the following eight scales: physical functioning, physical role, bodily pain, general health, vitality, social functioning, emotional role, and mental health. These eight scales can be consolidated into two broader dimensions: physical health and mental health. It is a self-rated instrument that can be completed in approximately 15 min. It provides two-component summary scores (physical and mental) and scores on each of the eight scales (see Table 5.1). Scores range from 0 to 100, with higher values indicating higher QoL.

A briefer form, The SF-12 Health Survey, appears to accomplish three objectives: (1) reproduction of more than 90 % of the variance in SF-36 physical and mental component summaries; (2) accurate reproduction of average scores for both SF-36 component summary scales, but less accurately for the eight-scale profile; and (3) sufficient reduction in length for self-administration in 2 min or less (Fervaha et al. 2014).

5.2.1.2 World Health Organization Quality of Life (WHOQOL-100) (Gaite et al. 2000)

This instrument was developed by the WHO to assess QoL in a wide range of physical and mental illnesses. It includes 96 items hierarchically structured to cover 24 facets and 4 extra items as a measurement of general health and QoL. These 24 facets account for 6 main domains (see Table 5.1):

1. Physical health: pain, energy, and sleep
2. Psychological health: positive and negative feelings, self-esteem, and body image
3. Level of independence: mobility, activities of daily living, medication or treatment dependence, and work capacity
4. Social relationships: personal relationships, social support, and activity as provider/supporter
5. Environment: physical safety, home, financial resources, access and quality of health and social care, physical environment, etc.
6. Spirituality/religion/personal beliefs: consists of this single facet

Table 5.1 Vital areas assessed by different quality-of-life psychometric instruments

| Domains | Type of quality-of-life instrument | | | | | | | | | | | | |
| | Generic | | | | Specific | | | | | | | | |
	SF-36	WHOQOL-BREF	EQ-5D	PROMIS	QLS	QoLI	LQoLP	MANSA	Q-LES-Q	SQLS-R4	S-QoL	SWN	PETiT
Activities of daily living	X		X		X	X	X		X				X
Self-control												X	
Self-care/autonomy		X	X								X		
Pain	X		X	X									
Finances						X		X					
Physical environment		X		X									
Place of residence						X	X	X					
Mobility			X	X									
Leisure						X		X	X				
Social participation	X			X									
Personal, family, and social relationships		X		X	X	X	X	X	X		X		X
Religion												X	
Physical health	X^a	X		X		X	X	X	X	X	X	X^b	X
Psychological health	X	X	X	X	X	X	X	X	X^c	X^d	X	X	X
Safety/legal aspects						X	X	X					
Work/academic issues					X	X	X	X	X				X

[a]Physical functioning and role
[b]Mental functioning and emotional regulation
[c]Subjective feelings
[d]Cognition and vitality

This tool has been demonstrated to have the reliability and validity to measure QoL in patients with schizophrenia (Garcia-Portilla et al. 2015), and, due to its large time requirement, in WHO (1998) developed a 26-item abbreviated form, the WHOQOL-BREF (Bobes et al. 2007) that assesses 4 of the 6 domains: physical and psychological health, social relationships, and environment.

5.2.1.3   EuroQoL-5 Dimensions (EQ-5D) (Gomez et al. 2000; Harvey 2013)

The EQ-5D is a generic, self-report, preference-based questionnaire (Hayhurst et al. 2014) consisting of three sections. The first is a descriptive system that assesses health-related QoL in the following five dimensions (see Table 5.1): mobility, self-care, usual activities, pain/discomfort, and anxiety/depression. Each dimension has three levels of severity, ranging from 1 (no problem) to 3 (extreme problem). Subjects have to choose the level that best describes their health status in each dimension on the day of administration. Each subject's health status is described as a combination of 5 digits (one for each dimension rated), and the EQ-5D descriptive system generates 243 different health states.

Prieto et al. (Heinrichs et al. 1984) investigated its construct validity in patients with schizophrenia in the context of the EFESO study ($n = 2657$ patients) (Insel 2010). They found a positive association between the scores on the GAF and CGI scales (clinician rated) and the scores on the EQ-5D scales (patient rated). In addition, the EQ-5D was able to identify differences in QoL among patients with different degrees of severity. They concluded that the EQ-5D appears to have acceptable construct validity in schizophrenia patients (Heinrichs et al. 1984).

5.2.1.4   Patient-Reported Outcome Measurement Information System (PROMIS) (Karow et al. 2014)

The PROMIS is a project sponsored by the NIMH with the aim of developing multiple item banks that offer PRO measures of physical, mental, and social functioning and well-being. The PROMIS has a multi-item bank for measuring each of the following three domains (see Table 5.1): physical, physical function, fatigue, pain intensity, pain interference, behavior and quality, sleep function, and sexual function; mental, depression, anxiety, anger, positive psychological function, and cognitive function; and social health, satisfaction with participation in social roles and with social roles and activities, social support, social isolation, and companionship. The multi-item banks can generate both fixed short-form scales and computerized adaptive testing.

This system of measurement is more efficient, flexible, and precise than the other available measures (Kind 1996).

5.2.2 Specific Quality-of-Life Instruments

5.2.2.1 The Heinrichs-Carpenter Quality of Life Scale (QLS) (Bullinger and Quitmann 2014)

Although this instrument was designed to evaluate the schizophrenia deficit syndrome, it is one of the most widely used instruments to evaluate QoL in patients with schizophrenia under different antipsychotic treatments. However, a more detailed examination of its items and the fact that is a "clinician-rated" instrument that does not incorporate the subjective views of patients suggest that this scale assesses real-world functioning rather than QoL.

Recently, the Heinrichs-Carpenter QLS has been conceptualized as an instrument that provides information on negative symptoms and level of functioning (Lehman et al. 1993). It is made up of 21 items grouped into the four following subscales (see Table 5.1): intrapsychic foundations (8 items), interpersonal relations (8 items), instrumental role (4 items), and common objects and activities (2 items). The intrapsychic foundation subscale assesses the negative symptoms of schizophrenia, and the other three subscales assess the level of functioning of these patients.

This is a semi-structured, clinician-rated interview that provides a global score and scores in each of the four categories. Higher scores reflect better functioning. It takes about 45 min, so two shorter versions have been developed.

The abbreviated QLS-7 includes items for assessing both negative symptoms and level of functioning: active acquaintances, social initiative, occupational functioning, motivation, anhedonia, commonplace objects, and empathy (Lehman 1988). These 7 items were selected as they demonstrated the largest correlation with the complete 21-item QLS compared with all other possible combinations of 7 items (Lehman 1988; Lehman 1983). A modified abbreviated 4-item QLS has been also developed, and it is scored as the mean of the 4 items that do not refer to the intrapsychic foundations domain (i.e., motivation, anhedonia, and empathy) (Lieberman et al. 2001).

5.2.2.2 The Quality of Life Interview (QoLI) (Naber et al. 2001)

The QoLI was developed to assess the life circumstances of severely mentally ill patients. It is based on information about personal characteristics, objective life conditions, and current subjective satisfaction with life. It consists of a global measure of life satisfaction and measures of objective and subjective QoL in the eight life domains (see Table 5.1): living situation, family relations, social relations, leisure, work, safety, finances, and physical health. For each life domain, objective measures of QoL are obtained first, followed by information regarding the subjective degree of satisfaction with life. It requires 45 min to complete its 143 items on:

1. Global, general life satisfaction
2. Objective scores in the eight life domains
3. Subjective scores in each of the eight life domains

5.2.2.3 The Lancashire Quality of Life Profile (LQoLP) (Naber 1995; Oliver et al. 1997)

This instrument was developed by Oliver et al. from the Lehman Quality of Life Interview (LQoLI) to assess the life circumstances of severely mentally ill patients (Insel 2010). It is a structured self-report interview with 105 items, which takes approximately 45 min.

It is based on information about personal characteristics, objective life conditions, and current subjective satisfaction with life. It consists of a global measure of life satisfaction and measures of objective and subjective QoL in eight life domains: living situation, daily activities, family relations, social relations, finances, job, safety, and health (see Table 5.1). The LQoLP also measures the following additional areas: positive and negative affect (with the Bradburn Affect Balance Scale), self-esteem, global well-being (Cantril's Ladder and Happiness Scale), perceived QoL, and the QoL of the patient independently of the patient's own opinion (with the Quality of Life Uniscale).

For each life domain, objective measures of QoL are obtained first, followed by information regarding the subjective degree of satisfaction with life. There is a European version, the LQoLP-EU, developed in the context of the EPSILON Study 8 (Oliver et al. 1997).

5.2.2.4 Manchester Short Assessment of Quality of Life (MANSA) (Orsel et al. 2004)

This is a modified version of the LQoLP that was intended to increase efficiency (the administration of the LQoLP takes nearly 30 min), construct validity (it assesses psychopathology), sensibility to change, and discriminant validity between samples.

The MANSA is a 25-item self-report measure that consists of three sections: personal information that is supposed to be consistent over time (gender, ethnicity, etc.), personal information that may vary (work status, monthly income, state benefits, living situation, etc.), and 16 questions (4 objective yes/no items and 12 subjective items rated by a 7-point Likert scale). The four objective items assess the existence of a "close friend," number of contacts with friends per week, accusation of a crime, and victimization of physical violence. The subjective questions obtain satisfaction with life as a whole, job (training, sheltered employment, or unemployed/retired status), financial situation, number and quality of friendships, leisure activities, accommodation, personal safety, people living with patient, sex life, relationship with family, and physical and mental health (see Table 5.1). It has demonstrated adequate reliability (Cronbach's alpha of 0.74) and validity (correlations with Lancashire QoL ranged from 0.83 to 0.99).

5.2.2.5 Quality of Life Enjoyment and Satisfaction Questionnaire (Q-LES-Q) (Calman 1984)

This is a 93-item self-report questionnaire designed to easily obtain sensitive measures of the degree of enjoyment and satisfaction experienced by subjects in various areas of daily functioning (see Table 5.1). Five of the eight summary scale scores are relevant to all patients (physical health, subjective feelings, leisure time activities, social relationships, and general activities), and the other three may be appropriate to certain subgroups (work, household duties, and school/academic functioning).

There is an abbreviated version (*Q-LES-Q-18*) (Cella et al. 2010) consisting of 18 items that predict the basic domains from the extended version (physical health, subjective feelings, leisure time activities, social relationships) and general index scores with adequate reliability (Cronbach's alpha ranging from 0.74 to 0.97), validity (compared with QLS and LQOLP), and stability of test-retest ratings (intraclass correlations ranging from 0.71 to 0.83).

5.2.2.6 The Schizophrenia Quality of Life Scale, Revision 4 (SQLS-R4) (Park et al. 2015)

Currently available in its most recent revised form, the SQLS-R4 was developed by (Wilkinson et al. 2000) for the measurement of health-related QoL in people with schizophrenia. It comprises 33 items in two domains (see Table 5.1): psychosocial feelings (22 items) and cognition and vitality (11 items). All items are scored on a five-point Likert-type scale. Individual domain and total scores are standardized by scoring algorithm to a 0–100 scale, with higher scores indicating comparatively lower QoL.

5.2.2.7 The Quality of Life Questionnaire in Schizophrenia (S-QoL) (Priebe et al. 1999)

Auquier et al. developed the S-QoL for assessing health-related QoL among people with schizophrenia. This questionnaire was based on Calman's approach (Prieto et al. 2004) where health-related QoL is defined as the discrepancies perceived by patients between their expectations and their current life experiences.

The questionnaire consists of 41 items grouped in 8 subscales (see Table 5.1): psychological well-being, self-esteem, family relationships, relationships with friends, resilience, physical well-being, autonomy, and sentimental life. It is a self-administered questionnaire that takes approximately 15 min. It provides a global quality-of-life index and scores on the 8 subscales.

5.2.2.8   The Subjective Well-Being Under Neuroleptics (SWN) (Endicott et al. 1993)

This scale was created to evaluate the clinical relevance of patient's perception of their health status, antipsychotic treatment, and other relevant vital aspects, as a subjective measure of illness and treatment experiences and overall life satisfaction among psychotic disorder patients.

The original version consists of 38 items (Endicott et al. 1993; Pukrop et al. 2003), but a 20-item short-form version, the SWN-K, is also available (Rabin and de Charro 2001). This instrument has been refined using a Rasch rating model (Revicki et al. 2014). The authors recommend omitting items 2 and 20 to improve construct validity, adding easier items related to individual ability estimates and reducing the number of response categories for the assessment of patients with schizophrenia.

The SWN has five subscores: mental functioning, self-control, emotional regulation, physical functioning, and social integration (see Table 5.1). One recent study conducted in a large sample of patients, their siblings and parents, and healthy controls determined that reliability within the four groups had a Cronbach's alpha between 0.88 and 0.92, thus concluding that this is a measure for subjective well-being that can also be used in relatives and healthy controls to investigate genetic and psychological dispositions of subjective well-being (Ritsner et al. 2005).

5.2.2.9   The Personal Evaluation of Transitions in Treatment (PETiT) (Auquier et al. 2003)

The PETiT was developed to evaluate subjective changes during antipsychotic treatment.

QoL is conceptualized as the patient's subjective perception of the interaction among severity of psychotic symptoms, medication side effects, and level of psychosocial performance.

The PETiT consists of 30 items grouped in 12 domains (see Table 5.1): psychological well-being, mood, energy level and activities, biological functions, self-esteem, coping abilities, subjective aspects of cognition, communication, aptitude for productivity, stigma, relationships and social functioning, and subjective responses and attitudes toward medication. It is a self-administered questionnaire that provides a total score.

5.3   Methodological Limitations of Current Measures and Future Directions in the Development of New Instruments

From our point of view, there are still some major challenges to assessing QoL in patients with schizophrenia that need to be addressed. These include (1) boundaries among concepts, (2) reliability of self-reports by patients with schizophrenia, and (3) goodness of the psychometric properties of the current measures.

In the last two decades, various related concepts have been developed without establishing clear boundaries among them, so researchers have sometimes used them interchangeably, leading to content validity problems (potential confounding elements between symptoms and functioning with respect to QoL). Among these concepts, we would like to highlight satisfaction, subjective well-being, quality of life, and even functionality. The clearest example related to this is the Heinrichs-Carpenter Quality of Life Scale as we commented in the previous section. It is one of the instruments most widely used for assessing QoL in patients with schizophrenia but one that actually evaluates negative symptoms and functioning.

With respect to the reliability of patient self-reports, there are still doubts concerning whether patients with schizophrenia, due to their lack of insight into their illness, the persistence of psychotic and depressive symptoms, their cognitive deficits, and their idiosyncratic views and values, are capable of self-assessing their QoL. Concerning the impact of patients' cognitive deficits on their ability to evaluate their QoL, Revicki et al. (Kind 1996) concluded that there is no consistent evidence to support it. The same can be applied to the other potentially disturbing factors. While some studies conclude that QoL is a consistent and homogeneous concept that can be measured by self-reports even in mentally ill populations (Schmidt et al. 2006; Skantze et al. 1992; Voruganti and Awad 2002; Vothknecht et al. 2013), other studies have found that scores on objectively and subjectively rated measures of QoL can differ markedly (Ware and Sherbourne 1992). In this regard, researchers recommend using both objectively and subjectively rated instruments, as complementary measures (Bobes 2001; Ware et al. 1996, 2002). In any case, questions about the validity of patient self-assessment of QoL should in no event deter us from our clinical duty to discuss and negotiate every aspect of treatment with patients and to take their views into account when developing services (Bobes et al. 2005).

Regarding psychometric properties, Evenson and Vieweg (WHO 1993) list some of the potential drawbacks of instruments for assessing QoL: lack of a theoretical basis, unclear and overlapping definitions, lack of data on the sensitivity of such measures as treatment outcome, and lack of norms in target populations. Readers should bear these limitations in mind when reading our review of the instruments most widely used for assessing QoL in patients with schizophrenia.

Finally, with respect to future directions in the development of new instruments, it would be advisable to incorporate recent psychometric advances, which can improve both the development of the test itself and the data analyses. To cite a couple of examples, the authors recommend incorporating technology such as differential item functioning (DIF) or computerized adaptive testing (CAT). In addition, it would be desirable to develop forms of assessment that better capture the inner experiences involved in patient perception of QoL.

5.4 Conclusions

The assessment of QoL in patients with schizophrenia is an area of growing importance since it is considered an essential distal outcome for clinical trials and patient management according to the patient-reported outcome movement in medicine.

Although a great deal of effort has been devoted to developing quality-of-life instruments with acceptable psychometric properties, there are still some major challenges that need to be addressed: boundaries among concepts, reliability of self-reporting, and goodness of psychometric properties. For this reason, the recent psychometric advances should be used when developing new instruments. In the meantime, several generic and specific instruments are now available to researchers and clinicians. The choice of the most appropriate instrument will depend upon the aim of the quality-of-life measurement, and, whenever possible, both generic and specific instruments should be combined.

References

Auquier P, Simeoni MC, Sapin C, Reine G, Aghababian V, Cramer J, et al. Development and validation of a patient-based health-related quality of life questionnaire in schizophrenia: the S-QoL. Schizophr Res. 2003;63(1–2):137–49.

Awad AG, Voruganti LN. Measuring quality of life in patients with schizophrenia: an update. Pharmacoeconomics. 2012;30(3):183–95.

Badia X, Roset M, Montserrat S, Herdman M, Segura A. The Spanish version of EuroQol: a description and its applications. European quality of life scale. Med Clin. 1999;112 Suppl 1:79–85.

Bilker WB, Brensinger C, Kurtz MM, Kohler C, Gur RC, Siegel SJ, et al. Development of an abbreviated schizophrenia quality of life scale using a new method. Neuropsychopharmacology. 2003;28(4):773–7.

Bobes J. Current status of quality of life assessment in schizophrenic patients. Eur Arch Psychiatry Clin Neurosci. 2001;251 Suppl 2:II38–42.

Bobes J, Garcia-Portilla P, Saiz PA, Bascaran T, Bousono M. Quality of life measures in schizophrenia. Eur Psychiatry. 2005;20 Suppl 3:S313–7.

Bobes J, Garcia-Portilla MP, Bascaran MT, Saiz PA, Bousono M. Quality of life in schizophrenic patients. Dialogues Clin Neurosci. 2007;9(2):215–26.

Brooks R. EuroQol: the current state of play. Health Policy. 1996;37:53–72.

Browne S, Roe M, Lane A, Gervin M, Morris M, Kinsella A, et al. Quality of life in schizophrenia: relationship to sociodemographic factors, symptomatology and tardive dyskinesia. Acta Psychiatr Scand. 1996;94(2):118–24.

Bullinger M, Quitmann J. Quality of life as patient-reported outcomes: principles of assessment. Dialogues Clin Neurosci. 2014;16(2):137–45.

Calman KC. Quality of life in cancer patients – an hypothesis. J Med Ethics. 1984;10(3):124–7.

Cella D, Riley W, Stone A, Rothrock N, Reeve B, Yount S, et al. The Patient-Reported Outcomes Measurement Information System (PROMIS) developed and tested its first wave of adult self-reported health outcome item banks: 2005–2008. J Clin Epidemiol. 2010;63(11):1179–94.

Endicott J, Nee J, Harrison W, Blumenthal R. Quality of Life Enjoyment and Satisfaction Questionnaire: a new measure. Psychopharmacol Bull. 1993;29(2):321–6.

Evenson RC, Vieweg BW. Using a quality of life measure to investigate outcome in outpatient treatment of severely impaired psychiatric clients. Compr Psychiatry. 1998;39(2):57–62.

Fervaha G, Remington G. Validation of an abbreviated quality of life scale for schizophrenia. Eur Neuropsychopharmacol. 2013;23(9):1072–7.

Fervaha G, Foussias G, Siddiqui I, Agid O, Remington G. Abbreviated quality of life scales for schizophrenia: comparison and utility of two brief community functioning measures. Schizophr Res. 2014;154(1–3):89–92.

Gaite L, Vazquez-Barquero JL, Arrizabalaga Arrizabalaga A, Schene AH, Welcher B, Thornicroft G, et al. Quality of life in schizophrenia: development, reliability and internal consistency of the Lancashire Quality of Life Profile – European version. EPSILON study 8. European Psychiatric Services: Inputs Linked to Outcome Domains and Needs. Br J Psychiatry Suppl. 2000;39:s49–54.

Garcia-Portilla MP, Garcia-Alvarez L, Menendez-Miranda I, Al-Halabi S, Bobes-Bascaran MT, Saiz-Martinez PA, et al. Escalas de funcionalidad, discapacidad y calidad de vida en esquizo-frenia. Drugs in context. Barcelona: J&C Ediciones Medicas, SL; 2015.

Gomez JC, Sacristan JA, Hernandez J, Breier A, Ruiz Carrasco P, Anton Saiz C, et al. The safety of olanzapine compared with other antipsychotic drugs: results of an observational prospective study in patients with schizophrenia (EFESO study). Pharmacoepidemiologic study of olan-zapine in schizophrenia. J Clin Psychiatry. 2000;61(5):335–43.

Harvey PD. Assessment of everyday functioning in schizophrenia: implications for treatments aimed at negative symptoms. Schizophr Res. 2013;150(2–3):353–5.

Hayhurst KP, Massie JA, Dunn G, Lewis SW, Drake RJ. Validity of subjective versus objective quality of life assessment in people with schizophrenia. BMC Psychiatry. 2014;14:365.

Heinrichs DW, Hanlon TE, Carpenter Jr WT. The quality of life scale: an instrument for rating the schizophrenic deficit syndrome. Schizophr Bull. 1984;10(3):388–98.

Insel TR. Rethinking schizophrenia. Nature. 2010;468:187–93.

Karow A, Wittmann L, Schottle D, Schafer I, Lambert M. The assessment of quality of life in clini-cal practice in patients with schizophrenia. Dialogues Clin Neurosci. 2014;16(2):185–95.

Kind P. The EuroQoL instrument: an index of HRQOL. In: Spilker B, editor. Quality of life and phar-macoeconomics in clinical trials. 2nd ed. Philadelphia: Lippincott-Raven; 1996. p. 191–201.

Lehman AF. The effects of psychiatric symptoms on quality of life assessments among the chronic mentally ill. Eval Program Plann. 1983;6(2):143–51.

Lehman AF. A quality of life interview for the chronically mentally ill. Eval Program Plann. 1988;11:51–62.

Lehman AF, Postrado LT, Rachuba LT. Convergent validation of quality of life assessments for persons with severe mental illnesses. Qual Life Res. 1993;2(5):327–33.

Lieberman JA, Perkins D, Belger A, Chakos M, Jarskog F, Boteva K, Gilmore J. The early stages of schizophrenia: speculations on pathogenesis, pathophysiology, and therapeutic approaches. Biol Psychiatry. 2001;50:884–97.

Naber D. A self-rating to measure subjective effects of neuroleptic drugs, relationships to objective psychopathology, quality of life, compliance and other clinical variables. Int Clin Psychopharmacol. 1995;10 Suppl 3:133–8.

Naber D, Moritz S, Lambert M, Pajonk FG, Holzbach R, Mass R, et al. Improvement of schizo-phrenic patients' subjective well-being under atypical antipsychotic drugs. Schizophr Res. 2001;50(1–2):79–88.

Oliver JP, Huxley PJ, Priebe S, Kaiser W. Measuring the quality of life of severely mentally ill people using the Lancashire quality of life profile. Soc Psychiatry Psychiatr Epidemiol. 1997;32(2):76–83.

Orsel S, Akdemir A, Dag I. The sensitivity of quality-of-life scale WHOQOL-100 to psychopatho-logical measures in schizophrenia. Compr Psychiatry. 2004;45(1):57–61.

Park IJ, Jung DC, Hwang SS, Jung HY, Yoon JS, Kim CE, et al. Refinement of the SWN-20 based on the Rasch rating model. Compr Psychiatry. 2015;60:134–41.

Priebe S, Huxley P, Knight S, Evans S. Application and results of the Manchester Short Assessment of Quality of Life (MANSA). Int J Soc Psychiatry. 1999;45(1):7–12.

Prieto L, Sacristan JA, Hormaechea JA, Casado A, Badia X, Gomez JC. Psychometric validation of a generic health-related quality of life measure (EQ-5D) in a sample of schizophrenic patients. Curr Med Res Opin. 2004;20(6):827–35.

Pukrop R, Schlaak V, Moller-Leimkuhler AM, Albus M, Czernik A, Klosterkotter J, et al. Reliability and validity of quality of life assessed by the short-form 36 and the modular system for quality of life in patients with schizophrenia and patients with depression. Psychiatry Res. 2003;119(1–2):63–79.

Rabin R, de Charro F. EQ-5D: a measure of health status from the EuroQol Group. Ann Med. 2001;33(5):337–43.

Revicki DA, Kleinman L, Cella D. A history of health-related quality of life outcomes in psychiatry. Dialogues Clin Neurosci. 2014;16(2):127–35.

Ritsner M, Kurs R, Gibel A, Ratner Y, Endicott J. Validity of an abbreviated quality of life enjoyment and satisfaction questionnaire (Q-LES-Q-18) for schizophrenia, schizoaffective, and mood disorder patients. Qual Life Res. 2005;14(7):1693–703.

Schmidt P, Clouth J, Haggenmuller L, Naber D, Reitberger U. Constructing an Index for the Subjective Well-being Under Neuroleptics scale (SWN), short form: applying structural equation modeling for testing reliability and validity of the index. Qual Life Res. 2006;15(7):1191–202.

Skantze K, Malm U, Dencker SJ, May PR, Corrigan P. Comparison of quality of life with standard of living in schizophrenic out-patients. Br J Psychiatry. 1992;161:797–801.

Voruganti LN, Awad AG. Personal evaluation of transitions in treatment (PETiT): a scale to measure subjective aspects of antipsychotic drug therapy in schizophrenia. Schizophr Res. 2002;56(1–2):37–46.

Vothknecht S, Meijer C, Zwinderman A, Kikkert M, Dekker J, van Beveren N, et al. Psychometric evaluation of the Subjective Well-being Under Neuroleptic Treatment Scale (SWN) in patients with schizophrenia, their relatives and controls. Psychiatry Res. 2013;206(1):62–7.

Ware Jr JE, Sherbourne CD. The MOS 36-item short-form health survey (SF-36). I. Conceptual framework and item selection. Med Care. 1992;30(6):473–83.

Ware Jr J, Kosinski M, Keller SD. A 12-item short-form health survey: construction of scales and preliminary tests of reliability and validity. Med Care. 1996;34(3):220–33.

Ware JE, Kosinski M, Turner-Bowker DM. User's manual for the SF-12v2 health survey with a supplement documenting SF-12 health survey. Lincoln: Quality Metric Incorporated; 2002.

WHO. Measuring quality of life. The development of the World Health Organization Quality of Life Instrument (WHOQOL-100). Genève: WHO; 1993.

WHO. Development of the World Health Organization WHOQOL-BREF quality of life assessment. The WHOQOL Group. Psychol Med. 1998;28:551–8.

Wilkinson G, Hesdon B, Wild D, Cookson R, Farina C, Sharma V, et al. Self-report quality of life measure for people with schizophrenia: the SQLS. Br J Psychiatry. 2000;177:42–6.

Chapter 6
Assessment of the Burden of Care and Quality of Life of Caregivers in Schizophrenia

Laurent Boyer, Karine Baumstarck, and Pascal Auquier

6.1 Introduction

As a disabling and severe psychiatric disorder with either episodic or continuous evolution, schizophrenia has a dramatic impact not only on patients suffering from it but also on their caregivers (Awad and Voruganti 2008; Caqueo-Urizar and Gutierrez-Maldonado 2006; Caqueo-Urizar et al. 2009; Testart et al. 2013; Zendjidjian and Boyer 2014), both on institutional and natural (family) caregivers (Van Humbeeck et al. 2002). Due to the move from traditional institutional care to community care of psychiatric patients, family caregivers now assume functions that were performed by psychiatric institutions in the past (Caqueo-Urizar and Gutierrez-Maldonado 2006; Caqueo-Urizar et al. 2009; Ochoa et al. 2008; Reine et al. 2003; Gutierrez-Maldonado et al. 2005). Caregivers are usually unpaid non-professionals who have significant input in the care and support of people affected by severe psychiatric illnesses. In the specific case of schizophrenia, the majority of caregivers are the parents of the patient, followed by brothers/sisters, and rarely friends who quickly lose interest in continuing the friendship (NAMI 2008). According to the preliminary results of the European Federation of Associations of Families of People with Mental Illness (EUFAMI) international survey, approximately three of four (72 %) caregivers living with individuals with schizophrenia are mainly or solely responsible for caring, placing a huge emotional and physical burden on them (EUFAMI 2014). Family caregivers perform their caregiver role for an average of 16 years, are likely to have to do so for the rest of their lives, and report an average of 23 h a week of caring. Having a family member with

L. Boyer, MD, PhD (✉) • K. Baumstarck, MD, PhD (✉) • P. Auquier, MD, PhD (✉)
Research Unit, Public Health, Chronic Diseases and Quality of Life,
Aix-Marseille Univ, EA 3279, Marseille 13284, France
e-mail: laurent.boyer@univ-amu.fr; karine.baumstarck@univ-amu.fr;
pascal.auquier@univ-amu.fr

© Springer International Publishing Switzerland 2016
A.G. Awad, L.N.P. Voruganti (eds.), *Beyond Assessment of Quality of Life in Schizophrenia*, DOI 10.1007/978-3-319-30061-0_6

schizophrenia results in care burden, stress, fear, and embarrassment about the illness signs and symptoms, including violence, uncertainty about the course of the disease, lack of social support, and stigma. This amount of care also equates to a part-time job (EUFAMI 2014). Family caregivers of people with schizophrenia give up employment or take time off work to provide care and support. The UK-SCAP study estimated that 4.8 % of family caregivers had terminated employment, and 15.5 % took a mean of 12.5 days off work per year specifically as a result of being a caregiver. This amount translates to a mean annual economic loss of £517 (707 Euros or 814 USD) per individual with schizophrenia in the household (Andrews et al. 2012). As in other chronic diseases, it is now well documented that caregiving may have an impact on both the patient suffering from schizophrenia and their family caregivers. Caregiving leads to a higher risk of mortality of the caregiver (Harvey et al. 2002) and to the deterioration of his own health (Caqueo-Urizar et al. 2009; Lua and Bakar 2011; Moller-Leimkuhler and Wiesheu 2011; Zamzam et al. 2011), and several studies have reported that caring for a patient with schizophrenia resulted in a significant and substantial burden (Glozman 2004; Li et al. 2007), lower quality of life (QoL) (Boyer et al. 2012; Caqueo-Urizar et al. 2012), restricted roles and activities, and increased psychosomatic, anxious, or depressive symptoms (Awad and Voruganti 2008; Schulz and Beach 1999). The family caregivers often experience grief and have to cope with stigma and social isolation, which leave them with a feeling of shame, embarrassment, or guilt. Caregiving was most often thought to be a negative phenomenon; however, it is increasingly recognized that caregiving is not only associated with negative consequences, but the caregivers also experience subjective gains and satisfaction (Cohen et al. 2002; Szmukler et al. 1996). The caregiving experience can promote a sense of accomplishment, companionship, fulfillment, enjoyment, and improved self-esteem, and some families can be brought closer together when someone is in need of care. However, according to the preliminary results of the EUFAMI survey, approximately one-third of caregivers report positive experiences of providing care, but positive caregiving experiences are eclipsed by the degree of dissatisfaction with the lack of support from care professionals (EUFAMI 2014).

Additionally, caregivers' experience, which can be positive or negative, may affect their ability to care for the patients. This factor is an important concern because the involvement of family caregivers is essential for the optimal treatment of patients by ensuring treatment compliance, continuity of care, and social support (Reine et al. 2003; Velligan et al. 2009). Several studies have shown that a lack of family involvement in treatment planning is associated with problems in treatment adherence (Ahn et al. 2008; Cooper et al. 2007; Valenstein et al. 2004). Therefore, considering the caregivers' experience is a noteworthy issue both for the caregivers themselves and indirectly for patients' health.

The assessment of caregiver experiences is considered increasingly important with regard to evaluating disease progression, treatment, and the management of care provided to schizophrenia patients and evaluating his/her own mental and physical health status. Despite the acknowledged need to consider caregiver experience issues, their assessment remains routinely underutilized. This review discusses several avenues to promote the use of caregiver experience assessment and convince clinicians and researchers of its clinical utility in clinical practice and clinical research.

6.2   How Can the Caregiver Experience Be Appropriately Assessed?

The EUFAMI survey highlights the family caregiver's desire to be more involved in treatment conversations and to be better equipped to influence care decisions. Healthcare professionals need to acknowledge that family caregivers can play a much stronger role, integrate them in treatment decisions, and work together to achieve better outcomes for the patient. The question of the assessment of caregiver experiences is thus crucial (EUFAMI 2014). Burden of care and QoL assessments can provide an outline of the real experiences of those who live directly with the illness—which includes families and other caregivers (NAMI 2008).

6.2.1   Caregivers' Burden of Care and QoL: Definitions and Measurement

The lack of consensus on a uniform definition of burden of care and QoL continues to be an issue in proposing a relevant measurement for caregivers (Awad and Voruganti 2012; Awad et al. 1997; Boyer et al. 2013, 2014a). Burden of care and QoL are complex constructs that elude any simple definition and measurement.

6.2.1.1   Definitions of the Concepts

Burden of care and QoL are considered by some authors as related constructs (Caqueo-Urizar et al. 2009). Indeed, several studies reported that the burden on family caregiver was associated with an important reduction in QoL (Gutierrez-Maldonado et al. 2005; Fadden et al. 1987). However, from a theoretical perspective, burden of care and QoL do not measure the same thing.

Caregivers' burden of care is usually defined by its impacts and consequences on caregivers and is a negative conceptualization of caregiving (Hunt 2003). According to the recommendations of Awad and Voruganti (Awad and Voruganti 2008), the definition of Hoenig and Hamilton of identifying subjective and objective components of burden of care is the most practical and encompassing (Hoenig and Hamilton 1966). Objective burden of care is meant to indicate the effects on the household (e.g., health, financial loss, and daily chores). In other words, it is the observable, concrete, and tangible cost to the caregiver resulting from the patients' illness (Jones 1996). Subjective burden represents the extent to which the caregivers perceive the burden of care (i.e., the positive or negative feelings that may be experienced in giving care) (Nijboer et al. 1999). Subjective burden is also defined as the person's appraisal of the situation (Maurin and Boyd 1990).

In contrast, QoL is not a direct conceptualization of caregiving and is a global assessment of the general well-being of individuals. QoL is originally a purely subjective construct eliciting patient's self-reports about their own quality of life. However, some authors have proposed to separate QoL into subjective (i.e., individual feeling and perception) and objective (i.e., quality of housing, economic sufficiency, employment, quantity and quality of relationships) components, but this separation is far from unanimous (Boyer et al. 2014a). Objective QoL is actually similar to burden and can explain the strong associations reported between these two concepts in the literature. Awad and Voruganti, following the work of Skantze et al. (1992), recommended to preserve the subjective nature of QoL, which was originally conceived in the development of the construct of QoL. Objective indicators related to standards of living (e.g., quality of housing, finance, employment) differ from QoL and should be considered as the "quality of living." From this perspective, it is now generally accepted that the content of QoL instruments should be based directly on relevant individuals' perspectives (patients, caregivers, etc.) (Slevin et al. 1988). Some authors have also recommended developing QoL measures using an emotional approach rather than based on the conditions of well-being (i.e., objective conditions and self-perceived functioning) because these conditions vary between individuals and thus reintroduce a normative approach (Boyer et al. 2014a). This approach would reaffirm the specificity of QoL in comparison with burden and other normative measures. Considering this emotional dimension in QoL measures may provide important information, which is more oriented toward patients' feelings and values, to clinicians.

6.2.1.2   Burden of Care and QoL Measurements

Caregiver experiences may be assessed from individual interviews (unstructured or semi-structured) performed by experienced professionals or from collective approaches including a group of caregivers (e.g., focus group). However, using measures as standardized questionnaires may be an interesting alternative approach in both clinical practice and research leading to objective and reproducible assessments and reducing the evaluation time. Burden and QoL are commonly assessed using self-reported questionnaires (Awad and Voruganti 2008; Caqueo-Urizar and Gutierrez-Maldonado 2006; Caqueo-Urizar et al. 2009; Testart et al. 2013; Zendjidjian and Boyer 2014). To fully understand and explore the caregivers' experience, it is important to have robust, valid, and reliable questionnaires. A major challenge in elaborating the content of a self-perceived (e.g., burden, QoL) questionnaire is to ensure that subjects' perceptions and perspectives are accurately taken into account (Slevin et al. 1988). Rat et al. showed that item generation based on patient perspectives (elaborated during interviews) was more valid than item generation based on isolated literature reviews or expert experiences (Patrick and

Deyo 1989). Other authors have also suggested that identifying the components of questionnaires based on face-to-face interviews strengthens the content validity of instruments (Platt 1985). It appears necessary to have a qualitative approach with caregivers as a first step in the construction of an instrument. Generic instruments are generally used to compare burden and QoL across various populations, whereas disease-specific instruments focus on particular health problems and are more sensitive in detecting and quantifying small changes (Patrick and Deyo 1989).

Burden

Several good reviews of instruments in measuring caregiver burden were provided (Awad and Voruganti 2008; Caqueo-Urizar and Gutierrez-Maldonado 2006; Caqueo-Urizar et al. 2009; Zendjidjian and Boyer 2014; Platt 1985; Schene et al. 1994). Multiple scales used in the literature are lengthy and comprise an extensive number of items, which would be cognitively taxing to an already distressed caregiver. A clinician contemplating these various rules and instruments may be overwhelmed by their level of complexity. Most of them rely on experts' perspectives or on previously published studies and, more rarely, on the caregivers' viewpoint. The content and domains explored by these instruments are variable. Their validity and reliability (considered to be the degree to which the tool measures what it claims to measure and the extent to which a measurement gives consistent results) were inhomogeneous and incompletely reported, which may compromise the robustness of the instrument. The validation process was most often performed on small sample size of less than 150 individuals. None of the individuals provided responsiveness, which is a core psychometric property in measuring an instrument and is defined as the ability to detect a meaningful change.

Some validated instruments are the Perceived Family Burden Scale (PFBS) (Levene et al. 1996), the Involvement Evaluation Questionnaire (IEQ) (Schene et al. 1994), and the Zarit Burden Interview (ZBI) (Zarit et al. 1980). The PFBS included the caregiver's perspective which is commonly considered as the best method to capture the patient's perceptions and to provide the content of the questionnaire. This questionnaire comprises 24 items exploring 2 dimensions: relatives' reactions to active/aggressive behaviors and withdrawn/passive behaviors. The sample size in the validation study was relatively small ($n=66$), but the psychometric properties were globally satisfactory (e.g., internal consistency $=0.83$).

The IEQ (Schene et al. 1994) was based on a review of the literature and previous existing instruments and comprises 36 items exploring 4 dimensions: tension, supervision, worrying, and urging. The sample size of the validation study was substantial ($n=480$), and the psychometric properties were satisfactory (e.g., internal consistency $=0.71–0.85$).

The last instrument, the Zarit Burden Interview (ZBI) (Zarit et al. 1980), had not been validated in this specific caregiver population in contrast with the two previous instruments but is widely used, allowing comparisons of burden across various caregiver populations. A recent work has begun to develop a revised version of the ZBI that is relevant to caregivers of people with schizophrenia (Gater et al. 2015). This revised version of the ZBI is now called the Schizophrenia Caregiver Questionnaire. Future work is ongoing to determine the reliability and validity of the instrument in this population and in several languages (Rofail et al. 2015).

Quality of Life

Among the numerous QoL questionnaires available in the literature, one is of particular interest: the Schizophrenia Caregiver Quality of Life (S-CGQoL) (Richieri et al. 2011). This questionnaire is the only QoL instrument specifically based on the perspective of caregivers of individuals with schizophrenia, whereas the other tools were based on experts' perspectives and were not specific to caregivers. The S-CGQoL is a short self-administered QoL and can be completed in 5 min, thereby fulfilling the goal of brevity sought in research and clinical practice. The sample size in the validation study was substantial ($n = 246$), and the psychometric properties were satisfactory. This questionnaire contains 25 items describing seven dimensions (psychological and physical well-being; psychological burden and daily life; relationships with spouse; relationships with the psychiatric team; relationships with family; relationships with friends; and material burden).

This measure is a multidimensional questionnaire that includes dimensions similar to other instruments (e.g., psychological and physical well-being, psychological burden and daily life, and material burden, as well as dimensions not explored elsewhere, including relationships with psychiatric teams, which are critical for caregivers of individuals with schizophrenia). The importance of relationships with psychiatric teams has been well established, especially in improving maintenance therapy and preventing relapse in schizophrenia. The focus on the various aspects of social life (i.e., relationships with spouses, family, and friends) also permits a precise description of the social dimension that is rarely explored in depth in other questionnaires for caregivers. The quality of life of caregivers is compromised if the person in charge has difficulties establishing and maintaining social contacts within the family group and other social institutions, as well as their ability to maintain a job. These data show the need to consider aspects related to the social and economic integration of patients and caregivers (Norman et al. 2005; Gutierrez-Maldonado et al. 2012). The S-CGQoL is presented in the appendix of this chapter.

Generic questionnaires are also used to assess the QoL of caregivers. The most widely used questionnaires are the WHOQOL (Power et al. 1999; Group 1998) and the Short-Form 36 (SF-36) (Ware and Sherbourne 1992). These questionnaires have been adapted for use in multiple languages, and norms are available for the two instruments (Hawthorne et al. 2006; Bowling et al. 1999), allowing comparisons across caregiver populations. These generic QoL instruments have been used in clinical studies in caregivers of people with various physical and mental disorders (Boyer et al. 2012; Zendjidjian et al. 2012; Gupta et al. 2015).

6.2.2 Synthesis of the Available Measurements and Choosing the Appropriate Measure

Several literature reviews have identified a large number of instruments that have been psychometrically validated with varying evidence (Awad and Voruganti 2008; Caqueo-Urizar and Gutierrez-Maldonado 2006; Caqueo-Urizar et al. 2009; Zendjidjian and Boyer 2014; Platt 1985; Schene et al. 1994). The selection of the "good" questionnaire is not easy for clinicians. In the previous sections, we proposed a selection of some useful questionnaires. However, other questionnaires may be used. Despite the absence of clear guidelines for selecting the most appropriate questionnaire, several issues should be considered. The concept underlying the caregivers' questionnaire elaboration is a key element of the questionnaire choice. Because of discrepancies between caregivers and experts' perspectives (Slevin et al. 1988), a questionnaire based on the subjects' perceptions and point of view should be preferred. Additionally, the validation process is particularly important for professionals seeking an effective instrument because it assures the questionnaire's performance (Boyer et al. 2009). Validation of metrological properties should integrate aspects such as internal consistency, construct validity, and responsiveness, but several instruments identified in literature reviews did not have information on internal consistency, construct validity, and responsiveness. Small sample size could have compromised the robustness of the instrument validation results because of the absence of representativeness of the caregiver population. This issue presents a problem because the limitations of these instruments are not known, and they may not be adapted to the objectives and assessment requirements of professionals. Moreover, the absence of information on responsiveness is problematic in evaluating psychoeducational or therapeutic programs (Yesufu-Udechuku et al. 2015). The lack of information about sensitivity to change is a major problem and should be studied in future research on instruments. Lastly, the language in which questionnaires were developed should be considered by clinicians. Translating questionnaires may be inappropriate because QoL and burden of care depend on cultural background (Boyer et al. 2012). Before using a translated foreign questionnaire, it is necessary to perform a transcultural validation according to specific rules and methods (Baider et al. 1995). It is thus preferable to use questionnaires devised in the country of origin. However, there is a lack of questionnaires that are psychometrically validated to appropriate standards and that are available in multiple languages.

6.3 Avenues of Research for the Clinical Utility of Caregivers' Burden of Care and QoL Assessments

According to previous authors (Boyer et al. 2013; Awad 2011; Baumstarck et al. 2013), burden of care and QoL assessment may be considered as an "unfulfilled promise" and remains underutilized in clinical practice and policy decision-making (Gilbody et al. 2002; Greenhalgh et al. 2005). This factor is true for patients and caregivers. Barriers to explain why these measures have not been routinely implemented have already been described. Some of them are discussed below.

6.3.1 The Acceptability of the Caregivers' Burden of Care and QoL Measurements

The acceptability of a questionnaire concerns the ergonomics of the questionnaire, such as the length of the questionnaire, a paper or electronic format, and the concept of computer adaptive testing (CAT). Providing shorter questionnaires or an electronic format may be appropriate and useful for use in clinical practice. However, the CAT appears as an attractive alternative approach allowing for the administration of only the items that will offer the most relevance for a given individual, reducing the length of the questionnaire and the completion time in addition to maintaining the test's precision (Weiss 2004; Reeve et al. 2007; Hill et al. 2007). To our knowledge, no CAT applied to caregivers, including burden of care and QoL measurements, is available.

6.3.2 Arguments for the Clinical Utility of the Caregivers' Measurements

Improving knowledge about the determinants of caregiver burden and QoL changes may reinforce the conviction of healthcare workers to use these measures in their clinical practice and assist them in choosing the most appropriate family interventions. Determinants of caregivers' QoL include caregivers' characteristics and patient characteristics. Sociodemographics (Bentsen et al. 1996; Parabiaghi et al. 2007; Lauber et al. 2003), personality traits (Geriani et al. 2015), cultural aspects (Boyer et al. 2012), finances (Awad and Voruganti 2008), coping strategies (Macleod et al. 2010), stress, objective burden, and social support are well-described determinants. The importance of stigma associated with severe mental illness (Dockery et al. 2015) is also an important determinant of caregivers' self-perceived burden/QoL given that it is associated with the cultural/ethnic aspects. The global functioning of the patient has also been described as a determinant of the caregiver's QoL (Flyckt et al. 2015; Kumar et al. 2014). Whereas some determinants appear relatively unchangeable, some of them appear interesting because specific assistance (Berglund et al. 2003) can be implemented to control some factors, allowing QoL improvement or burden reduction. For example, specific psychological assistance (Geriani et al. 2015) may be provided to vulnerable caregivers to employ positive coping strategies and help them face their situation. Currently, another interesting perspective may be related to the dyadic approach (i.e., incorporating the global patient-caregiver interaction). Previous researchers, specifically in people with dementia, showed that dyadic interventions—including a combination of intervention strategies and addressing both the patient and caregiver—may impact the mental and physical health of the patients (Teri et al. 2003; Prick et al. 2015). To our knowledge, no intervention was tested on the patient (with schizophrenia)-caregiver dyad, and few studies have specifically focused on the impact that family interventions have on the caregivers or on the function of the patient-caregiver dyad. Studies assessing a comprehensive dyadic intervention should be conducted in the future, and the burden/QoL of caregivers should be used as the endpoint.

6.3.3 Difficulties in Interpreting Burden of Care and QoL Scores

In some specific situations, clinicians can be perplexed in the interpretation of burden of care or QoL scores: (1) what does a score mean in the absence of normative/reference values and (2) what does a change in subjective burden or QoL score over time indicate?

6.3.3.1 The Lack of Norms in Burden and QoL Scores

The practical and clinical interpretations of burden and QoL data are difficult unless these data are presented with a reference system. A difficulty encountered in interpreting a score for clinicians is the lack of norm values. The widely generic QoL questionnaires, including SF-36 or WHOQOL, are commonly used because normative data from healthy adults and individuals with various illnesses are available (Leplege et al. 1998, 2001). However, to our knowledge, no norms are available for specific caregivers' QoL or burden questionnaires. Currently, the scores of the reference population described in the validation study of the instrument are implicitly used as norms. It is rare to have scores according to sex, gender, and other characteristics. Aggregating datasets may produce valid and robust norms. Each patient could then be compared to the norms, helping the interpretation of the score.

Another interesting option has been proposed in several recent studies (Michel et al. 2014, 2015). Instead of using norms to interpret QoL scores, these studies defined clusters of QoL levels from a specific questionnaire using a method of interpretable clustering based on unsupervised binary trees. The classification of patients into distinct QoL levels may thus be useful for translating dimension scores into meaningful and relevant categories (e.g., low, moderate, and high level of QoL), further aiding the interpretation of scores in clinical practice.

6.3.3.2 The Changes over Time: The Question of Response Shift

Another concern expressed by clinicians is the interpretation of subjective measures (subjective burden or QoL) in longitudinal studies because these measures, self-reported by the patient, might be influenced by psychological phenomena, such as adaptation to illness. Adaptation to illness is a potential explanation in cases in which, for example, the QoL of an individual who has experienced a serious health event or chronic condition is similar to the QoL of a healthy individual. An important mediator of this adaptation process is the "response shift" (RS), which involves changing internal standards, values, and the conceptualization of QoL (Schwartz and Sprangers 1999; Sprangers and Schwartz 1999). These changes do not allow comparing QoL changes over time. RS can be divided into (1) reconceptualization (i.e., a redefinition of QoL), (2) reprioritization (i.e., a change in the importance attributed to component domains constituting QoL), and (3) recalibration (i.e., a change in a patient's internal standards of measurements). True change may be over- or underestimated when RS is present, leading to biased estimates of the magnitude of change. A recent meta-analysis revealed a substantial body of literature on RS phenomena and concluded that RS was common and significant in QoL measurement (Schwartz et al. 2006). Some studies have already investigated this phenomenon in schizophrenia populations using the most established methods but more rarely for their caregivers (Boucekine et al. 2014). Recently, some studies explored the RS in family caregivers of patients in a vegetative state and of caregivers of stroke survivors (Bastianelli et al. 2014; Sajobi et al. 2014), but not in caregivers of patients with schizophrenia. Future studies should thus explore these phenomena for subjective burden and QoL in caregivers of individuals with schizophrenia.

Determining how to integrate the RS in the interpretation of burden and QoL scores will be an additional challenge. In another domain such as oncology, clinicians are often perplexed by an observed difference in QoL scores between two groups of treated patients (Boyer et al. 2014b). These clinicians need help interpreting the meaning of these differences and distinguish the part of the true change and the part of change related to RS. However, the true change of the QoL level can also be considered to be directly associated with the respondents' changing standards or values. Accordingly, RS cannot be considered in terms of measurement bias. Counterintuitive findings (e.g., the same QoL level before and after the occurrence of disease) can finally be paradoxical only for experts and not for patients, confirming the discrepancy between the views of patients and professionals.

6.4   Conclusion

Using burden of care and QoL measures may provide clinicians with information regarding the general health status of caregivers who might otherwise be unrecognized. Professionals should consider these measures for caregivers in the same way as routine objective measures. In this paper, we discussed several avenues to convince clinicians of the clinical relevance and accuracy of burden of care and QoL instruments for caregivers and to ultimately enhance the use of these measures in clinical practice.

Appendix: The Schizophrenia Caregiver Quality of Life Questionnaire (S-CGQoL)

The information contained in this questionnaire is strictly confidential. We are asking you to answer these questions because it will help us in assessing the quality of your daily life as well as the general state of your health. We would like to better understand the impact of caregiving on your quality of life.

Please answer each question by ticking the box that describes as closely as possible how you have felt for the last 12 months. Some questions concern your private life. They are necessary to evaluate all aspects of your state of health. However, if you feel that a question does not concern you or if you do not wish to answer it, skip it and go on to the next question.

Thank you

For each question, tick the box that corresponds to how you have felt for the last 12 months.

For the last 12 months, have you…	Never	Rarely	Sometimes	Often	Always
1 Felt sad, depressed?	☐	☐	☐	☐	☐
2 Felt overworked, burnt out?	☐	☐	☐	☐	☐
3 Lacked energy?	☐	☐	☐	☐	☐
4 Been tired, worn out?	☐	☐	☐	☐	☐
5 Felt anxious, worried?	☐	☐	☐	☐	☐
6 Had to give up doing things that you were very keen to do?	☐	☐	☐	☐	☐
7 Had to reduce the amount of time devoted to your leisure activities (outings, gardening, shopping, odd jobs…)?	☐	☐	☐	☐	☐
8 Been embarrassed to leave your child to attend your day or professional life?	☐	☐	☐	☐	☐
9 Had the feeling that you didn't devote enough time to the rest of your family?	☐	☐	☐	☐	☐
10 Had the feeling that you weren't free?	☐	☐	☐	☐	☐
11 Had the feeling that you led a day-to-day existence?	☐	☐	☐	☐	☐
12 Had difficulty in making professional or personal plans?	☐	☐	☐	☐	☐
13 Been helped, supported by your spouse?	☐	☐	☐	☐	☐
14 Been listened to, understood by your spouse?	☐	☐	☐	☐	☐

15 Had a satisfying emotional and sexual life?	☐	☐	☐	☐	☐
16 Been listened to, understood by doctors and nurses?	☐	☐	☐	☐	☐
17 Been helped, supported by doctors and nurses?	☐	☐	☐	☐	☐
18 Been satisfied with information given by doctors and nurses?	☐	☐	☐	☐	☐
19 Been helped, supported by your family?	☐	☐	☐	☐	☐
20 Been listened to, understood by your family?	☐	☐	☐	☐	☐
21 Been helped, supported by your friends?	☐	☐	☐	☐	☐
22 Been listened to, understood by your friends?	☐	☐	☐	☐	☐
23 Encountered difficulties because of your child's illness when applying to administration departments?	☐	☐	☐	☐	☐
24 Had financial troubles in facing your child's illness?	☐	☐	☐	☐	☐
25 Had material difficulties (housing, transportation…)?	☐	☐	☐	☐	☐

Thank you for your participation.

References

Ahn J, McCombs JS, Jung C, et al. Classifying patients by antipsychotic adherence patterns using latent class analysis: characteristics of nonadherent groups in the California Medicaid (Medi-Cal) program. Value Health. 2008;11(1):48–56.

Andrews A, Knapp M, McCrone P, Parsonage M, Trachtenberg M. Effective interventions in schizophrenia: the economic case. A report prepared for the Schizophrenia Commission. London: Rethink Mental illness; 2012. http://www.lse.ac.uk/LSEHealthAndSocialCare/pdf/LSE-economic-report-FINAL-12-Nov.pdf.

Awad AG. Quality-of-life assessment in schizophrenia: the unfulfilled promise. Expert Rev Pharmacoecon Outcomes Res. 2011;11(5):491–3.

Awad AG, Voruganti LN. The burden of schizophrenia on caregivers: a review. Pharmacoeconomics. 2008;26(2):149–62.

Awad AG, Voruganti LN. Measuring quality of life in patients with schizophrenia: an update. Pharmacoeconomics. 2012;30(3):183–95.

Awad AG, Voruganti LN, Heslegrave RJ. Measuring quality of life in patients with schizophrenia. Pharmacoeconomics. 1997;11(1):32–47.

Baider L, Ever-Hadani P, De-Nour AK. The impact of culture on perceptions of patient-physician satisfaction. Isr J Med Sci. 1995;31(2–3):179–85.

Bastianelli A, Gius E, Cipolletta S. Changes over time in the quality of life, prolonged grief and family strain of family caregivers of patients in vegetative state: a pilot study. J Health Psychol. 2014. pii: 1359105314539533. [Epub ahead of print]

Baumstarck K, Boyer L, Boucekine M, Michel P, Pelletier J, Auquier P. Measuring the quality of life in patients with multiple sclerosis in clinical practice: a necessary challenge. Mult Scler Int. 2013;2013:524894.

Bentsen H, Boye B, Munkvold OG, et al. Emotional over involvement in parents of patients with schizophrenia or related psychosis: demographic and clinical predictors. Br J Psychiatry. 1996;169(5):622–30.

Berglund N, Vahlne JO, Edman A. Family intervention in schizophrenia–impact on family burden and attitude. Soc Psychiatry Psychiatr Epidemiol. 2003;38(3):116–21.

Boucekine M, Boyer L, Baumstarck K, et al. Exploring the response shift effect on the quality of life of patients with schizophrenia: an application of the random forest method. Med Decis Making. 2014;35(3):388–97.

Bowling A, Bond M, Jenkinson C. Short Form 36 (SF-36) Health Survey questionnaire: which normative data should be used? Comparisons between the norms provided by the Omnibus Survey in Britain, the Health Survey for England and the Oxford Healthy Life Survey. J Public Health Med. 1999;21:255–70.

Boyer L, Baumstarck-Barrau K, Cano N, et al. Assessment of psychiatric inpatient satisfaction: a systematic review of self-reported instruments. Eur Psychiatry. 2009;24(8):540–9.

Boyer L, Caqueo-Urizar A, Richieri R, Lancon C, Gutierrez-Maldonado J, Auquier P. Quality of life among caregivers of patients with schizophrenia: a cross-cultural comparison of Chilean and French families. BMC Fam Pract. 2012;13:42.

Boyer L, Baumstarck K, Boucekine M, Blanc J, Lancon C, Auquier P. Measuring quality of life in patients with schizophrenia:an overview. Expert Rev Pharmacoecon Outcomes Res. 2013;13(3):343–9.

Boyer L, Baumstarck K, Guedj E, Auquier P. What's wrong with quality-of-life measures? A philosophical reflection and insights from neuroimaging. Expert Rev Pharmacoecon Outcomes Res. 2014a;14(6):767–9.

Boyer L, Baumstarck K, Michel P, et al. Statistical challenges of quality of life and cancer: new avenues for future research. Expert Rev Pharmacoecon Outcomes Res. 2014b;14(1):19–22.

Caqueo-Urizar A, Gutierrez-Maldonado J. Burden of care in families of patients with schizophrenia. Qual Life Res. 2006;15(4):719–24.

Caqueo-Urizar A, Gutierrez-Maldonado J, Miranda-Castillo C. Quality of life in caregivers of patients with schizophrenia: a literature review. Health Qual Life Outcomes. 2009;7:84.

Caqueo-Urizar A, Gutierrez-Maldonado J, Ferrer-Garcia M, Fernandez-Davila P. Quality of life of schizophrenia patients of Aymaran ethnic background in the north of Chile. Rev Psiquiatr Salud Ment. 2012;5(2):121–6.

Cohen CA, Colantonio A, Vernich L. Positive aspects of caregiving: rounding out the caregiver experience. Int J Geriatr Psychiatry. 2002;17(2):184–8.

Cooper C, Bebbington P, King M, et al. Why people do not take their psychotropic drugs as prescribed: results of the 2000 National Psychiatric Morbidity Survey. Acta Psychiatr Scand. 2007;116(1):47–53.

Dockery L, Jeffery D, Schauman O, et al. Stigma- and non-stigma-related treatment barriers to mental healthcare reported by service users and caregivers. Psychiatry Res. 2015;228(3):612–9.

EUFAMI. Family carers of people with schizophrenia are a hidden workforce at breaking point. European Federation of Associations of Families of People with Mental Illness; 2014.

Fadden G, Bebbington P, Kuipers L. The burden of care: the impact of functional psychiatric illness on the patient's family. Br J Psychiatry. 1987;150:285–92.

Flyckt L, Fatouros-Bergman H, Koernig T. Determinants of subjective and objective burden of informal caregiving of patients with psychotic disorders. Int J Soc Psychiatry. 2015;61(7):684–92.

Gater A, Rofail D, Marshall C, et al. Assessing the impact of caring for a person with schizophrenia: development of the schizophrenia caregiver questionnaire. Patient. 2015;8(6):507–20.

Geriani D, Savithry KS, Shivakumar S, Kanchan T. Burden of care on caregivers of schizophrenia patients: a correlation to personality and coping. J Clin Diagn Res. 2015;9(3):VC01–4.

Gilbody SM, House AO, Sheldon TA. Psychiatrists in the UK do not use outcomes measures. National survey. Br J Psychiatry. 2002;180:101–3.

Glozman JM. Quality of life of caregivers. Neuropsychol Rev. 2004;14(4):183–96.

Greenhalgh J, Long AF, Flynn R. The use of patient reported outcome measures in routine clinical practice: lack of impact or lack of theory? Soc Sci Med. 2005;60(4):833–43.

Group W. Development of the world health organization WHOQOL-BREF quality of life assessment. The WHOQOL group. Psychol Med. 1998;28(3):551–8.

Gupta S, Isherwood G, Jones K, Van Impe K. Assessing health status in informal schizophrenia caregivers compared with health status in non-caregivers and caregivers of other conditions. BMC Psychiatry. 2015;15:162.

Gutierrez-Maldonado J, Caqueo-Urizar A, Kavanagh DJ. Burden of care and general health in families of patients with schizophrenia. Soc Psychiatry Psychiatr Epidemiol. 2005;40(11):899–904.

Gutierrez-Maldonado J, Caqueo-Urizar A, Ferrer-Garcia M, Fernandez-Davila P. Influence of perceived social support and functioning on the quality of life of patients with schizophrenia and their caregivers. Psicothema. 2012;24(2):255–62.

Harvey K, Burns T, Fiander M, Huxley P, Manley C, Fahy T. The effect of intensive case management on the relatives of patients with severe mental illness. Psychiatr Serv. 2002;53(12):1580–5.

Hawthorne G, Herrman H, Murphy B. Interpreting the WHOQOL-Bref: preliminary population norms and effect sizes. In: Subjective well-being in mental health and human development research worldwide, Social indicators research, vol. 77(1). Dordrecht: Springer; 2006. p. 37–59.

Hill CD, Edwards MC, Thissen D, et al. Practical issues in the application of item response theory: a demonstration using items from the pediatric quality of life inventory (PedsQL) 4.0 generic core scales. Med Care. 2007;45(5 Suppl 1):S39–47.

Hoenig J, Hamilton MW. The schizophrenia patient in the community and his effect on the household. Int J Soc Psychiatry. 1966;12:165–76.

Hunt CK. Concepts in caregiver research. J Nurs Scholarsh. 2003;35(1):27–32.

Jones S. The association between objective and subjective caregiver burden. Arch Psychiatr Nurs. 1996;10(2):77–84.

Kumar CN, Suresha KK, Thirthalli J, Arunachala U, Gangadhar BN. Caregiver burden is associated with disability in schizophrenia: results of a study from a rural setting of south India. Int J Soc Psychiatry. 2014;61(2):157–63.

Lauber C, Eichenberger A, Luginbuhl P, Keller C, Rossler W. Determinants of burden in caregivers of patients with exacerbating schizophrenia. Eur Psychiatry. 2003;18(6):285–9.

Leplege A, Ecosse E, Verdier A, Perneger TV. The French SF-36 Health Survey: translation, cultural adaptation and preliminary psychometric evaluation. J Clin Epidemiol. 1998;51(11):1013–23.

Leplege A, Ecosse E, Pouchot J, Coste J, Perneger TV. MOS SF36 Questionnaire. Manual and guidelines for scores' interpretation. Estem: Vernouillet; 2001.

Levene JE, Lancee WJ, Seeman MV. The perceived family burden scale: measurement and validation. Schizophr Res. 1996;22(2):151–7.

Li J, Lambert CE, Lambert VA. Predictors of family caregivers' burden and quality of life when providing care for a family member with schizophrenia in the People's Republic of China. Nurs Health Sci. 2007;9(3):192–8.

Lua PL, Bakar ZA. Health-related quality of life profiles among family caregivers of patients with schizophrenia. Fam Community Health. 2011;34(4):331–9.

Macleod SH, Elliott L, Brown R. What support can community mental health nurses deliver to carers of people diagnosed with schizophrenia? Findings from a review of the literature. Int J Nurs Stud. 2010;48(1):100–20.

Maurin JT, Boyd CB. Burden of mental illness on the family: a critical review. Arch Psychiatr Nurs. 1990;4(2):99–107.

Michel P, Baumstarck K, Boyer L, et al. Defining quality of life levels to enhance clinical interpretation in multiple sclerosis: application of a novel clustering method. Med Care. 2014.

Michel P, Auquier P, Baumstarck K, et al. How to interpret multidimensional quality of life questionnaires for patients with schizophrenia? Qual Life Res. 2015;24(10):2483–92.

Moller-Leimkuhler AM, Wiesheu A. Caregiver burden in chronic mental illness: the role of patient and caregiver characteristics. Eur Arch Psychiatry Clin Neurosci. 2011;262(2):157–66.

NAMI. National Alliance on Mental Illness. Schizophrenia: public attitudes, personal needs. Views from people living with schizophrenia, caregivers, and the general public. Analysis and recommendations. 2008. http://www2.nami.org/SchizophreniaSurvey/SchizeExecSummary.pdf.

Nijboer C, Triemstra M, Tempelaar R, Sanderman R, van den Bos GA. Determinants of caregiving experiences and mental health of partners of cancer patients. Cancer. 1999;86(4):577–88.

Norman RM, Malla AK, Manchanda R, Harricharan R, Takhar J, Northcott S. Social support and three-year symptom and admission outcomes for first episode psychosis. Schizophr Res. 2005;80(2–3):227–34.

Ochoa S, Vilaplana M, Haro JM, et al. Do needs, symptoms or disability of outpatients with schizophrenia influence family burden? Soc Psychiatry Psychiatr Epidemiol. 2008;43(8):612–8.

Parabiaghi A, Lasalvia A, Bonetto C, et al. Predictors of changes in caregiving burden in people with schizophrenia: a 3-year follow-up study in a community mental health service. Acta Psychiatr Scand Suppl. 2007;437:66–76.

Patrick DL, Deyo RA. Generic and disease-specific measures in assessing health status and quality of life. Med Care. 1989;27(3 Suppl):S217–32.

Platt S. Measuring the burden of psychiatric illness on the family: an evaluation of some rating scales. Psychol Med. 1985;15(2):383–93.

Power M, Harper A, Bullinger M. The World Health Organization WHOQOL-100: tests of the universality of Quality of Life in 15 different cultural groups worldwide. Health Psychol. 1999;18(5):495–505.

Prick AE, de Lange J, Twisk J, Pot AM. The effects of a multi-component dyadic intervention on the psychological distress of family caregivers providing care to people with dementia: a randomized controlled trial. Int Psychogeriatr. 2015;27(12):2031–44.

Reeve BB, Hays RD, Bjorner JB, et al. Psychometric evaluation and calibration of health-related quality of life item banks: plans for the Patient-Reported Outcomes Measurement Information System (PROMIS). Med Care. 2007;45(5 Suppl 1):S22–31.

Reine G, Lancon C, Simeoni MC, Duplan S, Auquier P. Caregiver burden in relatives of persons with schizophrenia: an overview of measure instruments. Encéphale. 2003;29(2):137–47.

Richieri R, Boyer L, Reine G, et al. The Schizophrenia Caregiver Quality of Life questionnaire (S-CGQoL): development and validation of an instrument to measure quality of life of caregivers of individuals with schizophrenia. Schizophr Res. 2011;126(1–3):192–201.

Rofail D, Acquadro C, Izquierdo C, Regnault A, Zarit SH. Cross-cultural adaptation of the Schizophrenia Caregiver Questionnaire (SCQ) and the Caregiver Global Impression (CaGI) Scales in 11 languages. Health Qual Life Outcomes. 2015;13:76.

Sajobi TT, Lix LM, Singh G, Lowerison M, Engbers J, Mayo NE. Identifying reprioritization response shift in a stroke caregiver population: a comparison of missing data methods. Qual Life Res. 2014;24(3):529–40.

Schene AH, Tessler RC, Gamache GM. Instruments measuring family or caregiver burden in severe mental illness. Soc Psychiatry Psychiatr Epidemiol. 1994;29(5):228–40.

Schulz R, Beach SR. Caregiving as a risk factor for mortality: the Caregiver Health Effects Study. JAMA. 1999;282(23):2215–9.

Schwartz CE, Sprangers MA. Methodological approaches for assessing response shift in longitudinal health-related quality-of-life research. Soc Sci Med. 1999;48(11):1531–48.

Schwartz CE, Bode R, Repucci N, Becker J, Sprangers MA, Fayers PM. The clinical significance of adaptation to changing health: a meta-analysis of response shift. Qual Life Res. 2006;15(9):1533–50.

Skantze K, Malm U, Dencker SJ, May PR, Corrigan P. Comparison of quality of life with standard of living in schizophrenic out-patients. Br J Psychiatry. 1992;161:797–801.

Slevin ML, Plant H, Lynch D, Drinkwater J, Gregory WM. Who should measure quality of life, the doctor or the patient? Br J Cancer. 1988;57(1):109–12.

Sprangers MA, Schwartz CE. Integrating response shift into health-related quality of life research: a theoretical model. Soc Sci Med. 1999;48(11):1507–15.

Szmukler GI, Burgess P, Herrman H, Benson A, Colusa S, Bloch S. Caring for relatives with serious mental illness: the development of the Experience of Caregiving Inventory. Soc Psychiatry Psychiatr Epidemiol. 1996;31(3–4):137–48.

Teri L, Gibbons LE, McCurry SM, et al. Exercise plus behavioral management in patients with Alzheimer disease: a randomized controlled trial. JAMA. 2003;290(15):2015–22.

Testart J, Richieri R, Caqueo-Urizar A, Lancon C, Auquier P, Boyer L. Quality of life and other outcome measures in caregivers of patients with schizophrenia. Expert Rev Pharmacoecon Outcomes Res. 2013;13(5):641–9.

Valenstein M, Blow FC, Copeland LA, et al. Poor antipsychotic adherence among patients with schizophrenia: medication and patient factors. Schizophr Bull. 2004;30(2):255–64.

Van Humbeeck G, Van Audenhove C, Pieters G, et al. Expressed emotion in the client-professional caregiver dyad: are symptoms, coping strategies and personality related? Soc Psychiatry Psychiatr Epidemiol. 2002;37(8):364–71.

Velligan DI, Weiden PJ, Sajatovic M, et al. Adherence problems in patients with serious and persistent mental illness. The Expert Consensus Guideline Series. J Clin Psychiatry. 2009;70 Suppl 4:1-46; quiz 47–8.

Ware Jr JE, Sherbourne CD. The MOS 36-item short-form health survey (SF-36). I. Conceptual framework and item selection. Med Care. 1992;30(6):473–83.

Weiss DJ. Computerized adaptive testing for effective and efficient measurement in counseling and education. Meas Eval Couns Dev. 2004;37:70–84.

Yesufu-Udechuku A, Harrison B, Mayo-Wilson E, et al. Interventions to improve the experience of caring for people with severe mental illness: systematic review and meta-analysis. Br J Psychiatry. 2015;206(4):268–74.

Zamzam R, Midin M, Hooi LS, et al. Schizophrenia in Malaysian families: a study on factors associated with quality of life of primary family caregivers. Int J Ment Health Syst. 2011;5(1):16.

Zarit SH, Reever KE, Bach-Peterson J. Relatives of the impaired elderly: correlates of feelings of burden. Gerontologist. 1980;20:649–55.

Zendjidjian XY, Boyer L. Challenges in measuring outcomes for caregivers of people with mental health problems. Dialogues Clin Neurosci. 2014;16(2):159–69.

Zendjidjian X, Richieri R, Adida M, et al. Quality of life among caregivers of individuals with affective disorders. J Affect Disord. 2012;136(3):660–5.

Chapter 7
Electronic Technology and Advances in Assessment of Outcomes

Iris de Wit, Lieuwe de Haan, and Inez Myin-Germeys

7.1 Challenges of Traditional Measuring Instruments of Quality of Life

> Is quality of life a retrospective global appreciation of well-being by subjects with reference to the previous week or month, or is quality of life a concept that can be assessed by moment-to-moment prospective experiences? (Delespaul 1995)

The World Health Organization (WHO) defines quality of life as "individuals' perception of their position in life in the context of the culture and value system in which they live and in relation to their goals, expectations, standards and concerns" (WHOQoL Group 1998). This rather broad definition implies that quality of life is an overall appreciation of someone's satisfaction with their life. Traditional retrospective assessment methods based on this definition aim to measure "overall"

I. de Wit, MSc
Early Psychosis, AMC Psychiatry, Meibergdreef 5, Amsterdam, AZ 1105, The Netherlands

Department Early Psychosis, AMC, Academic Psychiatric Centre,
Meibergdreef 5, Amsterdam, AZ 1105, The Netherlands
e-mail: i.e.dewit@amc.uva.nl

L. de Haan (✉)
Early Psychosis, AMC Psychiatry, Meibergdreef 5, Amsterdam, AZ 1105, The Netherlands

Psychotic Disorders, AMC Academic Psychiatric Centre, Amsterdam, The Netherlands
e-mail: l.dehaan@amc.uva.nl

I. Myin-Germeys
Department of Psychiatry and Psychology, School of Mental Health and Neuroscience,
Maastricht University, PoBox 616 (VIJV), Maastricht, MD 6200, The Netherlands

Department of Neuroscience, Centre for Contextual Psychiatry, KU Leuven, Belgium
e-mail: i.germeys@maastrichtuniversity.nl; inez.germeys@kuleuven.be

© Springer International Publishing Switzerland 2016
A.G. Awad, L.N.P. Voruganti (eds.), *Beyond Assessment of Quality of Life in Schizophrenia*, DOI 10.1007/978-3-319-30061-0_7

well-being and thereby ignore momentary changes in mental status (Delespaul 1995). Answering the abovementioned question, we agree with Delespaul (1995) that the "building blocks" of quality of life are actually the moment-to-moment daily life experiences of patients and assessing those prospectively should have a central role in the assessment quality of life (Delespaul 1995). This view on quality of life consequences some challenges to the traditional measuring methods of quality of life.

Traditional measures do not take fluctuations or variability in daily life functioning into account in continuously changing contexts. This means that the natural occurrence of quality if life is not captured, limiting the *ecological validity*: the degree to which measurements represent real-life experiences and can be generalized to the real world. Secondly, because of their retrospective nature, traditional outcome measures of quality of life are vulnerable to *recall biases* (Kimhy et al. 2012) and to the affective state at the moment of questioning. Stone et al. (1998) compared the outcomes of in-the-moment measures with retrospective questionnaires (48 h later) regarding coping strategies. Limited concordance between the two methods was found, suggesting that even after 48-h time, a serious memory bias occurs (Stone et al. 1998). This may even be more problematic for patients with schizophrenia. Although research has shown that patients with schizophrenia are well capable of reliably reporting their "moment-to-moment" experiences (Delespaul 1995), there is evidence that due to cognitive impairments associated with this disorder, patients with schizophrenia in particular could experience problems recalling in retrospect (Lepage et al. 2007). This could result in a biased reflection of the actual daily life quality of patients with schizophrenia. For the reliability of quality of life measures, in-the-moment measures would therefore be preferable.

Abovementioned limitations of traditional retrospective methods ask for an alternative approach in assessing quality of life. Information on daily, moment-to-moment experiences would be a relevant addition to the current assessment methods. In conclusion, assessing quality of life "real time" directly in the life of patients with schizophrenia would be beneficial, but how could such an approach be operationalized?

7.2 Measuring Quality of Life in Daily Life: Momentary Assessment Strategies

7.2.1 Experience Sampling Methods

The answer can be found in experience sampling methods. Experience sampling methods (ESM) are momentary assessment strategies measuring experiences in real life (Myin-Germeys et al. 2009). ESM include structured *diary techniques* (Bolger et al. 2003): patients are instructed to fill out self-report questionnaires, at multiple random times a day in response to a signal ("beep") while performing their usual daily activities (Myin-Germeys et al. 2003). In contrast to the cross-sectional retro-spective traditional questionnaires, it provides real-time repeated measures with ecological validity. Therewith, ESM are promising for measuring quality of life in patients with schizophrenia.

Experience sampling was introduced in 1981 by Prescott and Csikszentmihalyi (1981). They described the purpose of using this new sampling method as the following:

> The present study represents a departure from previous studies since it introduces random time sampling of behavior and makes it possible to compare persons' reports of cognitive and affective states in a wide range of normal settings, including home, work, recreation, and transportation. (Prescott and Csikszentmihalyi 1981)

Participants were given a pager device ("beeper"), which randomly signaled 5–8 times a day, on 7 consecutive days, between 8 am and 11 pm. Participants were instructed to report their cognitive and affective states immediately in response to each "beep" by filling out a form with pen and paper (Prescott and Csikszentmihalyi 1981).

Nowadays, ESM designs are essentially similar, although the pen-and-paper reg-istration method has given way to electronic data collection. Patients are now able to report their behavior, experiences, and situational context on electronic devices, such as PDAs for which various ESM software packages have been developed (Kimhy et al. 2006). A device specifically designed to facilitate monitoring daily life experiences and behavior using mobile assessment is the *PsyMate* (Myin-Germeys et al. 2011) (Fig. 7.1). The small pocket-size device can be programmed to generate beeps, to which patients are instructed to respond by filling out question-naires about their current mood, place, activity, and social context directly on the device. The PsyMate stores data automatically and was used in several studies on schizophrenia since its development in 2011 (Myin-Germeys et al. 2011). Furthermore, the PsyMate is currently engaged in large longitudinal European stud-ies on schizophrenia (GROUP; EU-GEI).

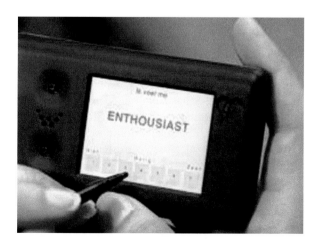

Fig. 7.1 The PsyMate Device (Myin-Germeys et al. 2011)

Moreover, several ESM apps are on the market for patients to install on their own smartphones, thus facilitating the usability of ESM. This may enhance the accessibility and therefore is promising for a wider implementation of this method. Evaluation of these new computerized technologies showed that they are less time-consuming for patients and have shown to be equally reliable compared with the diary method, showing similar response rates for patients with schizophrenia and healthy controls (Kimhy et al. 2006). Moreover, higher response rates were found for electronic ESM in comparison to diary methods (Stone et al. 2003).

7.2.2   How to Measure Quality of Life with ESM

Emotional experience (subjective well-being) is considered to be a determinant factor for psychological quality of life. Real-time measures of patient's emotional experiences (*positive and negative affect*) could therefore be the key to assessing subjective daily life quality in patients with schizophrenia. An example of recent research on subjective well-being, associated with quality of life in schizophrenia, is the study of Lataster et al. (2011). They examined the effect of theoretical dopamine D_2 occupancy of antipsychotics on emotional experience using ESM. The purpose of the study was to identify more subtle changes in emotional experiences associated with theoretical levels of D_2 occupancy, in an ecological valid way; hence, ESM was selected for data gathering. Emotional experiences were captured with ESM during 6 days. After each of the ten daily beeps, patients were expected to respond by filling out the ESM questionnaires regarding thoughts, context, and emotions. Experience of emotions was operationalized with four positive affect items (e.g., "I feel relaxed") and six negative affect items (e.g., "I feel down") on a 7-point Likert scale (Lataster et al. 2011). Results showed a significant increase of negative affect in the daily lives of patients in the group of antipsychotics with theoretically high levels of D_2 occupancy antipsychotics (Lataster et al. 2011). These findings added ecological validation to earlier laboratory finding showing that higher D_2 occupancy is associated with decreased emotional experience (De Haan et al. 2000, 2003; Mizrahi et al. 2007). This study demonstrated ESM's value in addition to traditional approaches by assessing outcomes of well-being in the reality of daily life as an indicator of subjective well-being and quality of life.

A second possibility is assessing *momentary* quality of life with ESM, as shown by a study of Barge-Schaapveld and Nicolson (2002). They examined the effects of antidepressant treatment on quality of life for patients with depression (Barge-Schaapveld et al. 2002). Quality of life was measured both retrospectively and with ESM. Retrospective measures consisted of the QoL VAS, a 100-mm visual analogue scale (Andrews and McKennell 1980), and satisfaction with life scale (SWLS) (Diener et al. 1985). The ESM (ten times a day, during 6 days) contained a *momentary* quality of life item (mQoL): "In general, how is it going with you right now?" Patients expressed their momentary quality of life on a 6-point Likert scale (very good to very bad). Moreover, ESM was also used to assess emotional experiences, with items measuring positive affect and negative affect. Results provided useful information regarding quality of life improvement associated with antidepressant treatment. Not only was it shown that the "overall" quality of life improved more in the treatment group (traditionally measured), also the *variability* in momentary QoL was more reduced in the treatment group, showing that patients in the treatment group were more "stable" in their momentary quality of life reports (Barge-Schaapveld et al. 2002). Also, side effects in relation to *momentary* QoL and drop-out were examined. They found a greater association between side effects measured with ESM in the group of patients who prematurely chose to discontinue their treatment. Moreover, dropped out patients reported more decrease in momentary QoL, suggesting that impact of side effects on momentary QoL leads to dropout (Barge-Schaapveld et al. 2002). Finally, ESM captured more reported side effects than were retrospectively weekly reported to their clinician (Barge-Schaapveld et al. 2002), underlining the gap between retrospective reports and measurements in real time.

In the last decades, ESM have proven to add ecologically valid knowledge to multiple research domains in psychopathology, providing valuable insights regarding phenomenology, etiology, psychological models, treatment outcomes, biological mechanisms, and gene-environment interactions (Myin-Germeys et al. 2009). For an overview of these findings, we refer to the article "Experience Sampling Research in Psychopathology: Opening the Black Box of Daily Life" (Myin-Germeys et al. 2009).

7.3   Using Experience Sampling Methods for Psychological Treatment

7.3.1   Ecological Momentary Interventions

ESM moreover offers opportunities for the psychological treatment of patients with schizophrenia by enabling *Ecological momentary interventions* (Heron and Smyth 2010; Myin-Germeys et al. 2011). Through ESM, personalized and patient-tailored interventions, as well as feedback on real-life behavior of patients, can be provided (Myin-Germeys et al. 2011).

An Example
Quality of life is, as earlier mentioned, related to affect. Patients with schizophrenia suffer from negative symptoms which can be reflected in a reduction of positive affect and increase of negative affect (Myin-Germeys et al. 2000). This is expected to lead to a reduction of quality of life. A recent study investigated emotional experience and behavior in schizophrenia using ESM (Oorschot et al. 2013). In comparison with a healthy control group, patients with schizophrenia experienced lower positive and higher negative affect (Oorschot et al. 2013). These findings were in concordance with earlier research on affect in schizophrenia patients (Myin-Germeys et al. 2000). However, ESM results showed contrary to the expectations

that patients with schizophrenia were equally able to enjoy pleasurable activities (Oorschot et al. 2013). But in contrast to healthy controls, this experienced pleasure did not lead to more motivation for this activity in the future in patients with schizophrenia (Oorschot et al. 2013).

These findings demonstrate opportunities provided by the use of ESM on emotional experience in the treatment:

1. Using ESM for monitoring within-patient patterns of emotional experiences and behavior helps individual patients to increase insight in which activities are pleasurable to them and encourages them to perform those (Myin-Germeys et al. 2011). Using ESM as a therapeutic application for treatment of depression was recently shown to be successful (Kramer et al. 2014).
2. People in general, and schizophrenia patients in specific, are often not conscious of what factors induce specific emotional experiences. ESM could help to generate more insight in these personal patterns (Myin-Germeys et al. 2011).
3. Through making patients active partners in treatment, they feel more empowered, which is likely to enhance compliance with treatment and recovery (Myin-Germeys et al. 2011).

7.4   Advantages and Limitations of Experience Sampling Methods

7.4.1   Advantages of ESM

To summarize, using ESM in addition to traditional measures assessing outcomes of quality of life has the following advantages:

- ESM's ecologically valid measures capture information about experiences in patients' everyday lives.
- ESM provide a minimization of recall biases due to measuring in the moment, which is particularly of value for patients with schizophrenia.
- ESM's repeated measure design generates detailed pictures of within-person patterns in daily lives of patients and allows studying fluctuations and patterns in quality of life, associated with interactions with the environment.
- New statistical approaches (e.g., multilevel models) can be used to analyze ESM data at both subject and at moment level (Myin-Germeys et al. 2009; Schwartz and Stone 1998; Hedeker et al. 2008).

7.4.2   Limitations

Despite the major advantages of ESM, it also has its limitations.

First of all, due to the frequency of the measurements, duration of the total assessment period (usually ten times a day, for 6 consecutive days (Myin-Germeys et al. 2009)), and the total of 60 measuring moments, this method is intensive and can be demanding for patients (Myin-Germeys et al. 2009). Second, there is a risk that using ESM evokes experiences, for instance, in acute phases of psychosis, which should be considered by researchers and clinicians beforehand (Myin-Germeys et al. 2009). Third, the uncontrolled setting of the assessments using ESM can result in noncompliance to the method. This however can be monitored with the use of electronic devices, which register the time of the reports. In case the time of the report differs more than 15 min from the "beep," it can be recommended to exclude the particular measure from the analysis (Myin-Germeys et al. 2009).

7.5   Conclusion

This chapter has provided an introduction in experience sampling methods and illustrated its valuable contribution to traditional methods assessing quality of life in schizophrenia. ESM are promising in elucidating the real daily life quality of patients with schizophrenia. Moreover, therapeutic interventions on improving quality of life can be monitored in real time, generating opportunities for personalized *ecological momentary interventions* (Myin-Germeys et al. 2011).

Delespaul (1995) proposed that the essence of quality of life actually lies in the daily life functioning of patients. We agree that ecological valid assessment is necessary to enrich the knowledge concerning real-life influences on the subjective quality of life of patients with schizophrenia.

References

Andrews FM, McKennell AC. Measures of self-reported well-being: their affective, cognitive, and other components. Soc Indic Res. 1980;8(2):127–55.

Barge-Schaapveld DQ, Nicolson NA. Effects of antidepressant treatment on the quality of daily life: an experience sampling study. J Clin Psychiatry. 2002;63(6):477–85.

Bolger N, Davis A, Rafaeli E. Diary methods: capturing life as it is lived. Annu Rev Psychol. 2003;54:579–616. doi:10.1146/annurev.psych.54.101601.145030.

De Haan L, Lavalaye J, Linszen D, et al. Subjective experience and striatal dopamine D(2) receptor occupancy in patients with schizophrenia stabilized by olanzapine or risperidone. Am J Psychiatry. 2000;157:1019–20. doi:10.1176/appi.ajp.157.6.1019.

De Haan L, Van Bruggen M, Lavalaye J, et al. Subjective experience and D 2 receptor occupancy in patients with recent-onset schizophrenia treated with low-dose olanzapine or haloperidol: a randomized, double-blind study. Am J Psychiatry. 2003;160:303–9. doi:10.1176/appi.ajp.160.2.303.

Delespaul PA. Assessing schizophrenia in daily life – the experience sampling method. Maastricht: University press; 1995.

Diener ED, Emmons RA, Larsen RJ, et al. The satisfaction with life scale. J Pers Assess. 1985;49(1):71–5.

Hedeker D, Mermelstein RJ, Demirtas H. An application of a mixed-effects location scale model for analysis of Ecological Momentary Assessment (EMA) data. Biometrics. 2008;64:627–34.

Heron KE, Smyth JM. Ecological momentary interventions: incorporating mobile technology into psychosocial and health behaviour treatments. Br J Health Psychol. 2010;15:1–39. doi:10.1348/135910709X466063.

Kramer I, Simons CJ, Hartmann JA, et al. A therapeutic application of the experience sampling method in the treatment of depression: a randomized controlled trial. World Psychiatry. 2014;13:68–77. doi:10.1002/wps.20090.

Kimhy D, Delespaul P, Corcoran C, et al. Computerized experience sampling method (ESMc): assessing feasibility and validity among individuals with schizophrenia. J Psychiatr Res. 2006;40:221–30. doi:10.1016/j.jpsychires.2005.09.007.

Kimhy D, Myin-Germeys I, Palmier-Claus J, Swendsen J. Mobile assessment guide for research in schizophrenia and severe mental disorders. Schizophr Bull. 2012;38:386–95. doi:10.1093/schbul/sbr186.

Lataster J, Van Os J, De Haan L, et al. Emotional experience and estimates of D2 receptor occupancy in psychotic patients treated with haloperidol, risperidone, or olanzapine: an experience sampling study. J Clin Psychiatry. 2011;72:1397–404. doi:10.4088/JCP.09m05466yel.

Lepage M, Sergerie K, Pelletier M, et al. Episodic memory bias and the symptoms of schizophrenia. Can J Psychiatry. 2007;52(11):702–9.

Mizrahi R, Rusjan P, Agid O, et al. Adverse subjective experience with antipsychotics and its relationship to striatal and extrastriatal D2 receptors: a PET study in schizophrenia. Am J Psychiatry. 2007;164:630–7. doi:10.1176/appi.ajp.164.4.630.

Myin-Germeys I, Birchwood M, Kwapil T. From environment to therapy in psychosis: a real-world momentary assessment approach. Schizophr Bull. 2011;37:244–7. doi:10.1093/schbul/sbq164.

Myin-Germeys I, Oorschot M, Collip D, et al. Experience sampling research in psychopathology: opening the black box of daily life. Psychol Med. 2009;39:1533–47. doi:10.1017/S0033291708004947.

Myin-Germeys I, Delespaul PA, Van Os J, et al. Experience sampling onderzoek bij psychose Een overzicht. 2003;45:131–140.

Myin-Germeys I, Delespaul PA, De Vries MW. Schizophrenia patients are more emotionally active than is assumed based on their behavior. Schizophr Bull. 2000;26:847–54.

Oorschot M, Lataster T, Thewissen V, et al. Emotional experience in negative symptoms of schizophrenia-no evidence for a generalized hedonic deficit. Schizophr Bull. 2013;39:217–25. doi:10.1093/schbul/sbr137.

Prescott S, Csikszentmihalyi M. Environmental effects on cognitive and affective states: the experiential time sampling approach. Soc Behav Personal Int J. 1981;9:23–32. doi:10.2224/sbp.1981.9.1.23.

Schwartz JE, Stone AA. Strategies for analyzing ecological momentary assessment data. Health Psychol. 1998;17:6–16.

Stone AA, Schwartz JE, Neale JM, et al. A comparison of coping assessed by ecological momentary assessment and retrospective recall. J Pers Soc Psychol. 1998;74(1670–1680):1670. doi:10.1037/0022-3514.74.6.

Stone AA, Shiffman S, Schwartz JE, et al. Patient compliance with paper and electronic diaries. Control Clin Trials. 2003;24:182–99. doi:10.1016/S0197-2456(02)00320-3.

WHOQoL Group. Development of the World Health Organization WHOQOL-BREF quality of life assessment. The WHOQOL Group. Psychol Med. 1998;28:551–8.

Chapter 8
Modern Psychometric Approaches to Analysis of Scales for Health-Related Quality of Life

Jakob Bue Bjorner and Per Bech

8.1 Introduction

In recent years, much effort has been invested in the development of new instruments for assessment of health-related quality of life (HRQOL). For many new instruments, modern psychometric methods, such as item response theory (IRT) models, have been used, either as supplemental to classical psychometric testing or as the primary methodological approach. We will use the term modern psychometric methods to refer to psychometric methods for multi-item scales that (1) examine the contribution of each item to the measurement properties of the overall scale and (2) recognize that items are categorical. The models include Rasch models (Rasch 1980; Fischer and Molenaar 1995), other IRT models (Samejima 1969; van der Linden and Hambleton 1997), and factor analytic models for categorical data (Muthén 1984). "Modern" psychometric methods have actually a rather long history within psychiatric research (both focusing on self-reported scales (Bech et al. 1978) and psychiatric outcome rating scales (Bech et al. 1984)). During the past 25 years, modern psychometric methods have increasingly been used in the analysis of patient-reported outcome measures (Teresi et al. 1989; Haley et al. 1994). For example, the NIH-sponsored Patient-Reported Outcomes Measurement Information System (PROMIS) project relies primarily on modern psychometric methods (Reeve et al. 2007). Similarly, modern psychometric analyses have started to be

J.B. Bjorner, MD, PhD (✉)
Patient Insights, Optum, 24 Albion Road, Lincoln, RI, USA

Department of Public Health, University of Copenhagen, Copenhagen, Denmark

National Research Centre for the Working Environment, Copenhagen, Denmark
e-mail: jbjorner@qualitymetric.com

P. Bech, MD, PhD
Psychiatric Research Unit, CCMH, Mental Health Centre North Zealand,
Copenhagen, Denmark

© Springer International Publishing Switzerland 2016
A.G. Awad, L.N.P. Voruganti (eds.), *Beyond Assessment of Quality of Life in Schizophrenia*, DOI 10.1007/978-3-319-30061-0_8

adopted for analysis of patient-reported HRQOL measures for patients with schizo-phrenia (D'haenen 1996; Pan et al. 2007; Boyer et al. 2010; Reise et al. 2011a; Laurens et al. 2012; Mojtabai et al. 2012; Chen et al. 2013; Michel et al. 2013; Park et al. 2015; Galindo-Garre et al. 2015; Norholm and Bech 2006). The present chap-ter provides an introduction to modern psychometric methods and discusses their potential use for analyses of HRQOL data from patients with schizophrenia. Rather than focusing on one particular approach, we will show what the methods have in common and how they can supplement each other.

A clear conceptual model of quality of life in schizophrenia is important for scale development and analysis (Awad et al. 1997). However, in order to focus on the psychometric models, we will take a pragmatic approach to the concept of HRQOL. We understand HRQOL as a multidimensional concept and discuss scales measuring domains that may contribute to or reflect parts of HRQOL, but do not constitute an exhaustive assessment of HRQOL (Connell et al. 2014). As a practical example, we will present IRT models for mental health items from the SF-36v2 questionnaire (Ware et al. 2007), a generic HRQOL instrument that is used also with schizophrenia patients (Boyer et al. 2013; Michel et al. 2015).

8.2   IRT Models

Figure 8.1 illustrates an IRT model, the generalized partial credit model (Muraki 1997), for an item measuring mental health: "How much of the time *during the past 4 weeks* did you feel downhearted and depressed?" Clinically, mental health is here considered as a rather narrow and unidimensional construct that can be represented with rather few items. The horizontal axis in this figure is mental health as it would have been measured by an ideal instrument, i.e., latent mental health. We have cali-brated this axis so that mental health has a mean score of 50 and a standard devia-tion of 10 in the US general population (Ware et al. 2007). Higher scores represent better mental health. The curved lines represent model predictions of the probability of selecting each response choice at each level of mental health. For example, a person with a score of 50 has a 0.53 probability of answering "None of the time," a 0.42 probability of answering "A little of the time," a 0.02 probability of answering "Some of the time," and negligible probabilities of other responses. The curved lines are termed *option characteristic curves* and represent item characteristics that are assumed to hold true regardless of the mental health status of the population.

8.3   IRT Score Estimation

Once an IRT model is established for an item, the model can be used to make infer-ences about the health level of a person, given his or her item response. For example, for a person answering "Most of the time" on the item "…did you feel downhearted

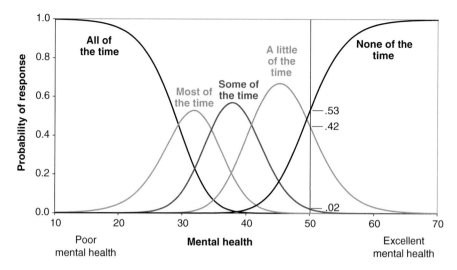

Fig. 8.1 Generalized partial credit IRT model for the item: "How much of the time *during the past 4 weeks* did you feel downhearted and depressed?" with the response choices "All of the time," "Most of the time," "Some of the time," "A little of the time," and "None of the time." Each curved line represents the probability of picking one of these response choices for a particular level of mental health. The mental health scale is standardized so the US adult population has an average score of 50 and a standard deviation of 10

and depressed?," the most likely mental health score is 32, since the option characteristic curve has its optimum at this score (Fig. 8.2). Furthermore, a 95 % confidence interval (CI) can be constructed based on the area under the option characteristic curve. For the example in Fig. 8.2, the 95 % CI is 20–40 – a fairly wide interval since a score estimate based on only a single item is bound to be imprecise.

A more precise score can be achieved by evaluating the pattern of responses to several mental health items. The top three left panes of Fig. 8.3 show the option characteristic curves for three items: "…downhearted and depressed (MH4)," "felt very nervous (MH1)," and "been a happy person (MH5)." To estimate a score for a person who chose the response "Most of the time" on the first two items and "A little of the time" on the last item (black lines), we calculate the probability of this response combination for each level of mental health by multiplying the values from the three functions. For example, for a score of 30, the probabilities are 0.49, 0.36, and 0.44, resulting in a likelihood of 0.076. Evaluation of this likelihood function results in a score estimate of 30 and a 95 % CI of 21–36. Thus, the score estimate has changed slightly and the confidence interval has narrowed – reflecting the added precision achieved by asking two more questions.

The approach presented above illustrates the general IRT approach to scoring. Several refinements to the procedure are available to allow scoring in situations where respondents have best (or worst) possible scores on all items (Warm 1989; Bock and Mislevy 1982) or where only the sum of the items is known and not the response pattern (Orlando et al. 2000).

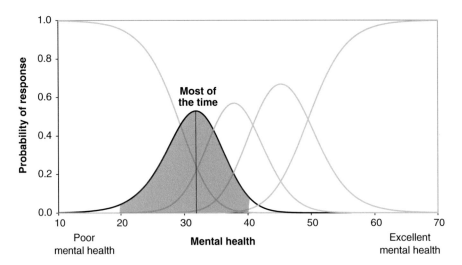

Fig. 8.2 Score estimate and 95 % confidence interval (CI) for the response "Most of the time" on the item "How much of the time during the past 4 weeks did you feel downhearted and depressed?" The score estimate (32) is indicated by the vertical black line and the 95 % CI (20–40) is indicated by the gray area. The 95 % CI is nonsymmetrical due to the slight negative skew of the option characteristic curve

    The right column in Fig. 8.3 illustrates score estimation for another combination of responses: the answer "Most of the time" on all three items. This combination of responses results in the likelihood function in the lower right pane, a score estimate of 34 and a 95 % CI of 26–40. However, the smaller area under the curve suggests that this response pattern is more unlikely than the response pattern seen in the left part of Fig. 8.3. While the response combination is not so unlikely as to cause serious concerns about the validity of the score, more extreme response combinations may suggest problems in the validity of the scale (such as the assumption that the three items are measuring the same construct) or in the ability of the respondent to answer the questionnaire. This idea has led to formal testing of response consistency (Drasgow et al. 1985). Such testing of response consistency may prove valuable in HRQOL scales for psychiatric research, where doubt is sometimes raised about the ability of patients to answer the questions (Awad et al. 1997).

8.4   Item Properties

A comparison of option characteristic curves for the different items (e.g., Fig. 8.3, left column) also reveals important item differences. For example, the option characteristic curves for MH1 are flatter than for MH4. If a score had to be estimated based on only the response "Most of the time" on item MH1, the score estimate would have been 28 and the 95 % CI would have been 4 to 42 – much wider than

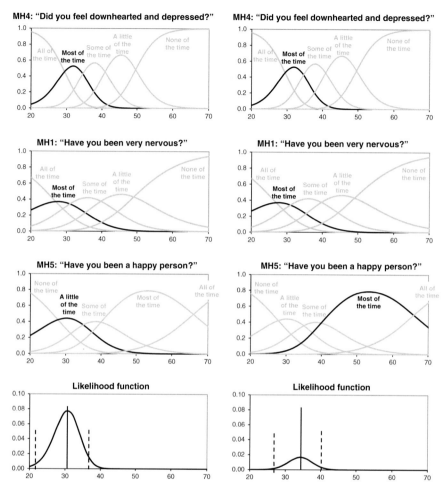

Fig. 8.3 Illustration of score estimation for two different combinations of responses to three items on mental health. In the *left column*, the responses "Most of the time," "Most of the time," and "A little of the time" (top 3 panes) result in a score estimate of 30 and a 95 % confidence interval of 21–36 (likelihood function in *bottom pane*). In the *right column*, the responses "Most of the time," "Most of the time," and "Most of the time" (top 3 panes) result in a score estimate of 34 and a 95 % confidence interval of 26–40 (likelihood function in *bottom pane*)

the confidence interval based only on MH4. In other words, for a person with a score around 30, MH1 provides less information about mental health than MH4. In IRT models, the steepness of the option characteristic curves is determined by a *discrimination parameter* – somewhat similar to the item-total correlations and factor loadings of classical psychometrics.

Another item property is illustrated by comparing the curves for the option indicating best mental health on each item ("None of the time" for MH1 and MH4, "All of the time" for MH5). Compared to MH1 and MH4, the curve for the best response

option on MH5 is shifted to the right – indicating that only a respondent with very
good mental health is likely to answer that he or she has been a happy person "All
of the time" during the past 4 weeks. Borrowing terminology from educational testing, MH5 can be said to be a difficult item in the sense that it is more difficult to
achieve the best possible score. In the IRT model used here, the generalized partial
credit model, item difficulties are modeled through *threshold parameters* that are
defined as the points on the latent scale where option characteristic curves for adja-
cent response choices overlap. Thus, for MH5, the threshold parameters are 28, 35,
40, and 66.

8.5 Item Information, Test Information, and Reliability

As we saw in the scoring examples, measurement precision can be evaluated directly
from the likelihood function for a particular response pattern. However, measurement precision can also be evaluated from *item information functions*. Item information functions are calculated from the option characteristic curves and represent
each item's contribution to the overall measurement precision for a particular level
of health. The right column of Fig. 8.4 shows the item information functions for
MH4, MH1, and MH5. A comparison with the option characteristic curves for each
item (left column) shows that item information is *high* when several responses are
possible for a particular level of mental health and *low* when one response option is
far more likely than the other responses. This is a mathematical formulation of the
principle that one achieves little information by asking questions with predictable
answers. Further, the item information functions have its maximum at a higher level
for an item with high discrimination (MH4) than for items with lower discrimination (MH1 and MH5).

The item information functions can be combined (by simple summation) into a
test information function that represents the precision of the test for each score
level. The test information function can be used to calculate a standard error of
measurement, an approximate 95 % CI, and a marginal reliability function (Fig. 8.4,
bottom right panel). The marginal reliability function is the scale reliability that corresponds to the standard error of measurement for the particular level of health. It
may be useful to compare IRT estimation of scale precision to classical reliability
estimates such a Cronbach's alpha. For the 3-item scale, an alpha of 0.78 was estimated in the same data set that was used for the IRT analyses. However, while classical test theory assumes that test precision is constant throughout the score range
(collected in a simple error term), IRT models differentiate error throughout the
score range and with respect to the individual items. Therefore, reliability tested by
Cronbach's alpha can be misleading. For people with very good mental health, the
test information function shows that we have limited measurement precision.

Another way of evaluating test information, popular among psychometricians
using Rasch models (see next section), are so-called item-person maps (Fig. 8.4,
fourth left pane). These plots compare the location of item threshold parameters

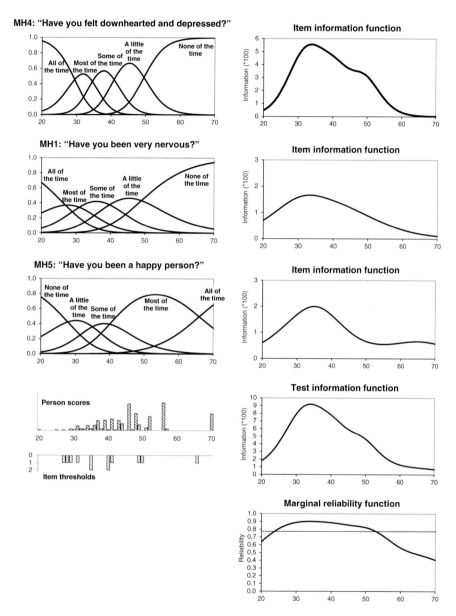

Fig. 8.4 Illustration of item information, test information, and marginal reliability functions. The *horizontal line* at 0.78 in the marginal reliability figure illustrates reliability as estimated through Cronbach's alpha

(lower part of the figure) to the distribution of IRT score estimates (upper part of the figure). To be perfectly targeted, the item threshold parameters should match the distribution of IRT scores. The item-person map in Fig. 8.4 shows less than perfect targeting due to a lack of items covering good mental health. When precise measurement of good mental health is important, e.g., in general population studies or when assessing recovery in schizophrenia, scales with more positive items should be considered, such as the full MH scale or the WHO-5 well-being scale, which contain items that are harder than the MH5 item (Bech 2015; Ellervik et al. 2016).

Comparison of the item map and the testing information function shows that test information is high in score ranges with many item thresholds. This is always the case for Rasch models and true with minor modifications for other IRT models.

8.6   Examples of Different Psychometric Models

Many different types of modern psychometric models are available for analysis of HRQOL data. We will provide a brief introduction to some of the standard models. Examples of option characteristic curves according to these models are provided in Fig. 8.5.

Nonparametric IRT models (Ramsay 1991; Mokken 1971; Sijtsma and Hemker 1998) do not assume a particular parametric form of the option characteristic curves. In one approach to nonparametric IRT, the item response probabilities are calculated as a function of the sum of all the other items in the scale. The option characteristic curves are then derived by a kernel smoothing approach (Ramsay 1991). This approach is illustrated in the left column of Fig. 8.5. Since these models stay close to the empirical data, the approach can be useful to check the assumptions of other IRT models. However, at score levels where there are few respondents, the models are not robust. Another approach to nonparametric IRT models defines some core requirements of items. The *monotone homogeneity model* assumes that the probability of a high score on a mental health item increases with increasing mental health (Mokken 1971; Sijtsma and Hemker 1998). This basic assumption of *monotonicity* applies to all the modern psychometric models that we will discuss

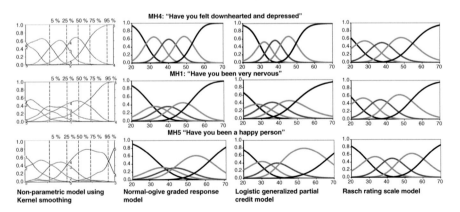

Fig. 8.5 Option characteristic curves for three items according to four different psychometric models

below. Thus, a test of the monotonicity can be used to evaluate whether any standard parametric IRT model can be used.

In the *normal-ogive IRT models*, the option characteristic curves are modeled using the cumulative distribution function of the normal distribution. For the typical HRQOL item with multiple rank-ordered responses, the normal-ogive *graded response* IRT model (Samejima 1997) is used. This model is illustrated in Fig. 8.5, second column. The normal-ogive graded response model is mathematically equivalent to a one-factor model for categorical data (Muthén 1984). This means that the normal-ogive graded response IRT model can be implemented using software for categorical data factor analysis (e.g., Muthén and Muthén 2014).

In *logistic IRT models*, the option characteristic curves are modeled using the logistic function. For HRQOL data, the most popular logistic IRT models are the *logistic graded response model* (Samejima 1997) and the *generalized partial credit model* (Muraki 1997). These models are similar in the sense that both models assume a rank order of the response choices and both models include a discrimination parameter and some threshold parameters (four threshold parameters for an item with five response choices). However, the models differ in the way the thresholds are defined (see, e.g., Bjorner et al. 2007). The option characteristic curves of the logistic graded response model are nearly identical to the option characteristic curves of the normal-ogive model. Option characteristic curves of the generalized partial credit model are shown in the third column in Fig. 8.5. Usually, the graded response model and the generalized partial credit model provide option characteristic curves that have a similar resemblance.

If the item response choices do not have a clear rank ordering, the *nominal categories model* (Bock 1997) may be used. This model has some similarity to the generalized partial credit model, but includes a separate discrimination parameter for each response choice. A comparison between the nominal category model and the generalized partial credit model can be used to test the rank order of the response choices.

Rasch models (Fischer and Molenaar 1995) can be seen as restricted versions of logistic IRT models. The Rasch models specify that all items have equal discrimination (usually set to 1). Thus, the *partial credit model* (Masters and Wright 1997), which belongs to the Rasch family of models, is similar to the *generalized partial credit model* except that all items are assumed to have equal discrimination. A more restricted Rasch model is the *rating scale model* (Andrich 1978), which specifies that the distance between item thresholds (e.g., the distance between thresholds 1 and 2) is the same across items. The rating scale model is illustrated in the fourth column in Fig. 8.5. The Rasch models were derived from theoretical requirements of valid measurement (Fischer and Molenaar 1995). For example, if the items in a mental health scale fit a Rasch model, the simple sum of the items encapsulates all the information in the items about mental health. This property (named *statistical sufficiency* (Fischer and Molenaar 1995)) is important, since HRQOL scales are very often scored as a simple sum of the items, thus implicitly assuming a Rasch model. Further, if the items fit the rating scale model, they can be consistently ordered in terms of difficulty. This property (named *invariant item ordering* (Sijtsma and Hemker 1998)) means that

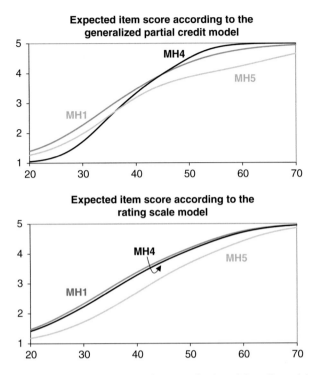

Fig. 8.6 Expected item scores according to the generalized partial credit model and the rating scale model. To calculate the expected score, each response choice is assigned a value (e.g., MH1: "All of the time" = 1…"None of the time" = 5). For a particular IRT score level, the expected item score is calculated by the sum of the response choice values weighted by the response choice probabilities. For example, for MH4 at an IRT score of 50, the expected item score according to the generalized partial credit model is calculated as $1*0.000 + 2*0.0002 + 3*0.02 + 4*0.42 + 5*0.53$ (see probabilities in Fig. 8.1)

throughout the IRT score range, the expected (average) score for an "easy" item is higher than the expected score for a "hard" item. Figure 8.6 illustrates the expected item scores according to the generalized partial credit and the rating scale model. According to the generalized partial credit model, MH4 is the "easiest" item for persons with an IRT score above 46, but the most "difficult" item for persons with an IRT score below 36. Thus according to the generalized partial credit model, MH4 cannot be consistently classified as easy or hard, relative to the other items. However, according to the rating scale model, MH5 is consistently the most "difficult" item, while MH1 is the "easiest" item, and MH4 is consistently in between (Fig. 8.6). Invariant item ordering provides important benefits in score interpretation and measurement of change over item (e.g., in a clinical trial) (Embretson 1991). In addition to the theoretical advantages described above, Rasch models have the practical advantage that they are more robust than the other models when the sample size is limited.

If the kernel smoothing model in the left column in Fig. 8.5 is taken as the truth, the other IRT models have various degrees of success in modeling the option characteristic curves. In particular, the rating scale model seems to provide a poor fit for MH5 – not capturing the broad range over which the response "Most of the time" is the most probable. A likely explanation for this misfit is that the response choices for this item have been "reverse coded" compared to the other items due to the positive item formulation ("happy person"). Thus, it is not reasonable to assume that the same rating scale model would apply to this item. A single rating scale model is usually only applied in situations where all the items share the same response choices (and direction of scoring). For an improved rating scale analysis of the current items, one rating scale model would be specified for MH1 and MH4 and another for MH5.

When comparing the option characteristic curves of the normal-ogive graded response model and the generalized partial credit model, the latter seems to provide a better fit. A possible reason for this is that the normal-ogive graded response model for illustration purposes was calculated based on the results of a categorical data factor analysis (Muthén and Muthén 2014). While this approach is correct in principle, a direct estimation of the normal-ogive graded response model would probably have resulted in a better fit.

8.7   Testing Model Assumptions

The above discussion illustrates the importance of evaluating the model assumptions and testing model fit. Typically, four major assumptions can be distinguished:

1. *Unidimensionality*: that all items in the scale measure the same underlying construct that can be expressed as one number. To illustrate, our example has assumed that mental health is a unidimensional construct and that it is not necessary to distinguish between anxiety, depression, and positive well-being.
2. *Local independence*: that the latent construct explains all covariation between items. Local dependence may occur for item pairs that share particular words (e.g., two items that both use the term "depressed"). While local dependence usually does not bias the score, it leads the analyst to overestimate test precision.
3. The particular form of the *option characteristic curves*. As illustrated in Fig. 8.5, the option characteristic curves may not always represent a good fit with the data. Such lack of fit will lead to misinterpretation of the item properties and can bias the score.
4. *Measurement invariance*: for a given item, we assume that the same measurement model applies to all respondents. Sometimes, however, some population subgroups may differ in their interpretation of an item. An example of such differential item functioning is shown in Fig. 8.7. The example is an item from the Mental Health Inventory (Veit and Ware 1983) asking: "How often have you felt like crying during the past month?" Calibration of a separate IRT model for men and women shows that this item is easier for men than for women with comparable level of mental health (as assessed by the rest of the items).

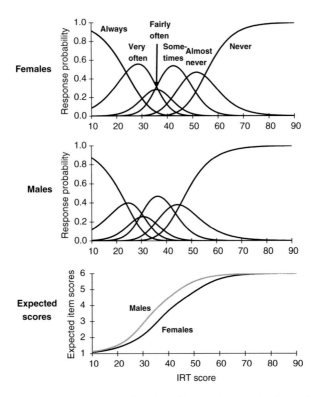

Fig. 8.7 Illustration of differential item function with regard to gender for an item on mental health: "How often have you felt like crying during the past month?"

Table 8.1 shows examples of different approaches to testing these four assumptions within each of the four modern psychometric approaches that we have discussed. While space does not permit a detailed discussion of these approaches, the table highlights that there are many different ways of accessing model fit. Fit tests often target particular types of misfit and are much less sensitive to other types of misfit. This is important since many studies often base claims of "good model fit" on tests that only cover a limited set of model assumptions. We would advise that a thorough model evaluation strategy should include tests of all the four types of model assumptions discussed above.

While most aspects of model fit can be evaluated within each of the four types of models, some fit test are more convenient or efficient than others. For example, categorical data factor analysis (listed under the normal-ogive models) offers powerful and flexible ways of assessing dimensionality and local independence. However, tests of whether the form of the implied option characteristic curves is a good fit to the data are very cumbersome, since they rely on evaluating all bivariate item frequency distributions. On the other hand, IRT models offer fit tests regarding the form of the option characteristic curve and tests for local independence. However, test of dimensionality through comparisons of uni- and multidimensional

Table 8.1 Examples of approaches to testing assumptions in modern psychometric models

	Nonparametric models	Normal-ogive models	General IRT models	Rasch models
Unidimensionality	Rosenbaum's test (Rosenbaum 1984) Poly-DIMTEST and DETECT index (Stout et al. 2001)	Eigen value analysis[a] CFA fit test (Hu and Bentler 1999) Bifactor models (Reise et al. 2007)	Multidimensional IRT (Muthén and Muthén 2014; Cai et al. 2011a)	Factor analysis of residuals Martin-Loef's test (Christensen et al. 2002)
Local independence		Residuals in CFA models Correlated error terms	Score test (Liu and Thissen 2014) Lagrange multiplier test (Glas 1999)	Generalized Tjur test (Kreiner and Christensen 2004)
Form of the option characteristic curve (item fit)	H coefficient (Mokken 1971) Kernel smoothing (Ramsay 1991)	Comparing expected and observed bivariate item distributions (Muthén and Muthén 2014)	S-X[b] (Orlando and Thissen 2003) Lagrange multiplier test (Glas 1999)	Conditional ML test (Andersen 1973) Infit and outfit statistics (Smith and Plackner 2008) R_{1c} test (Glas and Verhelst 1995)
Measurement invariance (lack of differential item function)	Logistic regression DIF test[b] (Zumbo 1999)	Multigroup CFA[a]	IRT-DIF tests[a]	Rasch-DIF test[a]

[a]Testing through general modeling approaches discussed by many authors

[b]Logistic regression DIF tests are listed under nonparametric models, since they use the sum of all items as control variable. However, the logistic regression in itself is a parametric technique and differs from the other tests mentioned under nonparametric models

models has so far been cumbersome, although better methods have become available in recent years (Muthén and Muthén 2014; Cai et al. 2011a). For these reasons, researchers often combine approaches from different types of models when evaluating a scale, e.g., evaluating dimensionality through categorical data factor analysis and then fitting and IRT models and testing item fit using the S-X^2 statistic (Bjorner et al. 2003). Published recommendations for comprehensive testing strategies (e.g., for IRT models (Reeve et al. 2007) and for Rasch models (Tennant and Conaghan 2007)) tend to cover the same aspects, although the specific tests may differ. Such comprehensive analyses can often lead to suggestions for scale revisions or shortenings (Khan et al. 2013; Reise et al. 2011a, b).

8.8   Advanced Models

While this review has focused on relatively standard application of modern psychometric models, the models can be expanded in many ways. We will briefly mention two types of advanced models that may be relevant for psychiatric research. In some situations – possibly our mental health example – an assumption of a unidimensional scale may be an unrealistic simplification. On the other hand, the subdimensions – anxiety, depression, and well-being in our example – may be so highly correlated that it is inappropriate to treat them as unrelated individual dimensions. Such situations may call for *multidimensional models* that could either be specified as a number of correlated dimensions or factors (e.g., Gardner et al. 2002; van den Berg et al. 2013) or as one global factor and a number of local factors (Cai et al. 2011b).

Rating scales are important tools in psychiatric research, and modern psychometric methods have made important contributions to the analyses of rating scales (e.g., Bech et al. 2014; Santor et al. 2007; Khan et al. 2013; van den Berg et al. 2013; Reise et al. 2011a, b; Østergaard et al. 2015). These analyses have usually used the ratings as individual items and analyzed them as described in this chapter. However, it is possible that different raters have slight differences in rating style making an item slightly harder if rated by rater A instead of rater B. Such rater effects can be built into the IRT model (Verhelst and Verstralen 2001), which may lead to a more efficient and realistic analysis (Stochl et al. 2015).

8.9   Conclusion

This review has only touched the surface of modern psychometric methods. We see a great potential for the application of these models in psychiatric research to evaluate and improve the validity of self-report and rating scales. The models can be used to evaluate and improve numerous aspects of measurement. There are many different ways of specifying the option characteristic curves leading to different types of psychometric models. However, the different approaches share a core set of assumptions: unidimensionality, local item independence, and measurement invariance. Consequently, it is important that these assumptions are carefully checked during the analysis.

References

Andersen EB. A goodness of fit test for the Rasch model. Psychometrika. 1973;38:123–40.
Andrich D. A rating formulation for ordered response categories. Psychometrika. 1978; 43:561–73.
Awad AG, Voruganti LN, Heslegrave RJ. A conceptual model of quality of life in schizophrenia: description and preliminary clinical validation. Qual Life Res. 1997;6:21–6.
Bech P. Clinical assessments of positive mental health. In: Jeste DV, Palmer BW, editors. Positive psychiatry: a clinician handbook. Washington DC: American Psychiatric Publishing; 2015. p. 127–43.
Bech P, Allerup P, Rosenberg R. The Marke-Nyman temperament scale. Evaluation of transferability using the Rasch item analysis. Acta Psychiatr Scand Suppl. 1978;57:49–58.
Bech P, Allerup P, Reisby N, Gram LF. Assessment of symptom change from improvement curves on the Hamilton depression scale in trials with antidepressants. Psychopharmacology (Berl). 1984;84:276–81.
Bech P, Allerup P, Larsen ER, Csillag C, Licht RW. The Hamilton Depression Scale (HAM-D) and the Montgomery-Asberg Depression Scale (MADRS). A psychometric re-analysis of the European genome-based therapeutic drugs for depression study using Rasch analysis. Psychiatry Res. 2014;217:226–32.
Bjorner JB, Kosinski M, Ware Jr JE. Calibration of an item pool for assessing the burden of headaches: an application of item response theory to the headache impact test (HIT). Qual Life Res. 2003;12:913–33.
Bjorner JB, Chang CH, Thissen D, Reeve BB. Developing tailored instruments: item banking and computerized adaptive assessment. Qual Life Res. 2007;16 Suppl 1:95–108.
Bock RD. The nominal categories model. In: van der Linden WJ, Hambleton RK, editors. Handbook of modern item response theory. Berlin: Springer; 1997. p. 3–50.
Bock RD, Mislevy RJ. Adaptive EAP estimation of ability in a microcomputer environment. Appl Psychol Meas. 1982;6:431–44.
Boyer L, Simeoni MC, Loundou A, D'Amato T, Reine G, Lancon C, et al. The development of the S-QoL 18: a shortened quality of life questionnaire for patients with schizophrenia. Schizophr Res. 2010;121:241–50.
Boyer L, Millier A, Perthame E, Aballea S, Auquier P, Toumi M. Quality of life is predictive of relapse in schizophrenia. BMC Psychiatry. 2013;13:15.
Cai L, Thissen D, du Troit SHC. IRTPRO for windows. [Computer software]. Lincolnwood: Scientific Software International; 2011a.
Cai L, Yang JS, Hansen M. Generalized full-information item bifactor analysis. Psychol Methods. 2011b;16:221–48.
Chen YL, Hsiung PC, Chung L, Chen SC, Pan AW. Psychometric properties of the mastery scale-Chinese version: applying classical test theory and Rasch analysis. Scand J Occup Ther. 2013;20:404–11.
Christensen KB, Bjorner JB, Kreiner S, Petersen JH. Tests for unidimensionality in polytomous Rasch models. Psychometrika. 2002;67:563–74.
Connell J, O'Cathain A, Brazier J. Measuring quality of life in mental health: are we asking the right questions? Soc Sci Med. 2014;120:12–20.
D'haenen H. Measurement of anhedonia. Eur Psychiat. 1996;11:335–43.

Drasgow F, Levine MV, Williams EA. Appropriateness measurement with polychotomous item response models and standardized indices. Br J Math Stat Psychol. 1985;38:67–86.

Ellervik C, Kvetny J, Bech P. The relationship between sleep length and restorative sleep in major depression. Results from the Danish General Suburban Population. Psychother Psychosom. 2016;85(1):45–6.

Embretson SE. Implications of a multidimensional latent trait model for measuring change. In: Collins LM, Horn J, editors. Best methods for the analysis of change. Washington DC: American Psychological Association; 1991. p. 184–203.

Fischer GH, Molenaar IW. Rasch models – foundations, recent developments, and applications. 1st ed. Berlin: Springer; 1995.

Galindo-Garre F, Hidalgo MD, Guilera G, Pino O, Rojo JE, Gomez-Benito J. Modeling the World Health Organization Disability Assessment Schedule II using non-parametric item response models. Int J Methods Psychiatr Res. 2015;24:1–10.

Gardner W, Kelleher KJ, Pajer KA. Multidimensional adaptive testing for mental health problems in primary care. Med Care. 2002;40:812–23.

Glas CAW. Modification indices for the 2-PL and the nominal response model. Psychometrika. 1999;64:273–94.

Glas CAW, Verhelst ND. Tests of fit for polytomous Rasch models. In: Fischer GH, Molenaar IW, editors. Rasch models – foundations, recent developments, and applications. Berlin: Springer; 1995. p. 325–52.

Haley SM, McHorney CA, Ware Jr JE. Evaluation of the MOS SF-36 physical functioning scale (PF-10): I. Unidimensionality and reproducibility of the Rasch item scale. J Clin Epidemiol. 1994;47:671–84.

Hu LT, Bentler PM. Cutoff criteria for fit indices in covariance structure analysis: conventional criteria versus new alternatives. Struct Eq Model. 1999;6:1–55.

Khan A, Lindenmayer JP, Opler M, Yavorsky C, Rothman B, Lucic L. A new Integrated Negative Symptom structure of the Positive and Negative Syndrome Scale (PANSS) in schizophrenia using item response analysis. Schizophr Res. 2013;150:185–96.

Kreiner S, Christensen KB. Analysis of local dependence and multidimensionality in graphical loglinear Rasch models. Commu Stat Theory Methods. 2004;33:1239–76.

Laurens KR, Hobbs MJ, Sunderland M, Green MJ, Mould GL. Psychotic-like experiences in a community sample of 8000 children aged 9 to 11 years: an item response theory analysis. Psychol Med. 2012;42:1495–506.

Liu Y, Thissen D. Comparing score tests and other local dependence diagnostics for the graded response model. Br J Math Stat Psychol. 2014;67:496–513.

Masters GN, Wright BD. The partial credit model. In: van der Linden WJ, Hambleton RK, editors. Handbook of modern item response theory. Berlin: Springer; 1997. p. 101–22.

Michel P, Baumstarck K, Auquier P, Amador X, Dumas R, Fernandez J, et al. Psychometric properties of the abbreviated version of the scale to assess unawareness in mental disorder in schizophrenia. BMC Psychiatry. 2013;13:1–10.

Michel P, Auquier P, Baumstarck K, Loundou A, Ghattas B, Lancon C, et al. How to interpret multidimensional quality of life questionnaires for patients with schizophrenia? Qual Life Res. 2015;24:2483–92.

Mojtabai R, Corey-Lisle PK, Ip EH, Kopeykina I, Haeri S, Cohen LJ, et al. The patient assessment questionnaire: initial validation of a measure of treatment effectiveness for patients with schizophrenia and schizoaffective disorder. Psychiatry Res. 2012;200:857–66.

Mokken RJ. A theory and procedure of scale analysis. Berlin: Mouton; 1971.

Muraki E. A generalized partial credit model. In: van der Linden WJ, Hambleton RK, editors. Handbook of modern item response theory. Berlin: Springer; 1997. p. 153–64.

Muthén BO. A general structural equation model with dichotomous, ordered categorical, and continuous latent variable indicators. Psychometrika. 1984;29:177–85.

Muthén BO, Muthén L. Mplus User's guide (version 7) [Computer software]. Los Angeles: Muthén & Muthén; 2014.

Norholm V, Bech P. Quality of life in schizophrenic patients: association with depressive symptoms. Nord J Psychiatry. 2006;60:32–7.

Orlando M, Thissen D. Further investigation of the performance of S – X2: an item fit index for use with dichotomous item response theory models. Appl Psychol Meas. 2003;27:289–98.

Orlando M, Sherbourne CD, Thissen D. Summed-score linking using item response theory: application to depression measurement. Psychol Assess. 2000;12:354–9.

Østergaard SD, Lemming OM, Mors O, Correll CU, Bech P. PANSS-6: a valid, brief rating scale for the measurement of symptom severity and cross-sectional remission in schizophrenia. Acta Psychiatrica Scandinavica. 2015. doi:10.1111/acps.12526.

Pan AW, Chung L, Fife BL, Hsiung PC. Evaluation of the psychometrics of the social impact scale: a measure of stigmatization. Int J Rehabil Res. 2007;30:235–8.

Park IJ, Jung DC, Hwang SS, Jung HY, Yoon JS, Kim CE, et al. Refinement of the SWN-20 based on the Rasch rating model. Compr Psychiatry. 2015;60:134–41.

Ramsay JO. Kernel smoothing approaches to nonparametric item characteristic curve estimation. Psychometrika. 1991;56:611–30.

Rasch G. Probabilistic models for some intelligence and attainment tests. 2nd ed. Chicago: University of Chicago Press; 1980.

Reeve BB, Hays RD, Bjorner JB, Cook KF, Crane PK, Teresi JA, et al. Psychometric evaluation and calibration of health-related quality of life item banks: plans for the Patient-Reported Outcomes Measurement Information System (PROMIS). Med Care. 2007;45:S22–31.

Reise SP, Morizot J, Hays RD. The role of the bifactor model in resolving dimensionality issues in health outcomes measures. Qual Life Res. 2007;16 Suppl 1:19–31.

Reise SP, Horan WP, Blanchard JJ. The challenges of fitting an item response theory model to the social anhedonia scale. J Pers Assess. 2011a;93:213–24.

Reise SP, Ventura J, Keefe RS, Baade LE, Gold JM, Green MF, et al. Bifactor and item response theory analyses of interviewer report scales of cognitive impairment in schizophrenia. Psychol Assess. 2011b;23:245–61.

Rosenbaum PR. Testing the conditional independence and monotonicity assumptions of item response theory. Psychometrika. 1984;49:425–35.

Samejima F. Estimation of latent ability using a response pattern of graded scores. Psy Mono Suppl. 1969;17:1–97.

Samejima F. Graded response model. In: van der Linden WJ, Hambleton RK, editors. Handbook of modern item response theory. Berlin: Springer; 1997. p. 85–100.

Santor DA, Ascher-Svanum H, Lindenmayer JP, Obenchain RL. Item response analysis of the positive and negative syndrome scale. BMC Psychiatry. 2007;7:66.

Sijtsma K, Hemker BT. Nonparametric polytomous IRT models for invariant item ordering, with results for parametric models. Psychometrika. 1998;63:183–200.

Smith RM, Plackner C. The family approach to assessing fit in Rasch measurement. J Appl Meas. 2008;10:424–37.

Stochl J, Jones, PB, Perez J, Khandaker GM, Böhnke JR, Croudace TJ. (2015). Effects of ignoring clustered data structure in confirmatory factor analysis of ordered polytomous items: a simulation study based on PANSS. Int J Methods Psychiatr Res.

Stout W, Habing B, Douglas J, Kim RH, Roussos L, Zhang J. Conditional covariance-based nonparametric multidimensionality assessment. Psychol Meas. 2001;20:331–54.

Tennant A, Conaghan PG. The Rasch measurement model in rheumatology: what is it and why use it? When should it be applied, and what should one look for in a Rasch paper? Arthritis Rheum. 2007;57:1358–62.

Teresi JA, Cross PS, Golden RR. Some applications of latent trait analysis to the measurement of ADL. J Gerontol. 1989;44:S196–204.

van den Berg SM, Paap MC, Derks EM. Using multidimensional modeling to combine self-report symptoms with clinical judgment of schizotypy. Psychiatry Res. 2013;206:75–80.

van der Linden WJ, Hambleton RK. Handbook of modern item response theory. Berlin: Springer; 1997.

Veit CL, Ware Jr JE. The structure of psychological distress and well-being in general populations. J Consult Clin Psychol. 1983;51:730–42.

Verhelst ND, Verstralen HHFM. An IRT model for multiple raters. In: Boomsma A, van Duijn M, Snijders T, editors. Essays on item response theory. New York: Springer; 2001. p. 89–108.

Ware Jr JE, Kosinski M, Bjorner JB, Turner-Bowker DM, Maruish M. SF-36 health survey. Manual and interpretation guide. 2nd ed. Lincoln: QualityMetric Incorporated; 2007.

Warm TA. Weighted likelihood estimation of ability in item response theory. Psychometrika. 1989;54:427–50.

Zumbo BD. A handbook on the theory and methods of Differential Item Functioning (DIF): logistic regression modeling as a unitary framework for binary and likert-type (ordinal) item scores. Ottawa: Directorate of Human Resources Research and Evaluation, Department of National Defense; 1999.

Part III
Beyond Assessment of Quality of Life in Schizophrenia

Chapter 9
Quality of Life as an Outcome and a Mediator of Other Outcomes in Patients with Schizophrenia

Anne Karow, Monika Bullinger, and Martin Lambert

9.1 Introduction

During the past decades subjective quality of life (hereafter QOL) has been proven to be a valid and useful outcome criterion in patients with schizophrenia besides the assessment of clinical parameters such as symptoms or daily functioning. Important predictors for a favorable outcome in patients with schizophrenia are a shorter duration of untreated psychosis, better premorbid functioning, an early treatment response, a lower level of psychopathology or illness severity, and better daily and social functioning at beginning of treatment (Lambert et al. 2010a). Clinical outcome is further compromised by a high risk of medication nonadherence and service disengagement (Velligan et al. 2009) and of comorbid disorders, especially substance use (Fleischhacker et al. 2008). All these factors directly or indirectly mediate QOL in patients with schizophrenia.

For a long time clinical outcome in patients with schizophrenia, especially the core symptoms of psychosis (positive, negative, and cognitive symptoms), has been seen as largely independent from subjective QOL (Schroeder et al. 2012). Meanwhile numerous studies, including meta-analyses, found higher levels of symptoms of psychosis being associated with less favorable QOL, while most sociodemographic factors show weaker associations with QOL, except that better QOL was consistently reported by females compared with males in patients with schizophrenia (Carpiniello et al. 2012; Eack and Newhill 2007; Vatne and Bjorkly 2008;

A. Karow, MD (✉) • M. Lambert, MD
Department of Psychiatry and Psychotherapy & Department of Child
and Adolescent Psychiatry, Centre for Psychosocial Medicine, University Medical
Centre Hamburg-Eppendorf, Martinistr. 52, Hamburg 20246, Germany
e-mail: karow@uke.de

M. Bullinger, PhD
Institute for Medical Psychology, Centre for Psychosocial Medicine,
University Medical Centre Hamburg-Eppendorf, Hamburg, Germany

© Springer International Publishing Switzerland 2016
A.G. Awad, L.N.P. Voruganti (eds.), *Beyond Assessment of Quality of Life in Schizophrenia*, DOI 10.1007/978-3-319-30061-0_9

Priebe et al. 2011; Galuppi et al. 2010). For example, in patients with chronic schizophrenia of the total variance in QOL, clinical symptoms explained around 50 % and social variables explained 16 % (Meesters et al. 2011).

Studies confirmed an important interrelation between changes in clinical outcome and QOL in patients with schizophrenia. Early QOL improvement predicted a better long-term symptomatic and functional outcome as well as early symptomatic response predicted better long-term QOL (Lambert et al. 2009; Boden et al. 2009). Pooled data of patients with schizophrenia showed that changes in all symptom areas were associated with changes in QOL. Especially symptoms of depression and social anxiety, self-stigma, and social cognition were major obstacles for QOL during long-term treatment. Multivariate analyses confirmed that a combination out of less depressive symptoms and a higher level of social functioning significantly predict better QOL, and explaining 53 % of the total variance (Meesters et al. 2011).

These and other findings have than led to suggestions that QOL scales in patients with schizophrenia might share too much variance with symptoms and therefore QOL might be not valid as an independent outcome criterion (Priebe et al. 2011). However, multivariate analyses demonstrated that QOL changes are influenced by symptom changes and vice versa, in particular by symptoms of depression and anxiety, but that the level of interrelation is not strong enough to compromise QOL as an independent outcome measure (Priebe et al. 2011).

Though QOL assessment visibly gained in importance since the introduction of the QOL concept in mental health research (WHO 1998), still few studies investigated how results of QOL research should best be turned into daily clinical practice to improve treatment and outcome of patients with schizophrenia (Awad and Voruganti 2012). A comprehensive understanding of the relationship between different domains of clinical outcome with QOL is needed because interventions that focus on psychotic symptoms or functioning alone may fail to improve subjective QOL at the same level. Or in other words, interventions, which focus on expert-rated parameters alone, may fail to address the patients' needs and perspective. Studies indicate that an adequate adaption of health-care structures to unmet needs of patients with schizophrenia has an important impact on clinical outcomes as well as on subjective QOL (Landolt et al. 2012a, b). The following passages may give an overview about QOL as an outcome and a mediator of clinical outcomes in patients with schizophrenia.

9.2   Clinical Outcome in Schizophrenia

Patients with schizophrenia have a high risk to develop a severe mental illness (hereafter SMI). SMI is defined by a considerable and persistent impaired functioning level (Delespaul 2013). Sixty percent of persons with SMI suffer from psychotic disorders. Ninety percent of patients with schizophrenia develop SMI, followed by psychosis spectrum disorders (60 %) and bipolar disorder/major depression with psychotic symptoms (40 %) (Ruggeri et al. 2000). Schizophrenia is diagnosed at initial contact in approximately 70 % of first-episode patients, and often already patients within the early stage of psychosis fulfill SMI criteria or display a high risk to develop them (Ruggeri et al. 2000). Several factors increase the SMI risk and consequently the risk for a poor response, non-remission, and non-recovery (e.g., a positive family history for psychosis, pregnancy or birth complications, early developmental disorders, childhood adversities, early and intensive cannabis use or use multiple drugs, mental disorders prior to the onset of the psychosis or psychosis onset in childhood or adolescence, poor premorbid functioning, early service disengagement, and medication nonadherence (Jaaskelainen et al. 2015)).

The symptomatic remission criterion for patients with schizophrenia is already well established, can be applied by clinicians at all stages of the disease, and facilitates cross-trial comparisons of therapeutic interventions (Lambert et al. 2010a; Andreasen et al. 2005). Symptomatic remission consists of two elements: a symptom-based criterion, which includes diagnostically relevant symptoms in the Positive and Negative Syndrome Scale (PANSS), the Brief Psychiatric Rating Scale (BPRS), or the Scales for Negative Symptoms/Scale for Positive Symptoms (SANS/SAPS), and a time criterion, which requires that an individual achieves the symptom-based criteria for a minimum of 6 months. Rates for a symptomatic remission in patients with schizophrenia depend highly on the sample selection and vary between 16–17 and 62–78 % (AlAqeel and Margolese 2012). Multiple-episode patients show lower remission rates compared with first-episode patients. Other variables being associated with higher rates of symptomatic remission were better premorbid functioning, lower symptoms at baseline (especially less negative symptoms), early treatment response, shorter duration of untreated psychosis, and treatment with long-acting and/or atypical antipsychotics (AlAqeel and Margolese 2012).

According to several authors, the concept of recovery in patients with schizophrenia still is poorly understood and further research is needed. Consumer-based groups often conceptualize recovery as a subjectively evaluated process of integration of illness into an individual's life (Harvey and Bellack 2009). Clinicians and researchers agree that ongoing clinical symptom remission is an important component of recovery in schizophrenia but that multidimensional measures should be combined in studies investigating recovery in schizophrenia. At least the combination of two domains, one related to clinical remission and another related to a broader outcome, e.g., social functioning or QOL, and the persistence of recovery for a minimum of 2 years have been recommended (Jaaskelainen et al. 2013; Faerden et al. 2008). Generic QOL scales often used in studies investigating patients with schizophrenia were (1) the WHO Quality of Life Interview (WHOQOL-Bref (WHO 1998)), (2) the Short Form 36 or Short Form 12 (SF-36/SF-12 (Ware 1993)), and the EuroQOL (EQ-5D (Brooks 1996); Table 9.1, Fig. 9.1). The most widely used schizophrenia-specific QOL scales were (1) the Heinrich-Carpenter Quality of Life Scale (QLS (Heinrichs et al. 1984)), (2) the Quality-of-Life Enjoyment and Satisfaction Questionnaire-18 (Q-LES-Q-18

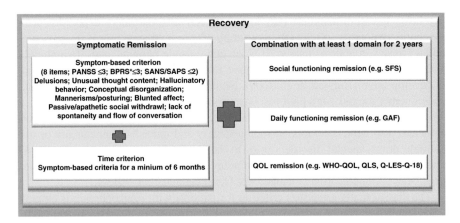

Fig. 9.1 Remission criteria as defined by Andreasen et al. (2005) and suggestions for recovery criteria (Jaaskelainen et al. 2013; Faerden et al. 2008) in patients with schizophrenia. (1) Scales: *PANSS* Positive and Negative Syndrome Scale, *BPRS* Brief Psychiatric Rating Scale, *SANS/SPAS* Scale for the Assessment of Negative/Positive Symptoms, *SFS* Social Functioning Scale, *GAF* Global Assessment of Functioning Scale, *QLS* Quality of Life Scale, *Q-LES-Q-18* Quality -of-Life Enjoyment and Satisfaction Questionnaire-18. (2) The two negative symptoms not included in the BPRS (i.e., "social withdrawal" and "lack of spontaneity") need to be additionally assessed with PANSS or SANS when BPRS is used

(Ritsner et al. 2005)), and (3) the Subjective Well-Being Under Neuroleptics (SWN (Naber 1995)) (Karow et al. 2015). A recent systematic review on 50 studies found that the median proportion of individuals with schizophrenia who met recovery in at least two outcome domains was 13.5 % (Jaaskelainen et al. 2013).

9.3   Symptomatic Remission and QOL

Different cross-sectional and longitudinal studies found significant associations between symptomatic remission and QOL. Patients with schizophrenia who ful-filled the criteria for symptomatic remission showed significant better QOL compared patients in non-remission (Brissos et al. 2011). Especially longitudinal studies found a significant association between QOL and symptomatic remission (Boden et al. 2009; Haynes et al. 2012). For example, Docherty and coworker found after 1 year of antipsychotic treatment a higher improvement in QOL and a better attitude toward treatment in patients who attained symptomatic remission compared with non-remitted patients (Docherty et al. 2007), and Haynes and coworker reported in a prospective observational study that the failure to achieve symptomatic remission after start of treatment was associated with impaired QOL and functional outcomes after 3 years and higher subsequent health-care costs (Haynes et al. 2012).

Baseline and early changes in QOL showed a high predictive validity for later symptomatic remission as well (Boden et al. 2009; Lambert et al. 2007). Boden and

Table 9.1 Relation of symptomatic remission according to Andreasen et al. (Lambert et al. 2010a) with QOL in patients with schizophrenia

Study	N	Assessment time points (baseline assessment [BA] and/or follow-up [in months])	Remission criteria assessed (SC = only severity criteria; STC = severity and time criteria)	Remitted vs. non-remitted patients[a,b] (NA = not assessed; NS = not specified; mc = mean change; ns = not significantly different)			
				Symptomatic or clinical remission	Functioning	Quality of life	Other outcome dimensions[c]
Studies comparing remitters with non-remitters							
Ciudad et al. (Landolt et al. 2012b)	1010	BA	SC	NS	SCOS: 8 vs. 11	MCS-12: 37 vs. 44	BSC[c]
Dunayevich et al. (Eack and Newhill 2007)	2771	6	SC	PANSS mc: −22 vs. −11	NA	QLS mc: +15 vs. +4	
Emsley et al. (Ruggeri et al. 2000)	462	12	STC	PANSS mc: −41 vs. −23	NA	WQLS mc: 0.7 vs. 0.3	NBC, LR[c]
Kelly et al. (Jaaskelainen et al. 2015)	43	12	STC	BPRS: 28 vs. 34	NA	QLS: 57 vs. 53 (ns)	
Wunderink et al. (Faerden et al. 2008)	125	24	STC	PANSS: 44 vs. 52	GSDS: 5 vs. 7	WHOQOL: 98 vs. 97 (ns)	
Addington and Addington (Brooks 1996) (LOCF)	240	36	STC	PANSS pos & neg: 19 vs. 35	NA	QLS: 85 vs. 57	
Haro et al. (2014)	6516	36	STC	CGI-SCH 38 % vs. 52 %	Sociodemographics	EQ5D-VAS: 77.3 vs. 61.4	
Lambert et al. (2010b)	529	18	STC	PANSS: 33 %	GAF	SF-36: 71.6 %	

(continued)

Table 9.1 (continued)

Study	N	Assessment time points (baseline assessment [BA] and/or follow-up [in months])	Remission criteria assessed (SC=only severity criteria; STC=severity and time criteria)	Remitted vs. non-remitted patients[a,b] (NA=not assessed; NS=not specified; mc=mean change; ns=not significantly different)			
				Symptomatic or clinical remission	Functioning	Quality of life	Other outcome dimensions[c]

Studies assessing the percentage of patients in symptomatic remission fulfilling QOL outcome criteria

Study	N	Assessment time points	Assessed criteria	Patients with adequate functioning in %	Functioning	Patients with adequate quality of life in %	Other outcome dimensions[c]
Lambert et al. (Docherty et al. 2007)	2960	36	STC	38		67	

[a]Data are only reported when already remitted patients were compared with non-remitters at baseline; data of baseline differences of patients who achieved remission or not at follow-up are not reported.

[b]Scales: PANSS Positive and Negative Syndrome Scale, BPRS Brief Psychiatric Rating Scale, CGI-I Clinical Global Impression-Improvement Scale, SCOS Strauss-Carpenter Outcomes Scale, GAF Global Assessment of Functioning Scale, GSDS Groningen Social Disability Schedule, QLS Quality of Life Scale, WQLS Wisconsin Quality of Life Scale, MCS-12 Mental Component Score of the Medical Outcomes Study 12-Item Short-Form Health Survey

[c]Other outcome dimensions: LCHC less consumption of health care, LR less relapse, BC better cognition, NBC no better cognition, BDA better drug attitude, LUN less unmet needs, BSC better social cognition

coworker found an early improvement of subjective well-being in schizophrenia significantly associated with enduring symptomatic remission (de Haan et al. 2008). This was confirmed by a study with severely ill patients with schizophrenia. Though rate and time to response differed markedly between expert- and self-rated measures, the combined symptomatic, functional, and subjective outcome was best predicted by an early response in QOL (Lambert et al. 2009).

However, though interventional studies confirmed that symptomatic remission could be reached at average by 40–60 % of patients with schizophrenia, remission frequencies differ markedly between different patient populations (e.g., acute versus stabilized patients or first versus multiple episodes of psychosis) (Lambert et al. 2006, 2008, 2010a, b; Bobes et al. 2009; Helldin et al. 2007; Cohen et al. 2009; Schennach-Wolff et al. 2009). Moreover, studies have shown that symptomatic remission is not necessarily associated with QOL improvement (Carpiniello et al. 2012; Karow et al. 2012a). The remission criteria explicitly focus the core symptoms of schizophrenia. Other symptom clusters such as affective symptoms of depression or anxiety, which exert a significant negative impact on all subjective outcomes across various studies and compromise QOL as reported previously, are not considered (Karow et al. 2005; Huppert et al. 2001; Hofer et al. 2004, 2006). Persisting symptoms of depression have been found in remitted patients with schizophrenia at almost the same level compared to non-remitted patients, which have ongoing negative effects on QOL as well (Carpiniello et al. 2012; Karow et al. 2012a). For example, in a prospectively investigated sample of never-treated patients with schizophrenia, 60 % of the patients were in symptomatic remission after 3 years, but only 28 % showed remission of both symptoms and QOL (Lambert et al. 2008). Studies assessing the frequency of remitted patients being in adequate QOL have found that only 60–70 % patients display a satisfying QOL. Moreover, self- and expert-rated outcomes differed markedly in an observational study, which compared symptomatic remission assessed by patients, family members, and psychiatrists, with a preference on the patients' side for subjective outcomes and on the psychiatrists' side for the expert-rated outcomes (Karow et al. 2012b).

9.4 Affective Symptoms and QOL

Various cross-sectional and longitudinal studies confirmed a close association between depressive symptoms with impaired QOL in patients with schizophrenia (Maurino et al. 2011). The higher the level of depression, the stronger is their negative impact on patients' QOL (Dan et al. 2011). A strong impact of depression on QOL was also found in the early course of illness or even prior to the first manifestation of a psychotic illness in high-risk populations (Rocca et al. 2009; Bechdolf et al. 2005). Beyond depression, symptoms of anxiety, especially social anxiety, and anhedonia were significantly associated with QOL (Ritsner and Grinshpoon 2013). For example, a prospective observational study found an increase in social anxiety over 5 years significantly associated with a decrease in QOL in remitted patients with schizophrenia after discharge through a deinstitutionalization project (Kumazaki et al. 2012).

Affective symptoms clearly outweigh positive psychotic symptoms as robust predictor of QOL in patients with schizophrenia (Renwick et al. 2012). In a long-term study over 10 years, improvement in QOL was best predicted by a reduction in self-reported symptoms of depression, sensitivity, or anxiety along with an increase in self-efficacy, social support, and emotion-oriented coping scores (Ritsner et al. 2014). In an 18-month trial, QOL was best predicted by anxiety, depression, and self-esteem and to a lesser extent by global functioning and social integration at both time intervals (Meijer et al. 2009). These findings are of major clinical relevance, as affective symptoms are amenable for specific therapeutic interventions, which need to be considered and included in integrative treatment approaches for patients with schizophrenia. With regard to clinical practice, future studies may focus the effectiveness of interventions addressing affective symptoms in patients with schizophrenia.

9.5   Negative Symptoms and QOL

The severity of negative symptoms is an important predictor of poor patient functioning. Negative symptoms (i.e., blunted affect, emotional and social withdrawal, poor rapport, lack of spontaneity and flow of conversation) affect the patient's ability to perform activities of daily living, to be socially active and maintain personal relationships, to live independently, and to work and study (Alonso et al. 2009; Harvey et al. 2012; Rabinowitz et al. 2012, 2013). Rabinowitz and coworker found in 1447 outpatients with schizophrenia that the coexistence of prominent negative symptoms was independently associated with a significant decline in functional mental health, health utility, and expert-rated QOL. The work status alone was of some, but minor, importance for QOL, whereas subjectively satisfying and valuable activities in daily life were consistently associated with QOL domains (Eklund 2009).

This is in line with previous studies, which reported significant associations between negative symptoms with functional impairment and expert-rated QOL, e.g., measured with the Heinrich-Carpenter Quality of Life Scale (QLS (Heinrichs et al. 1984)), and no significant associations with subjective (self-rated) QOL (Fujimaki et al. 2012a; Ojeda et al. 2012; Karadayi et al. 2012). There is a continuing debate whether QOL in patients with schizophrenia should best be assessed by self- or expert-rated scales or by a combination of both. The lack of association between negative and cognitive symptoms with their important negative impact on daily functioning with subjective QOL demonstrates the need for a combination of expert-rated with self-rated outcome measures in patients with schizophrenia. Most researchers consequently vote for a combination of self-rated QOL with expert-rated daily functioning for a comprehensive consideration of the different perspectives on clinical outcome (Karow et al. 2012b).

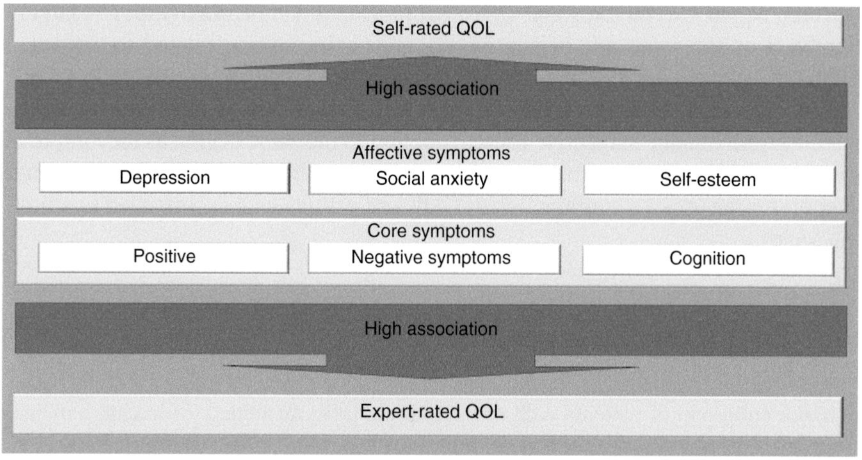

Fig. 9.2 Overview of the association between clinical outcomes and self- and expert-rated QOL in schizophrenia

9.6   Cognitive Dysfunction and QOL

Cognitive deficits are accepted as a core feature in schizophrenia spectrum disorders. Early and persistent cognitive dysfunctions are among the most critical determinants of daily functioning and are associated with higher levels of disability and worse occupational outcome (Nuechterlein et al. 2011; Reichenberg et al. 2010; Green et al. 2006). Studies on the relationship between cognitive function and QOL have shown contradictory results. Kurtz and Tolman (Kurtz and Tolman 2010) found QOL inversely related to crystallized verbal ability, attention, working memory, and problem-solving, while Boyer and coworker (Boyer et al. 2012) found no significant correlation between QOL and neuropsychological measures of attention, memory, or executive functioning in patients with schizophrenia. They proposed that functional outcomes might be mediated through metacognitive capacities, particularly theory of mind (TOM) abilities. One study found in patients with schizophrenia a significant relationship between decreased QOL and higher TOM skills, probably mediated by higher clinical symptom scores (Maat et al. 2012). However, a recent study could not replicate these findings (Urbach et al. 2013). The authors discussed an unreliable insight about cognitive capacities as possible reason and concluded that it is important to develop validated tools to improve social cognition and to provide rationales for therapies targeting cognitive skills in patients with schizophrenia. The importance of social cognition in patients with schizophrenia is further supported by results of studies, which found better insight into illness as well as higher self-stigma and anticipated discrimination associated with poor quality of life (Switaj et al. 2009; Ucok et al. 2013; Tang and Wu 2012; van Baars et al. 2013; Karow et al. 2008).

Results of a recent meta-analysis confirmed a positive link between neurocognition and expert-rated QOL (i.e., daily functioning) as found for the association between negative symptoms and QOL, but indicated that neurocognition is largely unrelated or for some neurocognitive domains even inverse related to self-rated QOL (i.e., worse cognition may sometimes be related with better subjective QOL). It was concluded that interventions targeting cognition need to ensure that they attend to individuals' subjective life satisfaction to the same degree as they improve expert-rated functioning (Tolman and Kurtz 2012). These findings provide further support for the use of a combination of QOL self-ratings with expert-rated functioning scales.

9.7   Insight into Illness and QOL

A major subgroup of patients with schizophrenia lacks awareness of having a mental disorder or symptoms of a mental disorder (Amador et al. 1993, 1994; McEvoy et al. 1989). Different studies found poor insight into illness related with clinical outcomes (Schwartz 1998; Sanz et al. 1998; Drake and Lewis 2003; Liraud et al. 2004; Whitty et al. 2004; Smith et al. 2004). Decreased insight was associated with higher positive symptom scores, especially persecutory delusions, more cognitive deficits, and comorbid substance abuse (Goldberg et al. 2001). On the other hand, an improvement of insight was related with lower self-esteem and an increase in depression, an enhanced risk to develop a postpsychotic depression, and suicide ideation (Hasson-Ohayon et al. 2006; Schwartz and Smith 2004; Drake et al. 2004; Mintz et al. 2004; Carroll et al. 1999; Iqbal et al. 2000; Kim et al. 2003). Moreover, higher insight was significantly related with better expert-rated social functioning and QOL (Schwartz 1998; Dickerson et al. 1997), but inversely related with subjective QOL (Karow et al. 2008; Hasson-Ohayon et al. 2006; Ritsner 2003; Sim et al. 2004). Especially in first-episode schizophrenia, patients' insight into illness, social consequences, and treatment efficacy was associated with lower subjective QOL, reduced emotional well-being, and higher levels of emotional distress (Hasson-Ohayon et al. 2006; Sim et al. 2004).

Improvement of insight requires social competence and the ability to evaluate the self from the perspective of others. An association of insight with theory of mind and social cognition has been expected (Bora et al. 2007). The increase of depression and suicidal ideation and the decrease in subjective QOL in patients with better insight underline the importance of insight for the clinical course in schizophrenia. Patients with good insight realize negative consequences caused by their illness, which has important implications for treatment adherence, service engagement, and satisfaction with treatment (Goldberg et al. 2001; Drake et al. 2004; Mintz et al. 2004; Koren et al. 2004; Subotnik et al. 2005; Gilleen and David 2005; Pedrelli et al. 2004). Obviously the stigmata of being mentally ill and being hospitalized are serious psychological strains. In addition delusions might serve as a defense strategy against low self-esteem and create alternative meanings of life (Moritz et al. 2006). Consequently the improvement of insight into illness without a deterioration of mood and QOL is an important therapeutic outcome in patients with schizophrenia (Cooke et al. 2005).

9.8   Antipsychotic Treatment and QOL

It is emphasized that outcome of antipsychotic treatment in patients with schizophrenia warrants a broader perspective than the reduction of core symptoms of psychosis alone. The measurement of QOL has been approved by the Food and Drug Administration as outcome parameter for the assessment of novel antipsychotic treatment (Andreasen et al. 2005; Lambert et al. 2006; (FDA) USFaDA 2006; Hofer et al. 2007). Various studies reported a significant QOL improvement under antipsychotic treatment, which is significantly associated with early treatment response, improvement in symptoms, subjective effectiveness, medication compliance, a low level of neuroleptic-induced dysphoria, and lower rates of antipsychotic side effects such as sedation, obesity, and sexual side effects (Lambert et al. 2007; Schimmelmann et al. 2005; Putzhammer et al. 2005; DeHaan et al. 2002; Karow et al. 2007; Sugawara et al. 2013). Patients with a first episode of psychosis reported lower levels of QOL at start of antipsychotic treatment and better QOL improvement during treatment compared with patients with multiple episodes (Yeh et al. 2013).

After the introduction of second-generation antipsychotics (SGAs), early comparison studies found better QOL improvement under treatment with SGAs compared with first-generation antipsychotics (FGAs). These results have been explained by differences in the side effect profiles, especially by a lower incidence of extrapyramidal side effects as neuroleptic-induced dysphoria under treatment with SGAs. Lately it has been discussed whether high dosages of FGAs, especially of haloperidol, in early studies may partly account for the QOL differences (Lewis et al. 2006; Fujimaki et al. 2012b). The latter is supported by the fact that comparison studies with different SGAs or studies comparing SGAs with low dosages of FGAs failed to reveal significant QOL differences (Hayhurst et al. 2013). Barnes and coworker, for example, showed a comparable improvement in self- and expert-rated QOL (daily functioning) under treatment with both FGAs and SGAs, especially if patients were switched from one oral antipsychotic to another oral antipsychotic at start of the study (Barnes et al. 2013). In addition, studies reported several side effects of SGAs during long-term treatment (e.g., weight gain, sedation, and sexual side effects (Rojo et al. 2015)) that may outweigh some of their positive effects on QOL. However, it should be noted that most comparison studies investigating antipsychotics in patients with schizophrenia used and still use the Heinrich Quality of Life Scale (QLS; (Heinrichs et al. 1984)), a scale originally designed to assess the negative syndrome and patients' functioning rather than QOL from the patients' perspective as defined by the WHO (WHO 1998; Harvey et al. 2009; Awad and Voruganti 2013).

In summary there is still no clear and enduring empirical evidence for the advantage of one antipsychotic beyond another antipsychotic in terms of QOL improvement, and studies investigating QOL under antipsychotic treatment should be interpreted carefully due to multiple factors affecting subjective QOL of each patient. However, from the patients' and the clinicians' perspective, effects and tolerability of the individual chosen antipsychotic drug could make a big difference in terms of subjective QOL improvement in daily clinical practice, which need to be considered.

9.9 Different Treatment Approaches and QOL

Two core prognostic interventions have proven to be effective in patients with schizophrenia: (1) improvement of early detection to shorten the duration of untreated psychosis (DUP) and (2) improvement of quality of care to improve outcome: (1) Previous studies showed that a sustained reduction of DUP can only be reached by multidimensional and long-term interventions including population-based improvement of mental health literacy, stigma reduction, and establishment of early detection services with assertive detection embedded in a catchment area detection network. (2) An increase of quality of care can be achieved by the implementation of service structures specifically created for patients with schizophrenia (Schöttle et al. 2013). They comprise on a structural-level team-based models of assertive outreach; early detection services; peer-to-peer counseling; support structures for school, education, work, finances, and living; and structures for the prevention and treatment of somatic illnesses. On the content level, such services should provide integrated care with individualized evidence-based diagnosis-specific psychological, social, and somatic interventions. Good evidence is available for the effectiveness of Assertive Community Treatment (ACT) (Schöttle et al. 2013) and it has been confirmed that ACT improves quality of care for patients with schizophrenia (Lambert et al. 2010c; Stein and Santos 2000; Marshall and Lockwood 2011). Key features mediating the effectiveness of ACT were the multidisciplinary team approach with a small client/staff ratio, home treatment, high-frequent treatment contacts, "no dropout policy," and the 24-h availability (Teague et al. 2012; Acta 2001). Compared to standard care, ACT was found to be superior in terms of QOL improvement, treatment retention, number of hospital admissions, accommodation status, employment, patient satisfaction, and cost-effectiveness by controlled trials (Lambert et al. 2010c; Karow et al. 2012c). The decrease of the number of hospitalizations and days spent in hospital may be critical, as it has been proven that (re-)hospitalizations especially in patients with a first episode of psychosis cause a decrease in QOL (Addington et al. 2012). The OPUS trial combined an intervention of early detection and integrated care for patients with schizophrenia. OPUS showed in comparison with standard care positive effects on psychotic symptoms, functioning, satisfaction with care, substance use, treatment adherence, family burden, costs, and quality of life (Nordentoft et al. 2010).

Various other therapeutic interventions (including cognitive behavioral psychotherapy, psychoeducation, physical activities (Chang et al. 2013; Penn et al. 2011; Pitkanen et al. 2012; Vancampfort et al. 2012a, b)) were investigated regarding their effects on QOL in patients with schizophrenia. In summary all studies on single therapeutic interventions found a QOL improvement in patients with schizophrenia undergoing their respective therapy. An example for a successful translation of QOL research into clinical practice may be a recent study of Boyer and coworker, who reported that QOL assessment in combination with a feedback for clinicians was able to improve QOL outcome in patients with schizophrenia (Boyer et al. 2013). However, only studies with complex and integrative interventions and high methodological standard were able to show robust long-term effects on QOL.

9.10   Cost Effectiveness of Different Treatment Approaches in Patients with Schizophrenia

Cost-effectiveness analyses are more and more used in the field of medicine, where it may not be appropriate to monetize health-care effects alone. The most commonly used outcome measure to compare the relative costs and outcomes of two or more therapeutic interventions in medical treatment is quality-adjusted life years (QALY) measured by standardized QOL scales (Kind 2003). "Cost-effective" treatments may save health-care costs, disability claims, and other societal costs. However, "cost-effective" is not similar with "cheap" but instead should describe treatments that are clinically and from the patients' perspective effective and their costs are considered as reasonable given the benefit they make. Different studies showed that integrative treatment concepts for patients with schizophrenia are able to lower medical costs, improve remission and recovery, and have positive effects on several other outcomes compared to similar patients not given comparable treatment options (Schöttle et al. 2013; Lambert et al. 2010c; Nordentoft et al. 2010). Moreover, cost-utility analyses confirmed that integrative treatment with ACT was comparably costly but more effective in terms of the gain of QALYs for patients with schizophrenia spectrum disorders (Karow et al. 2012c).

With respect to antipsychotic treatment, studies reported that SGAs (oral and long acting) were cost-effective compared with FGAs in patients with schizophrenia. Most studies found lower direct and indirect treatment costs under treatment with SGAs (oral or long acting) (O'Day et al. 2013; Citrome et al. 2014). Results of recent studies favored long-acting SGAs compared with oral SGAs (Einarson et al. 2014a, b; Rajagopalan et al. 2013). Different studies demonstrated that either risperidone, olanzapine, or paliperidone long-acting injection, relative to oral or other long-acting injectable drugs, was associated with cost savings and/or additional clinical benefits. Methodological aspects, e.g., that most studies included decision analytic models, average cost-effectiveness ratios, and the robustness of the results, have been discussed (Achilla and McCrone 2013).

However, due to health-care facts, patients with SMI often have limited access to appropriate multidimensional treatment approaches. Many patients, especially those who need extended and intensive psychiatric and psychotherapeutic treatment, are at risk of receiving substandard care with all negative consequences for remission, recovery, and QOL. Most studies investigating cost-effectiveness in patients with schizophrenia are still dominated by expert-rated outcomes (e.g., changes in clinical symptoms, relapse rates, hospitalizations). Only few cost-effectiveness studies (none of the studies investigating cost-effectiveness of antipsychotic treatment) included the patients' perspective (e.g., QALYs gained). Moreover, the variation of studies often restricts direct comparisons across populations. Consequently further studies investigating the cost-effectiveness of different treatment options are needed in order to regulate the health-care system in an appropriate way from the patients', payers', and a societal perspective.

9.11   Summary and Outlook

Important challenges for outcome improvement in patients with schizophrenia include the management of subobtimally controlled symptoms, enabling of better daily life functioning and better subjective QOL. Understanding the relationship between the different outcome domains with QOL is important because interventions that focus on psychotic symptoms or expert-rated functioning alone may fail to improve subjective QOL to the same level. Affective symptoms, namely, depression and social anxiety, self-stigma, and social cognition, are major obstacles for QOL improvement during long-term treatment in patients with schizophrenia. Though positive symptoms, negative symptoms, and cognitive functioning may be seen as largely independent from subjective QOL (Schroeder et al. 2012), long-term studies confirmed a critical impact of early QOL improvement on long-term symptomatic and functional remission and of early symptomatic response on long-term QOL (Lambert et al. 2009; Boden et al. 2009).

Approximately half of patients with schizophrenia in any kind of treatment achieve symptomatic remission, but only a minority reach recovery with a combination of QOL, functional, and symptomatic remission (Schennach-Wolff et al. 2009; Wunderink et al. 2007). Thus, achieving symptomatic remission should not mask the ongoing need for therapeutic efforts aimed at improving persisting negative, affective, and cognitive symptoms exerting a potential impact on functional status and long-term QOL. Moreover, patients and their relatives prefer a broader therapeutic view instead of a sole focus on symptomatic remission and antipsychotic treatment. Consequently, treatment outcome of patients with schizophrenia in clinical practice should be evaluated by a composite assessment of symptom severity, functioning, and QOL in order to guide early treatment decisions from a comprehensive and patient-orientated view (Lambert et al. 2010a; Ritsner and Grinshpoon 2013; Chen et al. 2011; Peuskens and Gorwood 2012; Naber et al. 2013). It has been demonstrated that coping strategies that deal with daily stressors and emotional upset also may be useful in diminishing the adverse impact of psychiatric symptoms on QOL. Thus, therapeutic approaches that have targeted the core symptoms of psychosis should be complemented by the strengthening of coping strategies that deal with general daily stressors. Moreover studies on empowerment in patients with schizophrenia showed mediating effects of symptoms on QOL and psychosocial interventions were able to increase the sense of empowerment and QOL (Chou et al. 2012; Marchinko and Clarke 2011). From a research perspective, longitudinal studies are needed to assess the long-term impact of different coping and empowerment strategies on outcome in patients with schizophrenia and to determine the relative merits of each strategy as well as their effectiveness compared with symptom-specific approaches (Cohen et al. 2011).

Different studies showed that early changes in QOL, as well as the clinical and functional status at entry to treatment programs, have an important impact on long-term QOL and clinical outcome in patients with schizophrenia (Lambert et al. 2010a). Not the reduction of symptoms alone but also treatment-related factors as the therapeutic alliance and the integration of care in multidimensional treatment approaches improve QOL continuously in patients with schizophrenia (Karow et al. 2012a; Schöttle et al. 2013). Promising approaches are diagnosis-specific team-based models of integrated care with a combination of early detection and assertive community treatment. Moreover, illness recovery models should be advocated which consider that especially chronically ill patients benefit from well-executed psychosocial rehabilitation and treatment programs (Briand et al. 2006). A close collaboration between clinicians, researchers, and economists and the consideration of different therapeutic interventions are required in order to translate QOL research into clinical practice (Awad and Voruganti 2012). For future research, the investigation of predictors for recovery and its relation to QOL in patients with schizophrenia have been recommended in order to understand how we finally could "get better in getting better our patients" (Jaaskelainen et al. 2013; Menezes et al. 2006).

References

Achilla E, McCrone P. The cost effectiveness of long-acting/extended-release antipsychotics for the treatment of schizophrenia: a systematic review of economic evaluations. Appl Health Econ Health Policy. 2013;11:95–106.

Acta. http://www.actassociation.org. Brighton; 2001–2012.

Addington DE, McKenzie E, Wang J. Validity of hospital admission as an outcome measure of services for first-episode psychosis. Psychiatr Serv (Washington, DC). 2012;63:280–2.

AlAqeel B, Margolese HC. Remission in schizophrenia: critical and systematic review. Harv Rev Psychiatry. 2012;20:281–97.

Alonso J, Croudace T, Brown J, et al. Health-related quality of life (HRQL) and continuous antipsychotic treatment: 3-year results from the Schizophrenia Health Outcomes (SOHO) study. Value Health. 2009;12:536–43.

Amador XF, Strauss DH, Yale SA, et al. Assessment of insight in psychosis. Am J Psychiatry. 1993;150:873–9.

Amador XF, Flaum M, Andreasen NC, et al. Awareness of illness in schizophrenia and schizoaffective and mood disorders. Arch Gen Psychiatry. 1994;51:826–36.

Andreasen NC, Carpenter Jr WT, Kane JM, et al. Remission in schizophrenia: proposed criteria and rationale for consensus. Am J Psychiatry. 2005;162:441–9.

Awad AG, Voruganti LN. Measuring quality of life in patients with schizophrenia: an update. Pharmacoeconomics. 2012;30:183–95.

Awad AG, Voruganti LN. The impact of newer atypical antipsychotics on patient-reported outcomes in schizophrenia. CNS Drugs. 2013;27:625–36.

Barnes TR, Drake RJ, Dunn G, et al. Effect of prior treatment with antipsychotic long-acting injection on randomised clinical trial treatment outcomes. Br J Psychiatry. 2013;203:215–20.

Bechdolf A, Pukrop R, Kohn D, et al. Subjective quality of life in subjects at risk for a first episode of psychosis: a comparison with first episode schizophrenia patients and healthy controls. Schizophr Res. 2005;79:137–43.

Bobes J, Ciudad A, Alvarez E, et al. Recovery from schizophrenia: results from a 1-year follow-up observational study of patients in symptomatic remission. Schizophr Res. 2009;115:58–66.

Boden R, Sundstrom J, Lindstrom E, Lindstrom L. Association between symptomatic remission and functional outcome in first-episode schizophrenia. Schizophr Res. 2009;107:232–7.

Bora E, Sehitoglu G, Aslier M, Atabay I, Veznedaroglu B. Theory of mind and unawareness of illness in schizophrenia: is poor insight a mentalizing deficit? Eur Arch Psychiatry Clin Neurosci. 2007;257:104–11.

Boyer L, Aghababian V, Richieri R, et al. Insight into illness, neurocognition and quality of life in schizophrenia. Prog Neuropsychopharmacol Biol Psychiatry. 2012;36:271–6.

Boyer L, Lancon C, Baumstarck K, et al. Evaluating the impact of a quality of life assessment with feedback to clinicians in patients with schizophrenia: randomised controlled trial. Br J Psychiatry. 2013;202:447–53.

Briand C, Vasiliadis HM, Lesage A, et al. Including integrated psychological treatment as part of standard medical therapy for patients with schizophrenia: clinical outcomes. J Nerv Ment Dis. 2006;194:463–70.

Brissos S, Dias VV, Balanza-Martinez V, Carita AI, Figueira ML. Symptomatic remission in schizophrenia patients: relationship with social functioning, quality of life, and neurocognitive performance. Schizophr Res. 2011;129:133–6.

Brooks R. EuroQol: the current state of play. Health Policy. 1996;37:5372.

Carpiniello B, Pinna F, Tusconi M, Zaccheddu E, Fatteri F. Gender differences in remission and recovery of schizophrenic and schizoaffective patients: preliminary results of a prospective cohort study. Schizophr Res Treatment. 2012;2012:576369.

Carroll A, Fattah S, Clyde Z, et al. Correlates of insight and insight change in schizophrenia. Schizophr Res. 1999;35:247–53.

Chang LR, Lin YH, Kuo TB, et al. Autonomic modulation and health-related quality of life among schizophrenic patients treated with non-intensive case management. PLoS One. 2013;6:e26378.

Chen EY, Tang JY, Hui CL, et al. Three-year outcome of phase-specific early intervention for first-episode psychosis: a cohort study in Hong Kong. Early Interv Psychiatry. 2011;5:315–23.

Chou KR, Shih YW, Chang C, et al. Psychosocial rehabilitation activities, empowerment, and quality of community-based life for people with schizophrenia. Arch Psychiatr Nurs. 2012;26:285–94.

Citrome L, Kamat SA, Sapin C, et al. Cost-effectiveness of aripiprazole once-monthly compared with paliperidone palmitate once-monthly injectable for the treatment of schizophrenia in the United States. J Med Econ. 2014;17:567–76.

Cohen CI, Pathak R, Ramirez PM, Vahia I. Outcome among community dwelling older adults with schizophrenia: results using five conceptual models. Community Ment Health J. 2009;45:151–6.

Cohen CI, Hassamal SK, Begum N. General coping strategies and their impact on quality of life in older adults with schizophrenia. Schizophr Res. 2011;127:223–8.

Cooke MA, Peters ER, Kuipers E, Kumari V. Disease, deficit or denial? Models of poor insight in psychosis. Acta Psychiatr Scand. 2005;112:4–17.

Dan A, Kumar S, Avasthi A, Grover S. A comparative study on quality of life of patients of schizophrenia with and without depression. Psychiatry Res. 2011;189:185–9.

de Haan L, Nimwegen L, Amelsvoort T, Dingemans P, Linszen D. Improvement of subjective well-being and enduring symptomatic remission, a 5-year follow-up of first episode schizophrenia. Pharmacopsychiatry. 2008;41:125–8.

DeHaan L, Weisfelt M, Dingemans PM, et al. Psychometric properties of the Subjective Well-Being Under Neuroleptics scale and the Subjective Deficit Syndrome Scale [Medico-economic study of Leponex (clozapine) in the Bordeaux Charles Perrens Hospital Center]. Psychopharmacology (Berl). 2002;162:24–8.

Delespaul PH. Consensus regarding the definition of persons with severe mental illness and the number of such persons in the Netherlands. Tijdschr Psychiatr. 2013;55:427–38.

Dickerson FB, Boronow JJ, Ringel N, Parente F. Lack of insight among outpatients with schizophrenia. Psychiatr Serv (Washington, DC). 1997;48:195–9.

Docherty JP, Bossie CA, Lachaux B, et al. Patient-based and clinician-based support for the remission criteria in schizophrenia. Int Clin Psychopharmacol. 2007;22:51–5.

Drake RJ, Lewis SW. Insight and neurocognition in schizophrenia. Schizophr Res. 2003;62:165–73.

Drake RJ, Pickles A, Bentall RP, et al. The evolution of insight, paranoia and depression during early schizophrenia. Psychol Med. 2004;34:285–92.

Eack S, Newhill C. Psychiatric symptoms and quality of life in schizophrenia: a meta-analysis. Schizophr Bull. 2007;33(5):1225–37.

Einarson TR, Vicente C, Zilbershtein R, et al. Pharmacoeconomics of depot antipsychotics for treating chronic schizophrenia in Sweden. Nord J Psychiatry. 2014a;68:416–27.

Einarson TR, Pudas H, Goswami P, van Impe K, Bereza BG. Pharmacoeconomics of long-acting atypical antipsychotics for acutely relapsed chronic schizophrenia in Finland. J Med Econ. 2014b,68:1–29.

Eklund M. Work status, daily activities and quality of life among people with severe mental illness. Qual Life Res. 2009;18:163–70.

Faerden A, Nesvag R, Marder SR. Definitions of the term 'recovered' in schizophrenia and other disorders. Psychopathology. 2008;41:271–8.

(FDA) USFaDA. Patient-reported outcome measures: use in medical product development to support labelling claims. In: Guidance for industry. FDA, US Government. 2006.

Fleischhacker WW, Cetkovich-Bakmas M, De Hert M, et al. Comorbid somatic illnesses in patients with severe mental disorders: clinical, policy, and research challenges. J Clin Psychiatry. 2008;69:514–9.

Fujimaki K, Morinobu S, Yamashita H, Takahashi T, Yamawaki S. Predictors of quality of life in inpatients with schizophrenia. Psychiatry Res. 2012a;197:199–205.

Fujimaki K, Takahashi T, Morinobu S. Association of typical versus atypical antipsychotics with symptoms and quality of life in schizophrenia. PLoS One. 2012b;7:e37087.

Galuppi A, Turola MC, Nanni MG, Mazzoni P, Grassi L. Schizophrenia and quality of life: how important are symptoms and functioning? Int J Ment Heal Syst. 2010;4:31.

Gilleen J, David AS. The cognitive neuropsychiatry of delusions: from psychopathology to neuropsychology and back again. Psychol Med. 2005;35:5–12.

Goldberg RW, Green-Paden LD, Lehman AF, Gold JM. Correlates of insight in serious mental illness. J Nerv Ment Dis. 2001;189:137–45.

Green C, Garety PA, Freeman D, et al. Content and affect in persecutory delusions. Br J Clin Psychol Br Psychol Soc. 2006;45:561–77.

Haro JM, Novick D, Perrin E, Bertsch J, Knapp M. Symptomatic remission and patient quality of life in an observational study of schizophrenia: is there a relationship? Psychiatry Res. 2014;220:163–9.

Harvey PD, Bellack AS. Toward a terminology for functional recovery in schizophrenia: is functional remission a viable concept? Schizophr Bull. 2009;35:300–6.

Harvey PD, Pappadopulos E, Lombardo I, Kremer CM. Reduction of functional disability with atypical antipsychotic treatment: a randomized long term comparison of ziprasidone and haloperidol. Schizophr Res. 2009;115:24–9.

Harvey PD, Sabbag S, Prestia D, et al. Functional milestones and clinician ratings of everyday functioning in people with schizophrenia: overlap between milestones and specificity of ratings. J Psychiatr Res. 2012;46:1546–52.

Hasson-Ohayon I, Kravetz S, Roe D, David AS, Weiser M. Insight into psychosis and quality of life. Compr Psychiatry. 2006;47:265–9.

Hayhurst KP, Drake RJ, Massie JA, et al. Improved quality of life over one year is associated with improved adherence in patients with schizophrenia. Eur Psychiatry. 2013;29:191–6.

Haynes VS, Zhu B, Stauffer VL, et al. Long-term healthcare costs and functional outcomes associated with lack of remission in schizophrenia: a post-hoc analysis of a prospective observational study. BMC Psychiatry. 2012;12:222.

Heinrichs DW, Hanlon TE, Carpenter Jr WT. The Quality of Life Scale: an instrument for rating the schizophrenic deficit syndrome. Schizophr Bull. 1984;10:388–98.

Helldin L, Kane JM, Karilampi U, Norlander T, Archer T. Remission in prognosis of functional outcome: a new dimension in the treatment of patients with psychotic disorders. Schizophr Res. 2007;93:160–8.

Hofer A, Kemmler G, Eder U, et al. Quality of life in schizophrenia: the impact of psychopathology, attitude toward medication, and side effects. J Clin Psychiatry. 2004;65:932–9.

Hofer A, Rettenbacher MA, Widschwendter CG, et al. Correlates of subjective and functional outcomes in outpatient clinic attendees with schizophrenia and schizoaffective disorder. Eur Arch Psychiatry Clin Neurosci. 2006;256(4):246–55.

Hofer A, Rettenbacher MA, Edlinger M, et al. Outcomes in schizophrenia outpatients treated with amisulpride or olanzapine. Pharmacopsychiatry. 2007;40:1–8.

Huppert JD, Weiss KA, Lim R, Pratt S, Smith TE. Quality of life in schizophrenia: contributions of anxiety and depression. Schizophr Res. 2001;51:171–80.

Iqbal Z, Birchwood M, Chadwick P, Trower P. Cognitive approach to depression and suicidal thinking in psychosis. 2. Testing the validity of a social ranking model. Br J Psychiatry. 2000; 177:522–8.

Jaaskelainen E, Juola P, Hirvonen N, et al. A systematic review and meta-analysis of recovery in schizophrenia. Schizophr Bull. 2013;39:1296–306.

Jaaskelainen E, Haapea M, Rautio N, et al. Twenty years of schizophrenia research in the Northern Finland Birth Cohort 1966: a systematic review. Schizophr Res Treatment. 2015;2015:524875.

Karadayi G, Emiroglu B, Ucok A. Relationship of symptomatic remission with quality of life and functionality in patients with schizophrenia. Compr Psychiatry. 2012;52:701–7.

Karow A, Moritz S, Lambert M, Schoder S, Krausz M. PANSS syndromes and quality of life in schizophrenia. Psychopathology. 2005;38:320–6.

Karow A, Czekalla J, Dittmann RW, et al. Association of subjective well-being, symptoms, and side effects with compliance after 12 months of treatment in schizophrenia. J Clin Psychiatry. 2007;68:75–80.

Karow A, Pajonk FG, Reimer J, et al. The dilemma of insight into illness in schizophrenia: self- and expert-rated insight and quality of life. Eur Arch Psychiatry Clin Neurosci. 2008; 258:152–9.

Karow A, Moritz S, Lambert M, Schottle D, Naber D. Remitted but still impaired? Symptomatic versus functional remission in patients with schizophrenia. Eur Psychiatry. 2012a;27: 401–5.

Karow A, Naber D, Lambert M, Moritz S. Remission as perceived by people with schizophrenia, family members and psychiatrists. Eur Psychiatry. 2012b;27(6):426–31.

Karow A, Reimer J, Konig HH, et al. Cost-effectiveness of 12-month therapeutic assertive community treatment as part of integrated care versus standard care in patients with schizophrenia treated with quetiapine immediate release (ACCESS trial). J Clin Psychiatry. 2012c;73:e402–8.

Karow A, Wittmann L, Schottle D, Schafer I, Lambert M. The assessment of quality of life in clinical practice in patients with schizophrenia. Dialogues Clin Neurosci. 2015;16:185–95.

Kim CH, Jayathilake K, Meltzer HY. Hopelessness, neurocognitive function, and insight in schizophrenia: relationship to suicidal behavior. Schizophr Res. 2003;60:71–80.

Kind P. Guidelines for value sets in economic and non-economic studies using EQ-5D. In: Brooks R, Rabin R, De Charro F, editors. The measurement and valuation of health status using EQ-5D: a European perspective. Dordrchet/Boston: Kluwer; 2003.

Koren D, Seidman LJ, Poyurovsky M, et al. The neuropsychological basis of insight in first-episode schizophrenia: a pilot metacognitive study. Schizophr Res. 2004;70:195–202.

Kumazaki H, Kobayashi H, Niimura H, et al. Lower subjective quality of life and the development of social anxiety symptoms after the discharge of elderly patients with remitted schizophrenia: a 5-year longitudinal study. Compr Psychiatry. 2012;53:946–51.

Kurtz MM, Tolman A. Neurocognition, insight into illness and subjective quality-of-life in schizophrenia: what is their relationship? Schizophr Res. 2010;127:157–62.

Lambert M, Schimmelmann BG, Naber D, et al. Prediction of remission as a combination of symptomatic and functional remission and adequate subjective well-being in 2960 patients with schizophrenia. J Clin Psychiatry. 2006;67:1690–7.

Lambert M, Naber D, Eich FX, et al. Remission of severely impaired subjective wellbeing in 727 patients with schizophrenia treated with amisulpride. Acta Psychiatr Scand. 2007;115:106–13.

Lambert M, Naber D, Schacht A, et al. Rates and predictors of remission and recovery during 3 years in 392 never-treated patients with schizophrenia. Acta Psychiatr Scand. 2008;118:220–9.

Lambert M, Schimmelmann BG, Naber D, et al. Early- and delayed antipsychotic response and prediction of outcome in 528 severely impaired patients with schizophrenia treated with amisulpride. Pharmacopsychiatry. 2009;42:277–83.

Lambert M, Karow A, Leucht S, Schimmelmann BG, Naber D. Remission in schizophrenia: validity, frequency, predictors, and patients' perspective 5 years later. Dialogues Clin Neurosci. 2010a;12:393–407.

Lambert M, De Marinis T, Pfeil J, Naber D, Schreiner A. Establishing remission and good clinical functioning in schizophrenia: predictors of best outcome with long-term risperidone long-acting injectable treatment. Eur Psychiatry. 2010b;25(4):220–9.

Lambert M, Bock T, Schottle D, et al. Assertive community treatment as part of integrated care versus standard care: a 12-month trial in patients with first- and multiple-episode schizophrenia spectrum disorders treated with quetiapine immediate release (ACCESS trial). J Clin Psychiatry. 2010c;71(10):1313–23.

Landolt K, Rossler W, Burns T, et al. The interrelation of needs and quality of life in first-episode schizophrenia. Eur Arch Psychiatry Clin Neurosci. 2012a;262:207–16.

Landolt K, Rossler W, Burns T, et al. Unmet needs in patients with first-episode schizophrenia: a longitudinal perspective. Psychol Med. 2012b;42:1461–73.

Lewis SW, Davies L, Jones PB, et al. Randomised controlled trials of conventional antipsychotic versus new atypical drugs, and new atypical drugs versus clozapine, in people with schizophrenia responding poorly to, or intolerant of, current drug treatment. Health Technol Assess (Winchester, England). 2006;10:iii–iv, ix–xi, 1–165.

Liraud F, Droulout T, Parrot M, Verdoux H. Agreement between self-rated and clinically assessed symptoms in subjects with psychosis. J Nerv Ment Dis. 2004;192:352–6.

Maat A, Fett AK, Derks E. Social cognition and quality of life in schizophrenia. Schizophr Res. 2012;137:212–8.

Marchinko S, Clarke D. The Wellness Planner: empowerment, quality of life, and continuity of care in mental illness. Arch Psychiatr Nurs. 2011;25:284–93.

Marshall M, Lockwood A. Assertive community treatment for people with severe mental disorders. Cochrane Database Syst Rev Online. 2011;(4):CD001089.

Maurino J, Sanjuan J, Haro JM, Diez T, Ballesteros J. Impact of depressive symptoms on subjective well-being: the importance of patient-reported outcomes in schizophrenia. Patient Prefer Adherence. 2011;5:471–4.

McEvoy JP, Apperson LJ, Appelbaum PS, et al. Insight in schizophrenia. Its relationship to acute psychopathology. J Nerv Ment Dis. 1989;177:43–7.

Meesters PD, Comijs HC, de Haan L, et al. Subjective quality of life and its determinants in a catchment area based population of elderly schizophrenia patients. Schizophr Res. 2011;147:275–80.

Meijer CJ, Koeter MW, Sprangers MA, Schene AH. Predictors of general quality of life and the mediating role of health related quality of life in patients with schizophrenia. Soc Psychiatry Psychiatr Epidemiol. 2009;44:361–8.

Menezes NM, Arenovich T, Zipursky RB. A systematic review of longitudinal outcome studies of first-episode psychosis. Psychol Med. 2006;36:1349–62.

Mintz AR, Addington J, Addington D. Insight in early psychosis: a 1-year follow-up. Schizophr Res. 2004;67:213–7.

Moritz S, Werner R, von Collani G. The inferiority complex in paranoia re-addressed. A study with the Implicit Association Test. Cogn Neuropsychiatry. 2006;11:402–15.

Naber D. A self-rating to measure subjective effects of neuroleptic drugs, relationships to objective psychopathology, quality of life, compliance and other clinical variables. Int Clin Psychopharmacol. 1995;10 Suppl 3:133–8.

Naber D, Kollack-Walker S, Chen J, et al. Predicting a 'combined treatment outcome' in chronic schizophrenia: the role of demographics, symptomatology, functioning and subjective well-being. Pharmacopsychiatry. 2013;46:114–9.

Nordentoft M, Ohlenschlaeger J, Thorup A, et al. Deinstitutionalization revisited: a 5-year follow-up of a randomized clinical trial of hospital-based rehabilitation versus specialized assertive intervention (OPUS) versus standard treatment for patients with first-episode schizophrenia spectrum disorders. Psychol Med. 2010;40:1619–26.

Nuechterlein KH, Subotnik KL, Green MF, et al. Neurocognitive predictors of work outcome in recent-onset schizophrenia. Schizophr Bull. 2011;37 Suppl 2:S33–40.

O'Day K, Rajagopalan K, Meyer K, Pikalov A, Loebel A. Long-term cost-effectiveness of atypical antipsychotics in the treatment of adults with schizophrenia in the US. Clinicoecon Outcomes Res. 2013;5:459–70.

Ojeda N, Sanchez P, Pena J, et al. An explanatory model of quality of life in schizophrenia: the role of processing speed and negative symptoms. Actas Esp Psiquiatr. 2012;40:10–8.

Pedrelli P, McQuaid JR, Granholm E, et al. Measuring cognitive insight in middle-aged and older patients with psychotic disorders. Schizophr Res. 2004;71:297–305.

Penn DL, Uzenoff SR, Perkins D, et al. A pilot investigation of the Graduated Recovery Intervention Program (GRIP) for first episode psychosis. Schizophr Res. 2011;125:247–56.

Peuskens J, Gorwood P. How are we assessing functioning in schizophrenia? A need for a consensus approach. Eur Psychiatry. 2012;27:391–5.

Pitkanen A, Valimaki M, Kuosmanen L, et al. Patient education methods to support quality of life and functional ability among patients with schizophrenia: a randomised clinical trial. Qual Life Res. 2012;21:247–56.

Priebe S, McCabe R, Junghan U, et al. Association between symptoms and quality of life in patients with schizophrenia: a pooled analysis of changes over time. Schizophr Res. 2011; 133:17–21.

Putzhammer A, Perfahl M, Pfeiff L, Hajak G. Correlation of subjective well-being in schizophrenic patients with gait parameters, expert-rated motor disturbances, and psychopathological status. Pharmacopsychiatry. 2005;38:132–8.

Rabinowitz J, Levine SZ, Garibaldi G, et al. Negative symptoms have greater impact on functioning than positive symptoms in schizophrenia: analysis of CATIE data. Schizophr Res. 2012;137:147–50.

Rabinowitz J, Berardo CG, Bugarski-Kirola D, Marder S. Association of prominent positive and prominent negative symptoms and functional health, well-being, healthcare-related quality of life and family burden: a CATIE analysis. Schizophr Res. 2013;150:339–42.

Rajagopalan K, Hassan M, O'Day K, Meyer K, Grossman F. Cost-effectiveness of lurasidone vs aripiprazole among patients with schizophrenia who have previously failed on an atypical antipsychotic: an indirect comparison of outcomes from clinical trial data. J Med Econ. 2013;16:951–61.

Reichenberg A, Caspi A, Harrington H, et al. Static and dynamic cognitive deficits in childhood preceding adult schizophrenia: a 30-year study. Am J Psychiatry. 2010;167:160–9.

Renwick L, Jackson D, Foley S, et al. Depression and quality of life in first-episode psychosis. Compr Psychiatry. 2012;53:451–5.

Ritsner M. Predicting changes in domain-specific quality of life of schizophrenia patients. J Nerv Ment Dis. 2003;191:287–94.

Ritsner MS, Grinshpoon A. Ten-year quality of life outcomes of patients with schizophrenia and schizoaffective disorders. Clin Schizophr Relat Psychoses. 2015, Fall issue, 125–134.

Ritsner M, Kurs R, Gibel A, Ratner Y, Endicott J. Validity of an abbreviated quality of life enjoyment and satisfaction questionnaire (Q-LES-Q-18) for schizophrenia, schizoaffective, and mood disorder patients. Qual Life Res. 2005;14:1693–703.

Ritsner MS, Lisker A, Arbitman M. Ten-year quality of life outcomes among patients with schizophrenia and schizoaffective disorders: I. Predictive value of disorder-related factors. Qual Life Res. 2014;21:837–47.

Rocca P, Giugiario M, Montemagni C, et al. Quality of life and psychopathology during the course of schizophrenia. Compr Psychiatry. 2009;50:542–8.

Rojo LE, Gaspar PA, Silva H, et al. Metabolic syndrome and obesity among users of second generation antipsychotics: a global challenge for modern psychopharmacology. Pharmacol Res. 2015;101:74–85.

Ruggeri M, Leese M, Thornicroft G, Bisoffi G, Tansella M. Definition and prevalence of severe and persistent mental illness. Br J Psychiatry. 2000;177:149–55.

Sanz M, Constable G, Lopez-Ibor I, Kemp R, David AS. A comparative study of insight scales and their relationship to psychopathological and clinical variables. Psychol Med. 1998;28: 437–46.

Schennach-Wolff R, Jager M, Seemuller F, et al. Defining and predicting functional outcome in schizophrenia and schizophrenia spectrum disorders. Schizophr Res. 2009;113:210–7.

Schimmelmann BG, Paulus S, Schacht M, et al. Subjective distress related to side effects and subjective well-being in first admitted adolescents with early-onset psychosis treated with atypical antipsychotics. J Child Adolesc Psychopharmacol. 2005;15:249–58.

Schöttle D, Karow A, Schimmelmann BG, Lambert M. Integrated care in patients with schizophrenia: results of trials published between 2011 and 2013 focusing on effectiveness and efficiency. Curr Opin Psychiatry. 2013;26:384–408.

Schroeder K, Huber CG, Jelinek L, Moritz S. Subjective well-being, but not subjective mental functioning shows positive associations with neuropsychological performance in schizophrenia-spectrum disorders. Compr Psychiatry. 2012;54:824–30.

Schwartz RC. Insight and illness in chronic schizophrenia. Compr Psychiatry. 1998;39:249–54.

Schwartz RC, Smith SD. Suicidality and psychosis: the predictive potential of symptomatology and insight into illness. J Psychiatr Res. 2004;38:185–91.

Sim K, Mahendran R, Siris SG, Heckers S, Chong SA. Subjective quality of life in first episode schizophrenia spectrum disorders with comorbid depression. Psychiatry Res. 2004;129: 141–7.

Smith TE, Hull JW, Huppert JD, et al. Insight and recovery from psychosis in chronic schizophrenia and schizoaffective disorder patients. J Psychiatr Res. 2004;38:169–76.

Stein LI, Santos AB. Assertive community treatment of persons with severe mental illness. New York: W. W. Norton & Company, Inc; 2000.

Subotnik KL, Nuechterlein KH, Irzhevsky V, et al. Is unawareness of psychotic disorder a neurocognitive or psychological defensiveness problem? Schizophr Res. 2005;75:147–57.

Sugawara N, Yasui-Furukori N, Sato Y, et al. Body mass index and quality of life among outpatients with schizophrenia in Japan. BMC Psychiatry. 2013;13:108.

Switaj P, Wciorka J, Smolarska-Switaj J, Grygiel P. Extent and predictors of stigma experienced by patients with schizophrenia. Eur Psychiatry. 2009;24:513–20.

Tang IC, Wu HC. Quality of life and self-stigma in individuals with schizophrenia. Psychiatry Q. 2012;83:497–507.

Teague GB, Mueser KT, Rapp CA. Advances in fidelity measurement for mental health services research: four measures. Psychiatr Serv (Washington, DC). 2012;63:765–71.

Tolman AW, Kurtz MM. Neurocognitive predictors of objective and subjective quality of life in individuals with schizophrenia: a meta-analytic investigation. Schizophr Bull. 2012;38: 304–15.

Ucok A, Karadayi G, Emiroglu B, Sartorius N. Anticipated discrimination is related to symptom severity, functionality and quality of life in schizophrenia. Psychiatry Res. 2013;209:333–9.

Urbach M, Brunet-Gouet E, Bazin N, Hardy-Bayle MC, Passerieux C. Correlations of theory of mind deficits with clinical patterns and quality of life in schizophrenia. Front Psychiatry. 2013;4:30.

van Baars AW, Wierdsma AI, Hengeveld MW, Mulder CL. Improved insight affects social outcomes in involuntarily committed psychotic patients: a longitudinal study in the Netherlands. Compr Psychiatry. 2013;54:873–9.

Vancampfort D, Vansteelandt K, Scheewe T, et al. Yoga in schizophrenia: a systematic review of randomised controlled trials. Acta Psychiatr Scand. 2012a;126:12–20.

Vancampfort D, Knapen J, Probst M, et al. A systematic review of correlates of physical activity in patients with schizophrenia. Acta Psychiatr Scand. 2012b;125:352–62.

Vatne S, Bjorkly S. Empirical evidence for using subjective quality of life as an outcome variable in clinical studies A meta-analysis of correlates and predictors in persons with a major mental disorder living in the community. Clin Psychol Rev. 2008;28:869–89.

Velligan DI, Weiden PJ, Sajatovic M, et al. The expert consensus guideline series: adherence problems in patients with serious and persistent mental illness. J Clin Psychiatry. 2009;70 Suppl 4:1–46; quiz 47–8.

Ware J. SF-36 health survey. Manual and interpretation guide. Boston: Health Institute, New England Medical Center; 1993.

Whitty P, Browne S, Clarke M, et al. Systematic comparison of subjective and objective measures of quality of life at 4-year follow-up subsequent to a first episode of psychosis. J Nerv Ment Dis. 2004;192:805–9.

WHO. Development of the World Health Organization WHOQOL-BREF quality of life assessment. The WHOQOL Group. Psychol Med. 1998;28:551–8.

Wunderink L, Nienhuis FJ, Sytema S, Wiersma D. Predictive validity of proposed remission criteria in first-episode schizophrenic patients responding to antipsychotics. Schizophr Bull. 2007;33:792–6.

Yeh CB, Huang YS, Tang CS, et al. Neurocognitive effects of aripiprazole in adolescents and young adults with schizophrenia. Nord J Psychiatry. 2013;68:219–24.

Chapter 10
Using Routine Quality of Life Assessment to Improve Effectiveness of Community Mental Health Care

Domenico Giacco and Stefan Priebe

10.1 Introduction

Quality of life (QoL) assessment taps into and highlights patients' current problems in real-life domains, such as personal relationships, housing, employment, and physical and mental health. For this reason, QoL assessment is meaningful not only for clinicians but also for patients and can be assessed from both perspectives during clinical meetings (McCabe and Priebe 2002).

In a usual clinical meeting, patients are seen by mental health professionals (psychiatrists, psychologists, nurses, or "care coordinators") who assess their needs and manage their care. Until recently, no research had been conducted on how to run these meetings so that they are therapeutically effective and best help patients in evaluating and improving their health and social situation.

In the last decade, research groups (including ours) have used these characteristics of QoL assessment to develop interventions for improving the effectiveness of patient-clinician meetings in community mental health care.

A regular QoL assessment may help patients and clinicians to select which problems are most important for the patients and should be addressed during the clinical meetings. This can be used to make clinical meetings more patient centered, promote the active participation of patients in clinical decision-making, and help both clinicians and patients to arrive at decisions that are better targeted at improving the most prominent problems in the patients' lives.

In this chapter we provide an overview of the conceptual development, evidence base, and structural components of interventions using routine QoL to improve outcomes of community mental health care.

D. Giacco, MD, PhD (✉) • S. Priebe, DiplPsych, DrMedHabil, FRCPsych
Unit for Social and Community Psychiatry, (WHO Centre for Mental Health Service Development), Queen Mary University of London, East London NHS Foundation Trust, Newham Centre for Mental Health, Glen Road, London E13 8SP, UK
e-mail: d.giacco@qmul.ac.uk; s.priebe@qmul.ac.uk

© Springer International Publishing Switzerland 2016
A.G. Awad, L.N.P. Voruganti (eds.), *Beyond Assessment of Quality of Life in Schizophrenia*, DOI 10.1007/978-3-319-30061-0_10

Table 10.1 Components of the interventions using routine QoL assessment to improve care

	Structured psychosocial assessment		Active patient involvement in care	Use of ITs	Brief psychological intervention
	Prior to the meeting	During the meeting			
FOCUS	√	–	–	–	–
DIALOG	–	√	√	√	–
DIALOG+	–	√	√	√	√

10.2 Intervention Models

The intervention models using routine QoL assessment for improving treatment outcomes have built on each other and can be considered as different steps of a constant refinement process over time. In the first intervention model (the FOCUS intervention), the QoL assessment is made by patients, and then the results and the progress over time are reported to them and to clinicians outside of the clinical meetings. In the subsequent models (DIALOG and DIALOG+), the QoL assessment is carried out collaboratively by patients and clinicians during the clinical meeting. In DIALOG and DIALOG+, information technologies are used to facilitate the assessment. As part of DIALOG+ – the most recent intervention model – clinicians are trained in a brief psychological intervention so they can address the identified concerns and agree on actions that can improve these concerns.

See Table 10.1 for a summary of the structural components for each intervention, which will be then discussed in detail in a specific paragraph (see Sect. 10.6).

10.3 The FOCUS Intervention

The FOCUS intervention was the first to use routine QoL assessment with the aim of influencing interactions between patients and clinicians and improving outcomes (Slade et al. 2006).

FOCUS was developed by Slade and colleagues (2006). QoL was assessed from the patient perspective, and the results were fed back by researchers to clinicians and patients separately at regular intervals, outside of the clinical meetings. Their expectation was that providing feeding back on the patient's QoL would generate cognitive dissonance – an awareness of discrepancy between actual QoL and ideal QoL. It was hoped this would prompt a discussion and consequent changes of the care plans and clinical decisions. In turn, this process would – in itself or through an enhancement of the patient-clinician alliance – improve patients' QoL (Slade 2002a, b).

The FOCUS intervention involves asking patients to rate monthly a QoL measure (the Manchester Short Assessment of quality of life, Priebe et al. 1999) delivered through the post. The researchers then collect the results of the assessments and meet the patients and the clinicians separately every 3 months. At these meetings researchers provide identical feedback of the assessment results to both patients and clinicians. The intervention goes on for 6 months.

FOCUS was tested in a randomized controlled trial and compared to standard mental health care (Slade et al. 2006). The trial did not find a positive effect of FOCUS on QoL.

The lack of effectiveness of the intervention in improving QoL and reducing health and social needs was attributed to the absence of any behavioral change in patients or clinicians as a consequence of the intervention. Although both patient and clinician knew the results of the QoL assessment, this awareness did not change what decisions the patient and clinician made during their meetings, nor did it lead to any novel action being taken to improve the results. A process evaluation suggested that the intervention did not impact on clinical decisions and care plans (Slade et al. 2006), despite clinicians and patients recognizing that they had been prompted to consider the process and content of care.

The evaluation of the FOCUS intervention showed that just providing regular feedback to patients and clinicians on the assessment of QoL can stimulate a reflection on patients' problems in different life domains or concerns about treatment aspects. However, FOCUS did not manage to translate such reflection into actions or changes to treatment.

10.4   The DIALOG Intervention

The DIALOG intervention used a different strategy from FOCUS; QoL assessments were made collaboratively between patients and clinicians during their clinical consultation, providing opportunity for a patient-centered assessment. Patients were able to decide which issues should be prioritized and discussed in the clinical meeting and thus feel more involved in decisions being made about their treatment. The intervention focused on looking to the future, i.e., on what additional help patients feel they need for their current difficulties, rather than on what has caused those difficulties.

As part of the DIALOG intervention, every 2 months for 1 year, patients rate, in collaboration with clinicians, their satisfaction with various life domains and treatment aspects. Once patient satisfaction is established for each life domain or treatment aspect, they are asked by the clinicians whether they feel they need help in that area.

Eight life domains (mental health, physical health, accommodation, job situation, leisure activities, friendships, relationship with family/partner, personal safety) and three treatment domains (practical help, psychological help, and medication) are part of the evaluation. The life domains are derived from the MANSA (Priebe et al. 1999).

Satisfaction with life domains is measured through a Likert scale from 1 ("couldn't be worse") to 7 ("couldn't be better") (Priebe et al. 1999, 2007). The ratings are made on a handheld computer or laptop, either by the patient or the clinician using a software program with the option of passing the computer between the pairs to enable a more collaborative process. Ratings can be shown individually or as an overview of all ratings and can be compared with previous ratings to visualize changes and improvements over different periods of time. The ratings and the comparison with previous ratings are discussed during the meeting.

In a multicenter trial including patients with psychotic disorders in six European countries, the regular use of DIALOG over a 1-year period led to better QoL, fewer unmet needs, and a higher treatment satisfaction. This was achieved despite symptom levels not significantly improving compared to a standard care control group (Priebe et al. 2007).

The improvement in QoL independently from symptom change was in line with findings of previous large-scale studies in schizophrenia and other severe mental disorders, which showed that QoL is only partially influenced by symptoms (Priebe et al. 2010, 2011a). To improve QoL, the clinical consultations need to have a broader focus than just symptom management, which was demonstrated comprehensively through DIALOG.

However, the effect size of the improvement in outcomes was small, and a few challenges were identified. Firstly, there was no model or guidance for clinicians on how to respond to patients' concerns or how to establish a plan of action. Secondly, the relatively long duration of the intervention (1 year) might not have been applicable to patients who were treated by the services for a shorter time.

These considerations led to further refinement of the DIALOG intervention and to the development of DIALOG+.

10.5   The DIALOG+ Intervention

Similarly to previous interventions, DIALOG+ aimed to use QoL ratings to prompt a discussion between patients and clinicians, hence influencing care planning and clinical decisions. The main innovation in DIALOG+ was that clinicians were trained in a brief and simple psychological intervention informed by the principles of solution-focused therapy (SFT) (De Shazer 1988; Bavelas et al. 2013). This psychological intervention helps clinicians to respond to patients' current concerns and encourage them to "look forward," generating ideas and viable solutions for their difficulties. The brief psychological intervention was developed based on experiences with DIALOG in practice, consultations with clinicians in community mental health teams, leading practitioners in SFT, and focus groups with patients.

DIALOG+ is used in monthly sessions for a period of 6 months. Each DIALOG+ session begins with the same assessment of topics as in the original DIALOG intervention, whereby patients are asked to rate their satisfaction with the same 11 life domains or treatment aspects (see Fig. 10.1). Each satisfaction item is rated on a scale from 1 ("totally dissatisfied") to 7 ("totally satisfied") and is followed by a question on whether the patient wants additional help in the given domain. The ratings are then summarized on the screen allowing for comparisons with previous ratings from past meetings.

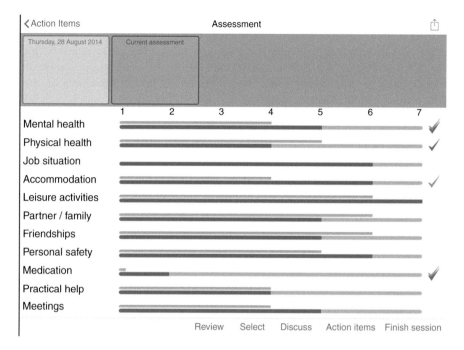

Fig. 10.1   DIALOG+ interface

In DIALOG+, a tablet was used instead of a computer for the assessment. The tablet was easier to pass between patient and clinician and, as such, helped facilitate the collaborative process. Clinicians are instructed to offer positive feedback on any improving or high-scoring domains. The summary is then used to inform a joint decision about which domains should be discussed in greater depth. Figure 10.1 shows a snapshot of the DIALOG+ interface.

Clinicians are also trained to address each of the domains chosen for further discussion in a 4-step approach informed by principles of SFT. This involves (1) understanding the patient's concerns and previous effective coping strategies; (2) identifying best-case scenarios and smallest steps for improvement; (3) exploring options available to the patient, including the patient's own resources, the clinician's, and those of others in the patient's life; and finally (4) agreeing on actions to address the identified concerns. Agreed actions are later reviewed at the start of the following meeting.

The effectiveness and cost-effectiveness of DIALOG+ were compared to standard care in a randomized controlled trial conducted in the United Kingdom including patients with psychotic disorders (Priebe et al. 2015). DIALOG+ improved QoL independently from symptoms, similarly to DIALOG. In addition DIALOG+ helped improve objective social outcomes relating to housing, employment, and social contacts up to 1 year after the start of the intervention. The intervention was found to be potentially cost saving; costs related to buying IT tools (in this case, tablets) and to the training of clinicians were much smaller than the treatment costs in the treatment group, mainly due to higher rehospitalization rates.

The analysis of care plans showed that DIALOG+ achieved the desired goal of helping patients to take an active role in clinical decision-making and in resulting actions as recorded in the care plan (Omer et al. in press). The improvement in QoL was often in the domains that were discussed during the meeting, but sometimes also extended to other life domains. Thus, it can be assumed that decisions on specific actions had an effect in the given life domain, but there was also a general encouragement for patients to take action and address other issues in life to improve their QoL.

As such, DIALOG+ proved to be effective in improving outcomes such as QoL and objective social outcomes, which are very difficult to change with any mental health-care intervention (Priebe et al. 2008) and has also potential for cost savings. Provided that such findings can be replicated in different trials, they would indicate that efforts for a more widespread implementation may be justified.

Yet, what are the structural components of the intervention that are particularly important for its acceptability and effectiveness in practice? We examined this as part of the DIALOG+ process evaluation.

10.6 What Are the "Active" Structural Components of the Interventions Using Routine QoL Assessment to Improve Care?

DIALOG+, being the most recent and advanced model, includes structural components which were already part of the previous models (FOCUS and DIALOG) and new ones, in particularly the training of clinicians to a brief psychological intervention (see Table 10.1). Overall, four structural active components can be described: (a) a structured psychosocial assessment within routine clinical meetings, (b) involvement of patients in clinical decision-making, (c) use of information technology tools to facilitate assessment and visualization of progress, and (d) training clinicians to a brief psychological intervention to help steer the discussion toward generating solutions to patients' problems.

These active components will be illustrated, below, with quotes taken from interviews and focus groups with patients and clinicians who used DIALOG+.

10.6.1 A Structured Psychosocial Assessment Within Routine Clinical Meetings

The QoL assessment provides a holistic structure that covers all aspects of the patient's life, not just their mental health. This can favor a shared understanding of problems and increase collaborative care planning (Slade 2002b; Priebe et al. 2015). The assessment is more likely to influence clinician and patient behaviors if conducted collaboratively during the clinical meetings (as opposed to separately outside of the clinical meeting).

> Every month, once a month. Talking about my, my medication… Talking about my accommodation… Talking about my family… They were talking about so many things in my life. I've been enjoying it … My family. My future. How my future will be. Talking about so many things." (Patient)
>
> It is actually very beneficial because you have your questionnaire that has been structured in such a way that you can cover almost everything that you need to cover with a client, from the psychosocial intervention to other things like their physical health, their mental health, their social life, their relationships… (Clinician)

10.6.2   Involving Patients in Clinical Decisions

Both patients and clinicians reported that routine QoL assessment can increase awareness of problems and provide a way to measure progress. This can empower a patient to be more actively involved in clinical decisions. Patient involvement in clinical decisions during mental health treatment has shown, in different studies, positive effects on satisfaction with care (Coulter 2010; Beitinger et al. 2014), adherence to treatment (Joosten et al. 2008; McCabe et al. 2013), and long-term clinical outcomes (Joosten et al. 2008; Puschner et al. 2016).

> You start improving yourself because you're aware of it now… It made me realise what I needed to do. And then if I needed that assistance, I would approach my care coordinator and let him know that, "you know what, I'm lacking in this department", or "I'm doing well in this department, so, what can we do to improve myself." (Patient)
>
> The client has been a part of a process that is good and there's an output… That's kind of engaging with services instead of just using the service… They liked the idea of seeing what they were doing and what they were achieving … Having quite clear ideas of what we are working on that feels much more recovery-orientated and more belonging to the client. (Clinician)
>
> Making the individual like he was in a position of power… whereby he can feel the service is meeting his needs, I'm not … dictating how this service should be led … I'd say the approach to this has enabled [my patients] to see mental health services in a different light. (Clinician)

10.6.3   Use of Information Technologies

Information technologies (ITs) help routine QoL assessment and its use for individual patients' care in different ways (Priebe et al. 2012).

ITs enable a clear, immediate, and user-friendly observation of treatment progress, which can be discussed during the clinical meeting.

An additional advantage is that ITs can be mobile (e.g., tablets) and can be used flexibly in the different settings of community mental health care, i.e., not only in office-based consultations but also at the home of the patient. This mobility also allows the assessment to be passed easily between patient and clinician so both can work together on establishing the patient's concerns and solutions to improve these.

Despite concerns that some patients with psychosis might have shown difficulties in using ITs, conducting the joint assessment through IT tools was found to be a medium that enhanced the collaboration. Patients and clinicians would help each other in using the tablets which was often viewed an "icebreaker" especially during initial meetings.

> It helped me track my progress…. On a monthly basis… My lifestyle, my accommodation, my safety, medication, all those things. (Patient)
>
> It kind of showed me… You kind of get to see what you said before and if you kind of made any improvements. (Patient)
>
> Also the whole fact that you are doing it on computer or [Tablet], is a novelty as well… So it's something to, to play around with, 'cause you can use it, or they can use it and it's a form of interaction. So if the person is not really interacting with you and you've got that possibly you can break the ice. (Clinician)

10.6.4 Training Clinicians to a Brief Psychological Intervention

A structured psychosocial assessment is at the core of different psychological approaches such as cognitive-behavioral therapy (Grant et al. 2010), solution-focused therapy (De Shazer 1988; Bavelas et al. 2013), or motivational interviewing (Levensky et al. 2007).

Hence, routine QoL assessment can be a starting point for brief psychological interventions within the routine clinical meetings, which may increase the therapeutic value of such meetings (Priebe et al. 2015). In particular, it has been suggested that having a psychological model of reference improves the communication between patients and clinicians (Priebe et al. 2011b).

The introduction of a solution-focused intervention to DIALOG+ was particularly appreciated by clinicians.

> Normally some of them will want you to do everything for them but with this solution focused therapy it did help them to see how to actually help themselves rather than being spoon-fed by the care coordinator … It did help them to understand how to actually come up with a solution rather than me saying "this is how to do it." (Clinician)
>
> A few of them recognised that actually they're more independent in themselves … It's just that sometimes they have this sort of … sudden anxiety, erases all the things that they could've done easily… [My patient] is able to change his overall insight into things that will benefit him, his strengths really, because he's got a lot of strengths really which he didn't recognise, but that him to recognise a lot of strengths. (Clinician)

Patients may recognize an increased therapeutic value of the consultations more indirectly. The solution-focused approach was sometimes interiorized by the patients leading to feelings of increased empowerment and confidence in their strengths:

> It was like mind stimulating that you could build upon something that might have started off as negative and no options. (Patient)
>
> It does help you because you can find positive things about a negative thing even. (Patient)

>It can make you think about what you're going to do for your life, obviously when you're asked questions it can make you think about what you can do for yourself as well. (Patient)

A clinical vignette is provided to give an example of the use of DIALOG+ in a routine consultation between a clinician (care coordinator) and a patient:

Clinical Vignette

M met his care coordinator for a routine meeting. They used DIALOG+ for their consultation. M rated two domains lower than "4" which indicated dissatisfaction in those domains. He rated his satisfaction with the place he was living in as two (dissatisfied) and his satisfaction with his friendships as three (slightly dissatisfied). Therefore, they both agreed to focus the consultation of these two domains.

M decided to start with his housing situation. M was living in a supported accommodation, which was a flat he shared with some flatmates who also had mental health problems. The care coordinator asked M why he rated this domain as two. He said that his flat was untidy and his flatmates would not help him with cleaning the flat.

He believed his flatmates, whom he also regarded as friends, should have helped him more in taking care of the flat (which explained the rating 3 for friendships).

The care coordinator started by considering why the rating for satisfaction with the place was not given a lower rating of 1 ("What works?"). M responded that the flat was in good condition, and if it was not untidy, it would have been a nice place to live. He also got along well with his flatmates apart from the frustration of them not helping as much as he needed for household chores.

The care coordinator then started a discussion on what would be a realistic improvement that could be achieved in a short time and how M could use the resources available to him to achieve this. M mentioned that he would be able to ask his friends to be more involved in household chores. He would also be happy to clearly explain to his friends how they could help. He reflected on how creating a clear timetable for household chores with indication of "who does what" might be an option to engage his flatmates more in the care of the flat. Therefore, M and his care coordinator agreed on the following action: M should have a meeting with his flatmates and mention the problem and propose they create a weekly rota for household chores.

Comment:

The assessment of life domains identified a problem for the patient that could be clearly described and assessed in detail. Two life domains were affected by the problem. The patient was encouraged to identify a solution based on personal resources (the good relationship with his flatmates) and his strengths (he put forward a viable solution, i.e., a rota for household chores and was able to be in charge of the rota). A clear and reviewable action was established following the discussion. Notably, the action was proposed and was going to be carried out by the patient.

10.7 Conclusions

In the last decade, novel intervention models have used the potential of routine QoL assessment to improve care of patients with schizophrenia. The evaluation of these interventions showed that routine QoL assessment and provision of feedback to clinicians and patients do not improve outcomes in itself and have no impact on clinical decisions. However, routine QoL assessment can be a component of more complex interventions, including a patient-centered approach, use of information technologies, and brief psychological interventions focused on finding solutions to patients' concerns.

Rigorous randomized controlled trials showed that the use of DIALOG and DIALOG+ improved QoL of patients. DIALOG+ was also effective in improving objective social outcomes and showed potential for saving costs of mental health care. The improvement of these outcomes was independent from symptom change. Hence, these interventions may be an important addition to symptom management.

Although the experimental evaluations of these interventions have yielded promising results, there is scope for further research in this field.

No replication studies have been carried out thus far in Europe nor have any been conducted outside of Europe. There is a need for further trials to be conducted by research groups that have not taken part in the development of the interventions.

DIALOG and DIALOG+ were tested only in patients with schizophrenia and in community mental health care. However, their structural components are not specific to schizophrenia or to community mental health care. They may help clinical interactions with other patients – for example, those with depression or anxiety disorders – and in other settings, such as hospital care or primary care.

At the moment, the only trial in a different setting of which we have knowledge, the ComQUOL trial, is currently ongoing to assess the effectiveness of DIALOG in forensic psychiatric wards (MacInnes et al. 2013).

Replication of findings by different trials, testing the potential of these models for the care of other patient populations, and the identification of strategies for a successful implementation in different mental health-care settings may be potential avenues for further research.

These endeavors are likely to offer interventions that can be easily implemented in clinical practice. Such interventions may substantially contribute to mental health services' efforts to improve patients' quality of life.

References

Bavelas J, De Jong P, Franklin C, et al. Solution focused therapy treatment manual for working with individuals (2nd version). Santa Fe: Solution Focused Brief Therapy Association; 2013.
Beitinger R, Kissling W, Hamann J. Trends and perspectives of shared decision-making in schizophrenia and related disorders. Curr Opin Psychiatry. 2014;27:222–9.
Coulter A. Implementing shared decision making in the UK. London: Health Foundation; 2010. Retrieved at: http://www.health.org.uk/sites/default/files/ImplementingSharedDecisionMaking InTheUK.pdf.

De Shazer S. Clues: investigating solutions in brief therapy. New York: Norton; 1988.

Grant A, Townend M, Mulhern R, Short N. Cognitive behavioural therapy in mental health care. London: SAGE Publications; 2010.

Joosten EA, DeFuentes-Merillas L, de Weert GH, Sensky T, van der Staak CP, de Jong CA. Systematic review of the effects of shared decision-making on patient satisfaction, treatment adherence and health status. Psychother Psychosom. 2008;77:219–26.

Levensky ER, Forcehimes A, O'Donohue WT, Beitz K. Motivational Interviewing: an evidence-based approach to counseling helps patients follow treatment recommendations. Am J Nurs. 2007;107:50–8.

MacInnes D, Kinane C, Beer D, et al. Study to assess the effect of a structured communication approach on quality of life in secure mental health settings (Comquol): study protocol for a pilot cluster randomized trial. Trials. 2013;14:257.

McCabe RM, Priebe S. Focussing on quality of life in treatment. Int Rev Psychiatry. 2002;14:225–30.

McCabe R, Healey PG, Priebe S, Lavelle M, Dodwell D, Laugharne R, Snell A, Bremner S. Shared understanding in psychiatrist-patient communication: association with treatment adherence in schizophrenia. Patient Educ Couns. 2013;93:73–9.

Omer S, Golden E, Priebe S. Exploring the mechanisms of a patient-centred assessment with a solution focused approach (DIALOG+) in the community treatment of patients with psychosis: a process evaluation within a cluster-randomised controlled trial. PLoS One. 2016;11:e0148415.

Priebe S, Huxley P, Knight S, Evans S. Application and results of the Manchester Short Assessment of Quality of Life (MANSA). Int J Soc Psychiat. 1999;45:7–12.

Priebe S, McCabe R, Bullenkamp J, et al. Structured patient-clinician communication and 1-year outcome in community mental healthcare. Cluster randomised controlled trial. Br J Psychiat. 2007;191:420–6.

Priebe S, Watzke S, Hansson L, Burns T. Objective social outcomes index (SIX): a method to summarise objective indicators of social outcomes in mental health care. Acta Psychiatr Scand. 2008;118:57–63.

Priebe S, Reininghaus U, McCabe R, Burns T, Eklund M, Hansson L, Junghan U, Kallert T, van Nieuwenhuizen C, Ruggeri M, Slade M, Wang D. Factors influencing subjective quality of life in patients with schizophrenia and other mental disorders: a pooled analysis. Schizophr Res. 2010;121:251–8.

Priebe S, McCabe R, Junghan U, Kallert T, Ruggeri M, Slade M, Reininghaus U. Association between symptoms and quality of life in patients with schizophrenia: a pooled analysis of changes over time. Schizophr Res. 2011a;133:17–21.

Priebe S, Dimic S, Wildgrube C, Jankovic J, Cushing A, McCabe R. Good communication in psychiatry–a conceptual review. Eur Psychiatry. 2011b;26:403–7.

Priebe S, Golden E, McCabe R, Reininghaus U. Patient-reported outcome data generated in a clinical intervention in community mental health care–psychometric properties. BMC Psychiatry. 2012;12:113.

Priebe S, Kelley L, Golden EM, et al. The effectiveness of a patient-centred assessment with a solution focused approach (DIALOG+) for patients with psychosis – a pragmatic cluster randomised controlled trial in community care. Psychother Psychosom. 2015;84:304–13.

Puschner B, Becker T, Mayer B, et al. Clinical decision making and outcome in the routine care of people with severe mental illness across Europe (CEDAR). Epidemiol Psychiatr Sci. 2016;25(1):69–79.

Slade M. Routine outcome assessment in mental health services. Psychol Med. 2002a;32:1339–43.

Slade M. What outcomes to measure in routine mental health services, and how to assess them: a systematic review. Aus New Zealand J Psychiat. 2002b;36:743–53.

Slade M, McCrone P, Kuipers E, Leese M, Cahill S, Parabiaghi A, Priebe S, Thornicroft G. Use of standardised outcome measures in adult mental health services: randomised controlled trial. Br J Psychiat. 2006;18:330–6.

Chapter 11
Quality of Life Assessments in the Development and Clinical Trials of New Antipsychotics: Pharmaceutical Industry Perspective

Raimund Buller and Christophe Sapin

11.1 Introduction

For more than 50 years, pharmacotherapy of schizophrenia has focused primarily on the treatment of positive symptoms (i.e., hallucinations, delusions, excitement, and hostility) and on the prevention of exacerbations and re-hospitalizations (maintenance treatment). The aspect of quality of life (QoL) has only recently found to be critical for clinical trials in patients with severe mental disorders and important as a target for therapeutic interventions, in spite of the fact that schizophrenia is associated with significant reductions in QoL. Historical milestones for the introduction of quality of life into mental health can be found in a paper by Bobes and Gonzales (1997).

Clinical practice has had little influence on QoL as shown in a clinical study following patients over 10 years. Poor outcomes were found in 76 % of the patients, and only 24 % reported that they had improved or remained satisfied with their QoL (Ritsner et al. 2012). Now an increasing number of trials also include quality of life assessments, although in most cases still only as secondary or exploratory outcome parameters. Results from these trials are often difficult to interpret due to a number of methodological shortcomings. This may also have contributed to the fact that quality of life measures have not yet made a large impact on clinical care (Awad and Voruganti 2012).

R. Buller, MD (✉)
Clinical Development, Lundbeck, 37 – 45 Quai du Président Roosevelt,
Issy-les-Moulineaux F-92445, France
e-mail: rabu@lundbeck.com

C. Sapin, MSc
Global Analytics, Lundbeck A/S,
37 – 45 Quai du Président Roosevelt, Issy-les-Moulineaux F-92445, France
e-mail: chsa@lundbeck.com

© Springer International Publishing Switzerland 2016
A.G. Awad, L.N.P. Voruganti (eds.), *Beyond Assessment of Quality of Life in Schizophrenia*, DOI 10.1007/978-3-319-30061-0_11

157

11.2 Methodological Aspects of Quality of Life Assessments in Drug Development Trials

There is no universally accepted operational definition of quality of life and various authors have proposed different concepts. This lack of consensus is a major problem for research and has a serious impact on the assessment of QoL in the context of drug development. However, there appears to be general agreement that QoL is primarily subjective in nature and represents the patient's personal view or feelings ("well-being," "happiness," or "life satisfaction") but also has important objective facets related to the environment and to social functioning. QoL assessments therefore cover several dimensions like the patients' overall functioning, their psychological well-being, their perceived quality of life, and the impact of the environment on their quality of life.

11.2.1 Selection of Assessment Instruments

Since there is no "gold standard" instrument for the assessment of QoL, the selection of one or more specific QoL measurements for use in a clinical trial will depend on the type of questions that are to be addressed. Investigators, who design a trial, should be familiar with the theoretical construct that the authors of a particular instrument have applied and with results from the use in situations similar to the intended research. In general, measurements should have documented adequate psychometric properties in the particular populations for which they will be used. As an example, reliability data established in chronic stable outpatients may not be extrapolated to acutely exacerbated hospitalized patients.

Social and environmental factors are critical for QoL; however, they are not targets for interventions in clinical trials where the emphasis is mainly on health and illness. The FDA 2009 Guidance for Industry on Patient-Reported Outcome Measures: Use in Medical Product Development to Support Labeling Claims discusses quality of life and explains in the glossary: Quality of life is "a general concept that implies an evaluation of the effect of all aspects of life on general well-being. Because this term implies the evaluation of non-health-related aspects of life, and because the term generally is accepted to mean *what the patient thinks it is*, it is too general and undefined to be considered appropriate for a medical product claim." However, the FDA accepts claims based on health-related quality of life (HRQL) which the agency defines as follows: "HRQL is a multi-domain concept that represents the patient's general perception of the effect of illness and treatment on physical, psychological, and social aspects of life."

Assessment of QoL or HRQL in mental disorders is faced with several methodological challenges, not least due to the fact that QoL to a large extent involves psychological aspects. As a consequence, there may be an overlap between items that are directly linked to psychopathology and those that are assessed in the context of QoL, like depressed mood, anxiety, somatic concerns, sleep disturbances, and pain – to name only a few. On the other hand, mental states like depression, dysphoria or euphoria, as well as cognitive impairment may lead to bias in subjective assessment, over- or underestimating the level of QoL. Measurements based on "subjective" patient-reported QoL have been accepted in conditions like cancer or chronic pulmonary diseases but have been met with skepticism in the case of schizophrenia (and even depression), since there were doubts whether patients could provide reliable and valid information on their QoL.

There are several instruments with a particular focus on health-related quality of life (HRQL) covering important general domains like physical health, mental health, cognitive functioning, sexual functioning, and role performance in work or school. The SF-36 (Ware and Sherbourne 1992), a generic QoL measure, contains 36 items which are grouped into 8 scales. These are physical functioning, role physical, bodily pain, general health, vitality, social functioning, and role emotional and mental health; they can be summarized into two broad dimensions, physical health and mental health. The instrument has been widely used in various physical illnesses but also in depression and schizophrenia (Nasrallah et al. 2004). The scale differentiated between patients with schizophrenia and healthy controls and showed improvements in patients with schizophrenia from admission to discharge (Pukrop et al. 2003). Several other generic scales that have been used in samples with schizophrenia, like the WHOQoL (The Whoqol Group 1998) and the EQ-5D (Brooks et al. 2013), are discussed by Bobes and colleagues (2005), who summarize findings supporting their use as the two instruments discriminated between patients with schizophrenia and healthy subjects and showed that higher severity was related to lower QoL scores. Generic instruments can be used for cost-utility analysis since they can refer to sets of preference-based utility values and may allow for comparisons across diseases, but will not necessarily capture all important aspects of a specific condition. Furthermore, it remains questionable whether similar scores on a generic instrument have the same meaning and relevance in different diseases like pulmonary disease, cancer, diabetes, or schizophrenia.

For this reason specific instruments have been developed for use in schizophrenia. Initially, mainly "objective" clinician-rated instruments were applied, like the QLS (Heinrichs et al. 1984). This scale has been widely used, but it was originally intended for the assessment of a deficit syndrome and as such rather measures the impact of negative symptoms. Several other clinician-administered instruments also exist, like the Quality of Life Interview, QoLI (Lehman et al. 1982), and the Lancashire Quality of Life Profile, LQoLP (Oliver et al. 1996).

Like healthy subjects, psychiatric patients can be prone to various reporting biases known also as "social desirability." In spite of these potential limitations in assessments, a number of studies (e.g., Wehmeier et al. 2007) have provided empirical evidence demonstrating that a vast majority of patients with schizophrenia, particularly chronic stable and treatment-adherent patients with moderate severity, can in fact reliably assess their QoL and that tools based on self-reports are useful in clinical trials and outcome studies. However, patients with acute exacerbations, severe psychotic symptoms or hostility, profound lack of insight, or substantial cognitive impairment may be unable to fill in self-reports or to respond adequately to a QoL interview.

Several patient-rated instruments for schizophrenia are now available, including the Schizophrenia Quality of Life Scale (SQLS) (Wilkinson et al. 2000), the Sevilla Quality of Life Questionnaire (Ibáñez et al. 1997), the Personal Evaluation of Transitions in Treatment (PETiT) (Voruganti and Awad 2002), and the Auquier Schizophrenia Quality of Life Questionnaire S-QoL (Auquier et al. 2003). None of these instruments have so far been widely used in clinical trials so that there is only limited experience with their ability to measure treatment effects. Bobes et al. (2005) discuss several instruments, which are all based on different theoretical approaches and dimensions, contain between 21 and 143 items, and take between 2 and 45 min to complete: QLS, clinician-rated only with focus on deficit syndrome; QoLI and LoLP, patient-rated, based on a general QoL model; SQLQ, patient-rated favorable and unfavorable aspects of life; PETiT, patient-rated changes of symptoms, side effect, and performance during treatment; and the S-QoL, patient-rated with focus on discrepancies between their expectations and their current experiences. The authors conclude that the choice of the most appropriate instrument depends on the aim of the research and that generic and specific instruments should be combined.

A scale worth mentioning, which has demonstrated sensitivity to change and assesses side effects of antipsychotic treatment rather than the impact of schizophrenia per se on QoL, is the Subjective Well-Being Under Neuroleptic Scale (SWN) (Naber 1995). With regard to a broader concept of well-being, Schrank et al. (2013) comment that this is still "ill-defined" although it has conceptual overlaps with HRQL. It depends on the environment, the economy, relationships and family connections, activities, finances, general and mental health, as well as satisfaction.

At present there is not one single "optimal" instrument for the "objective" or "subjective" assessment of QoL that would be useful for all kinds of clinical trials. In fact, a selection of several instruments adapted to the research aim may provide a better fit. However, discrepancies between results from "objective" clinician-rated measures of QoL and from "subjective" patient-rated rated measures have been observed and may be explained by the fact that instruments are based on different constructs and tap into different domains. Patients and clinicians also appear to differ in their valuation of aspects like symptom profile, adverse events, living situation, and role functioning. Thus it is unclear if and how well objective and subjective measures should correlate. According to Wehmeier et al. (2007), QoL is perceived more similarly by clinicians and patients in more severely ill patients, in patients with lack of tolerability or in need of a treatment change, in younger patients, and in patients who have received psychotherapy; on the other hand, QoL in women with schizophrenia was rated higher by clinicians than by the patients themselves. In fact, there have been observations that self-rated benefits of treatment have not been captured by clinician-rated measures (Awad and Voruganti 2004). Since QoL in the case of schizophrenia is also essentially a subjective construct, assessments should always include subjective, self-report-based assessments as well as objective measures.

11.2.2   Factors with Potential Impact on Quality of Life Assessments in Clinical Trials with Antipsychotics

Clinical development programs are increasingly conducted on a global scale. However, the relevance of diverse cultural backgrounds for the assessment of QoL in schizophrenia in multinational clinical trials has not been systematically explored in the literature. The World Health Organization (WHO) has made an effort to develop methods that are acceptable across various cultures based on the idea that QoL is what individuals perceive as their position in life related to their goals and values. In a review of health-related quality of life measures in Arabic-speaking populations, Al Sayah et al. (2013) pointed out that most instruments have originally been developed in the English language for a specific culture and that cross-cultural adaptation techniques are needed to preserve aspects of equivalence when comparing populations from different geographical regions. On a similar note, Xiang et al. (2010) reviewed the literature on trials with Chinese patients with schizophrenia and concluded that cultural factors play an important role and that assessment tools derived from Western sources may not have sufficient sensitivity to eliminate cultural bias.

Ratings of QoL may be influenced by several other factors unrelated to treatment, like demographics, education, social status, living conditions, employment status, psychopathology, and comorbidity – to name just some. These factors and their potential interactions with treatment also need to be taken into consideration when designing trials and selecting populations in order to correctly interpret the potential impact of treatment effects on QoL measures.

In general, younger patients, women, married persons, those with lower levels of education, and patients participating in support programs or psychotherapy report better quality of life. Negative correlations with QoL are reported for duration of illness, duration of untreated psychosis, and levels of negative and depressive symptoms (Bobes et al. (2005). Caron et al. (2005) reviewed the literature on sociodemographic and clinical predictors for various QoL domains in schizophrenia. Higher age (i.e., 40–49 years) was related to better QoL. Women reported higher QoL total scores and better QoL related to activities of daily living. The relation between the level of education and QoL may not always be straightforward. Although in general patients with higher education levels report higher degrees of satisfaction with life and psychological well-being, there are some patients with an inverse relation between higher education and higher premorbid social status and reported satisfaction, possibly due to an illness-related downward shift in status.

There is still limited data on the relevance for QoL of factors like employment status, ability to work, income, and social relations, legal problems, and premorbid adjustment and results vary between samples. Homeless people with schizophrenia generally report low QoL except when showing significant lack of insight or neurocognitive impairment. Nilsson and Levander (1998) found no subjective differences in quality of life discontent scores among four other living conditions (mental hospital, group home, treatment collective, and patients' own flats). Although the four groups had relevant differences in psychopathology, the finding could indicate that patients felt that their personal needs were adequately met in the respective institutions.

Several specific clinical variables have been consistently found to have an impact on QoL ratings – although the degrees varied between studies. Lower QoL is associated with the level of depression and negative symptoms, although there could be an overlap in measures of QoL with negative symptoms since both tap into the same construct, as is the case with the QLS, originally developed to assess deficit schizophrenia. Negative symptoms may explain up to 45 % of the variance in QoL in stable patients but only around 15 % during acute exacerbations (Bow-Thomas et al. 1999). Negative symptoms are usually present to a significant extent in acutely exacerbated patients, but the severity of positive symptoms may overshadow the clinical picture. Hayhurst et al. (2014) identified depression as the main driver for patient-rated reduced QoL whereas negative symptoms were the main driver for clinician-rated low QoL. Unsurprisingly, lack of insight was the main driver for discrepancies between clinician- and patient-rated QoL assessments. The role of positive symptoms for QoL is less clear. Most authors have found no strong relation between positive symptoms and QoL, although there are some reports that see them as predominant factors for QoL. In a meta-analysis Eack and Newhill (2007) reported that positive and negative symptoms were significantly negatively related to both composite and domain-specific indicators of QoL, although the relationships between positive symptoms and QoL were not particularly strong, except for health-related QoL. General psychopathology, which includes symptoms like depression and anxiety, was significantly negatively related to QoL. The lack of a uniform relation between positive symptoms and QoL can also be seen in a paper by Xiang et al. (2012) who reported on a sample of community-dwelling Chinese patients with schizophrenia. More severe positive symptoms predicted worse QoL in psychological and environmental domains and better social support independently predicted higher QoL in all domains. Overall psychopathology predicted both worse physical and psychological domains; depressive symptoms and being married predicted worse physical and social QoL, respectively.

The level of insight and cognitive impairment are of specific importance as they may introduce biases into ratings and reduce their reliability. This may be the case in patients with severe symptomatology and during acute exacerbations. As an example, Siu et al. (2015 in press) showed that the level of insight and cognitive performance had moderating effects on the reported level of subjective life satisfaction.

Some general factors related to treatment have also been found to have an impact on QoL. A recent hospitalization during the previous 12 months is associated with lower QoL although this could also be an indirect effect of higher severity or a less favorable course of the illness. Patients with longer duration of the illness may report increased quality of life, possibly due to better adjustment to treatment or greater autonomy. There appears to be an interaction between treatment adherence and QoL. Those with higher QoL are more adherent, and those with better adherence report higher QoL and subjective well-being. Finally the quality of the patient-doctor relationship is directly related to QoL.

A general model linking clinical variables with health-related quality of life has been proposed by Wilson and Cleary (1995). Based on a classification scheme for different measures of health outcome, divided into five levels (biological factors, symptoms, functioning, general health perception, and overall quality of life), the authors suggest to analyze the causal relationships between them and to determine the size of their effects on outcome with statistical tools. Being able to identify how symptomatology, functional status, and other domains are interrelated may help with the interpretation of the observed effects of therapeutics on QoL measures. Several authors have attempted to develop a concept for QoL in schizophrenia. In their paper Awad et al. (1997) proposed and tested an integrative model, where QoL in schizophrenia is seen as the subject's perception of the outcome of an interaction between three major determinants: the severity of psychotic symptoms, side effects including subjective responses to antipsychotic drugs, and the level of psychosocial performance. This may be modulated by other factors like personality and premorbid adjustment that influence the outcome. In a cross-sectional study, the symptoms of schizophrenia, assessed with the Positive and Negative Syndrome Scale (PANSS), and the subjective distress due to adverse events like akathisia and neuroleptic dysphoria were found to explain nearly half of the variance in QoL in this population of stable patients. Ritsner and colleagues (2000) translated findings from several HRQL studies into a Distress/Protection Vulnerability model, which postulated dissatisfaction with HRQL as a particular syndrome linked to severe mental disorders, like schizophrenia. This syndrome was the result of an interaction between distressing factors and factors protecting against stress. The level of dissatisfaction with quality of life increases when distressing factors overweigh protective factors.

The ways how antipsychotic medications interact with QoL have been debated over time. Awad and Voruganti (2004) postulated that medications by themselves cannot raise the level of QoL in patients with schizophrenia; this would also require other interventions, such as rehabilitation or psychosocial skills training. However, several studies have now shown that QoL can actually improve during treatment with antipsychotics although the exact mechanism by which this is achieved is not clear and may actually differ between drugs and from trial to trial. As an example, Phillips et al. (2006) reported on significant correlations between changes in PANSS scores and changes on the SF-36 as well as on the QLS. In their sample there were a 30.72 % improvement on the PANSS total score and a 28.55 % improvement on the QLS total score.

In a meta-analysis paper, Leucht et al. (2009a) report differences between first- and second-generation antipsychotic effects on quality of life based, however, on merely 17 studies. For most compounds (amisulpride, aripiprazole, clozapine, sertindole, ziprasidone, and zotepine), the authors could actually only rely on one study with sample sizes between 72 and 311 subjects. For olanzapine there were 5 studies with a total of 1450 patients included, for risperidone 4 studies with a total of 330 patients, and for quetiapine 2 studies with a total of 166 patients. Only amisulpride, clozapine, and sertindole were better than the comparators on QoL measures with effect sizes between −0.24 and −0.44 (Hedges' g), but these results were based on a single trial and neither the specific measures of quality of life, nor the effects of the first-generation comparators on these measures were discussed in detail in the paper.

Antipsychotic medications can cause a wide range of adverse events that may negatively affect QoL, especially when assessed with subject, patient-rated instruments. Still, the amount of variance in QoL explained by adverse events appears to be relatively small. In a multiple regression analysis, the amount of variance in QoL ratings explained was 20.9 % for psychosocial factors, 10.1 % for clinical symptoms and associated distress, and only 3.2 % for adverse effects (Ritsner et al. 2002).

The results are particularly contradictory when looking at extrapyramidal symptoms (EPS), a potentially major differentiator between typical and atypical antipsychotics. Two large effectiveness trials, CATIE (Swartz et al. 2007) and CUtLASS (Jones et al. 2006) found no differences in QoL between the two types of antipsychotics in spite of differences in the AE profiles. This could be due to methodological limitations in the two trials, as several other controlled studies and effectiveness trials have reported on better QoL outcomes with atypical antipsychotics, when assessed by subjective instruments (Naber and Lambert 2009). The total adverse event load also appears to be correlated with QoL as well as some individual adverse events like sexual side effects, sleep disturbances, tachycardia, dizziness, and fatigue. On the other hand, metabolic syndrome and weight gain have not been consistently identified as a source of reduced QoL.

There have been suggestions that improvement in QoL takes longer than symptomatic improvement. However, in a 12-week study to assess the effects of early response to an antipsychotic, Kinon et al. (2010) found that patients with an early improvement in their psychiatric symptoms also showed an early and consistent improvement in functioning, quality of life (QLS), and subjective well-being (SWN-K). This is of great relevance since early improvement in symptoms and in QoL has an important impact on long-term QoL (Karow et al. 2014). In this context it is important to assess how much change is actually needed to represent a "detectable change" in QoL. A clinician rating of "improved" appears to correspond to a 21 % decrease in PANSS score and to a 26 % increase of the QLS score. A rating of "much better" corresponds to a 45 % decrease of the PANSS total score and a 50 % increase on the QLS (Cramer et al. 2001). This information may also be useful for sample size calculations in order to ensure not only statistical significance but also clinical relevance and to identify "responder rates" which can then be used to calculate "numbers needed to treat" (NNT). In general, it is desirable to refer to a defined "minimal clinically important difference" (MCID) for a given QoL scale which can be derived either from a distribution-based method or from an anchor-based method described in detail by McLeod et al. (2011) and shown for the QLS by Falissard et al. (2015).

Besides the effects of treatment on QoL, the final outcome in a therapeutic trial most likely depends on additional factors and their interactions. These factors are, among others, the clinical features, adverse events and the distress they cause, distress-protective factors, the quality of the therapeutic relation, and elements of psychosocial support.

11.2.3 Clinical Trials with Focus on Quality of Life

As is the case for clinical research in general, there are several design features that also apply to clinical trials which focus on QoL. Assessments of QoL can be included in a wide variety of studies, ranging from cross-sectional and observational studies that investigate characteristics of relevant patient populations or current standards of care and patients' needs to naturalistic and interventional trials of various durations that provide comparative data for different drugs or interventions. The target audiences for these trials are clinicians, Health Technology Assessment (HTA) bodies, and regulatory agencies like the Food and Drug Administration (FDA) and the European Medicines Agency (EMA). So far most studies are sponsored by the pharmaceutical industry; however, there have been calls for more independent, well-designed, and adequately powered, comparative, controlled studies.

In all cases, assessment tools should be chosen carefully with regard to their psychometric properties and corresponding to aim and design of the trial. When used in multinational trials, not only translations but also cultural adaptions may be needed to allow for valid comparisons, interpretation of the results, or pooling of the data. Trials should have adequate sample sizes and sample size calculations should take into consideration the reliability of the chosen instruments.

When there is more than one primary end point, the sample size needs to be adjusted for multiplicity. Underpowering should be avoided in comparative studies since it could lead to false conclusions about a lack of difference while there is actually just a lack of evidence for a truly existing difference. Trials should be of a sufficient duration to allow for changes, but especially in populations with schizophrenia, longer duration may be associated with substantial discontinuation rates and thus leads to the question of how best to handle the potential impact of missing data on the estimates of a potential treatment effect.

QoL is not only an outcome but also a factor that may work as a mediator of outcomes: Higher QoL is associated with better treatment adherence, improved community functioning, or lower relapse rates. QoL assessments should thus always be included in trials, even if this is only to more fully characterize the patient population. Baseline differences in QoL measures between patients or sites may lead to different outcomes between sites and could result from differences in sampling, treatment settings, or basic background care for the patients.

In efficacy or effectiveness studies, the inclusion of subjective and objective QoL measures provides important information to clinicians on relevant positive or negative properties of specific compounds that would not be illustrated by classical outcome measures based on recording symptom change. In this respect, any discrepancies between results from patient-rated and clinician-rated instruments should be discussed and explained (e.g., due to different underlying concepts). The guidelines of the World Federation of Societies of Biological Psychiatry (WFSBP) on long-term treatment of schizophrenia (Hasan et al. 2013) highlight the relevance of QoL since one of the declared main goals of treatment during the stable phase is to ensure that the patients are maintaining or improving their level of functioning and quality of life. Psychopharmacological management should be individually tailored to the needs and preferences of the patient, focusing, among others, on improvement of subjective well-being and quality of life. In general, clinicians will benefit from reliable information about the degree with which compounds improve or negatively interfere with aspects of QoL in schizophrenia. So far, based on the available literature, the guideline makes no recommendations for specific treatments as they have found "no evidence that would favor one particular antipsychotic drug or a group."

After the introduction of second-generation antipsychotics, several studies have been conducted that included measures of QoL. With the difficulties in demonstrating superior efficacy versus first-generation compounds, the comparisons eventually focused on safety and tolerability as well as on quality of life. Advantages of the newer drugs were their improved subjective tolerability and a more favorable side-effect profile with respect to extrapyramidal symptoms and neuroleptic dysphoria leading to inquiries of how these differences might translate into improved quality of life. Initially, the target audiences were clinicians (prescribers) and later also agencies involved in pricing and reimbursement, but often the assessment of QoL was not the primary target of the studies. Many of these studies also did not allow for clear conclusions due to significant methodological shortcomings – discussed in more detail by Awad and Voruganti (2004). The authors criticize that "frequently the inclusion of quality of life assessments in clinical trials seems to be an afterthought. Many of the studies are short term lasting only a few weeks with no long-term follow up. The use of several measurement scales based upon different theoretical constructs seems to limit any reliable comparative analysis. Some of the instruments used are of unknown psychometric properties and maybe inappropriate for use in the schizophrenia population or are not sensitive enough to detect small changes in quality of life as expected in such relatively short term trials."

In recent years, studies have been conducted for submissions to Health Technology Assessment (HTA) bodies in order to secure satisfactory pricing and reimbursement for newly introduced compounds. From a HTA perspective, HRQL is one of three important factors (together with mortality and morbidity) for relative effectiveness assessment of new drugs. Both generic HRQL and disease (or population)-specific questionnaires are useful and effects should be investigated in comparative, interventional trials, taking into consideration that the trial conduct itself may influence QoL results ("trial effect"). For cost-utility assessment health gains are normally presented in terms of quality-adjusted life years (QALYs). HRQL findings are then translated into utility and entered into the calculation of the QALY. This process will be greatly facilitated when selecting a HRQL measure, for which a set of preference-based utility values has been elicited. Cost-utility analyses have been successful in various indications, but their applicability to schizophrenia appears to be still a challenge in view of the heterogeneity of the condition and the complex clinical picture. The timing of these studies is still debated. Results from phase II trials may have limited utility for HTA assessments but could provide relevant information for further clinical development and the choice of QoL measures when designing the phase III trials.

As an example for HTA assessments, the National Institute for Health and Care Excellence (NICE) appraises the evidence of all the clinical benefits and costs of an intervention in the broadest sense, including the impact on quality of life. Data on final clinical outcomes such as life years gained and changes in patient quality of life are actually preferred to intermediate clinical outcomes. NICE is primarily interested in "clinical effectiveness" which encompasses benefits to patients including reductions in morbidity and mortality but also improved quality of life. The ideal source of effectiveness data is from prospective, randomized, controlled trials with a naturalistic design and minimal restrictions on the normal decision-making processes of health-care professionals and patients.

Regulatory claims based on health-related quality of life (HRQL) measures are accepted by both the FDA and EMA. While the patients' perspective is gaining importance in clinical research for the EMA and FDA, HR-QoL end points are still playing a minor role in product claims with psychiatry products, possibly due to methodological weaknesses of the trials submitted which have been criticized for an "unscientific practice of including any vaguely relevant PRO instrument in a clinical trial at the eleventh hour" (Speight and Barendse 2010).

Over the years, the FDA also appears to have become more critical of instruments used to measure patient-reported outcomes (PROs) in clinical trials. In 2006 the agency has sent out the draft of a guidance document on patient-reported outcomes which covers assessment of QoL and was finally issued in 2009 (FDA 2009). In 2014 the agency has also provided guidance on the qualification process for drug development tools which describes the framework for how drug developers and manufacturers may submit and seek qualification approval for tools like PROs that may be used for HRQL claims (FDA 2014). After the release of the draft guidance in 2006 on PROs, the number of successful PRO-based product labeling claims has actually fallen compared with the preceding 5 years although the guidance document now outlines a clear strategy for the inclusion of PROs in clinical trials, similar to that for other clinical end points. In order to make valid PRO claims for new compounds, drug companies will need to start collecting evidence in support of the PRO already as early as phases I–II and to carefully consider the development of appropriate PRO measures. According to the FDA, claiming a statistical and meaningful improvement in HRQL implies (1) that all HRQL domains that are important to interpreting change in how the clinical trial's population feels or functions as a result of the targeted disease and its treatment were measured, (2) that a general improvement was demonstrated, and (3) that no decrement was demonstrated in any domain.

The EMA, unlike the FDA, has not issued formal guidelines specific to PROs but has instead published a reflection paper (EMA 2005) to provide broad recommendations on health-related quality of life (HRQL) evaluation in the context of clinical trials. So far, the EMA has been more likely to grant PRO claims and is more likely to grant claims for higher order constructs such as HRQL. The EMA also accepts existing measures, including global assessment and diaries, provided the assessments are supported by peer-reviewed publications covering the development and validity of the instruments. This difference in acceptance rates possibly results from the way both agencies treat HRQL measures. The EMA recommends specific, validated instruments for use within the therapeutic area, whereas the FDA typically recommends the identification of concepts and does not endorse specific measures.

A paper by Marquis et al. (2011) summarizes the current situation as follows: 15 guidance documents from the FDA and 34 guidance documents from the EMA contain recommendations for the inclusion of PRO end points in clinical trials. However, the FDA referred to HRQL (as a secondary end point) in only 3 guidance documents, whereas the EMA recommended use of HRQL end points in 22 guidance documents. The FDA approved 8 products with PRO end points documenting treatment benefits characterized as HRQL and the EMA approved 16 products with a PRO claim reflecting HRQL data, but none of these HRQL claims were granted in the context of a schizophrenia indication.

With regard to the timing of HRQL assessment in relation to the marketing authorization, the EMA reflection paper on HRQL describes broadly two situations: When the medicinal product has not yet received a marketing authorization, the sponsor company may choose to study the effects on HRQL simultaneously to the efficacy/safety of the medicinal product in pivotal (phase III) trials. Studies should be powered to test both for the efficacy of the test drug versus placebo and/or active comparator as appropriate and for the HRQL change. Efficacy and HRQL are co-primary end points, or alternatively, a hierarchical testing of end points could be applied. When the medicinal product has already obtained a marketing authorization, and if HRQL is planned to be studied once efficacy and safety of the test drug have already been shown in the target population, it may be difficult to perform a study versus placebo. In this case HRQL change due to the test drug may be compared to HRQL change due to an active comparator, and a study incorporating both efficacy and HRQL change (e.g., non-inferiority for efficacy and superiority for HRQL) may be an appropriate design for including data in the label.

A significant limitation is of course that HRQL findings from controlled clinical trials with their structured environment, frequent visits, and more intensive interaction with clinical staff may not be easily transferable to routine practice. Study participants usually have to meet highly selective inclusion and exclusion criteria and their clinical characteristics may vary significantly from those common in routine clinical practice, like higher severity, psychiatric and medical comorbidities, more intensive cognitive impairment, or polypharmacy.

11.3   Some History and then Back to the Future: Quality of Life in Schizophrenia as a Specific Target for Drug Development

Following the initial serendipitous discovery of the first antipsychotic, chlorpromazine, there are now more than 60 first- and second-generation antipsychotics globally available, the vast majority of them already as generics. All antipsychotics are different with respect to their heterogeneous receptor profiles but they are mainly distinguished by their safety and tolerability, while efficacy differences between them tend to be small in magnitude (except for clozapine which has superior efficacy in treatment-resistant schizophrenia). Antipsychotic drugs primarily target positive symptoms, but there is a significant level of treatment resistance, and many patients do not even respond to clozapine, the only approved drug for this indication. Antipsychotics also have, at best, marginal effects on other, but probably more significant, aspects of the schizophrenia syndrome, as there are negative symptoms, depressive features, and cognitive impairment. In this sense, all available compounds are still only "antipsychotics" and none can yet claim to be an "antischizophrenia" treatment although the label claim is usually "for the treatment of schizophrenia."

The choice of positive symptoms as the primary target for treatment has not simply been a consequence of the discovery of chlorpromazine and the development of compounds with a comparable mode of action, but was also due to changes in the concept of schizophrenia over time. When Eugen Bleuler introduced the term "schizophrenia," in his famous monograph from 1911 "Dementia praecox oder Gruppe der Schizophrenien," he stressed that this was not a single entity but a group of disorders sharing a set of basic or fundamental symptoms like loosening of association, blunt or incongruous affect, ambivalence, and autism which he considered unique to schizophrenia. Today, several of the basic symptoms would be identified as negative symptoms or cognitive impairment. Bleuler did not believe that delusions and hallucinations were essential to schizophrenia. In fact, he regarded them as "accessory symptoms" as they more likely represented failed attempts at dealing with the illness.

Kurt Schneider (1959) proposed a new diagnostic approach to schizophrenia based on features that could be more easily identified than Bleuler's basic or fundamental symptoms. The new criteria were restricted to particular types of hallucinations and delusions and have been known as "first rank symptoms." They show improved inter-rater reliability and were integrated into the classification system of DSM-III (American Psychiatric Association 1980). Although Schneider stated that the primacy of first rank symptoms was not a theoretical matter but that they were "primary" only in the practical diagnostic decision making, hallucinations and delusions (also referred to as "positive symptoms") eventually were treated as the core features of schizophrenia. Supported by the specific efficacy of antipsychotic compounds, positive symptoms became the main targets for pharmacotherapy and for drug development. However, a number of meta-analyses have illustrated the important limitations of antipsychotics in the treatment of schizophrenia (Leucht et al. 2009b, 2013). The lack of significant improvements in course and outcome of schizophrenia over the past 100 years for the majority of patients, in spite of the availability of medications, has been discussed extensively (Hegarty et al. 1994; Jääskeläinen et al. 2013).

Even at present, medications for schizophrenia continue to be approved by regulatory agencies based on their antipsychotic efficacy (and safety) that is usually demonstrated in samples with acutely exacerbations. Antipsychotics will certainly remain useful for symptom reduction in many patients and for reducing the risk of relapse. Their limitations have, however, led to a shift in goal posts. The field is now aiming at remission (Andreasen et al. 2005) and recovery (Andresen et al. 2003; Silverstein and Bellack 2008; Zipursky and Agid 2015). For schizophrenia, complete recovery implies the ability to function in the community, socially and vocationally, as well as being relatively free of disease-related psychopathology. Therefore, QoL can be considered an increasingly important objective for treatment in schizophrenia, since improvements in QoL would be a significant step forward in reaching recovery.

This should stimulate research and drug development and will obviously require novel approaches and targets for treatments that have different or additional pharmacological effects. More focus needs to be placed on aspects like cognitive impairment, negative symptoms and motivational deficits, depressive symptoms, and anxiety as well as comorbid conditions like substance abuse. Unmet medical needs in schizophrenia are still very high and drug development that seeks treatments for better outcomes will probably need to undergo dramatic changes. Many companies have seen this as too risky and too costly and have therefore left the field or terminated their activities of treatments for schizophrenia. But with the movement of consumerism, there are now clear expectations of better therapies also for schizophrenia that will deliver "value for money." This then provides important commercial opportunities for those companies, who continue their development activities and succeed in finding compounds with improved therapeutic activity and low side-effect burden. New compounds should then be tested in well-designed studies with external validity and a focus on QoL so that they can already bridge the "efficacy-effectiveness gap" (Eichler et al. 2011) during clinical development. Although these trials come with an increased cost, they will have more weight with regulators, HTAs, and payers.

With an increasing shift in psychiatric practice from reducing psychotic symptoms to improving quality of life and with an emphasis on evidence-based medicine, quality of life can play a central role and may become a key target for future drug development in schizophrenia.

References

Al Sayah F, Ishaque S, Lau D, Johnson JA. Health related quality of life measures in Arabic speaking populations: a systematic review on cross-cultural adaptation and measurement properties. Qual Life Res. 2013;22:213–29.

American Psychiatric Association. Diagnostic and statistical manual of mental disorders. 3rd ed. Washington, DC: American Psychiatric Association; 1980.

Andreasen N, Carpenter W, Kane J, Lasser RA, Marder SR, Weinberger DR. Remission in schizophrenia: proposed criteria and rationale for consensus. Am J Psychiatry. 2005;162:441–9.

Andresen R, Oades L, Caputi P. The experience of recovery from schizophrenia: towards an empirically validated stage model. Aust N Z J Psychiatry. 2003;37:586–94.

Auquier P, Simeoni MC, Sapin C, Reine G, Aghababian V, Cramer J, Lancon C. Development and validation of a patient-based health-related quality of life questionnaire in schizophrenia: the S-QoL. Schizophr Res. 2003;63:137–49.

Awad AG, Voruganti LNP. Impact of atypical antipsychotics on quality of life in patients with schizophrenia. CNS Drugs. 2004;18:877–93.

Awad AG, Voruganti LNP. Measuring quality of life in patients with schizophrenia – an update. Pharmacoeconomics. 2012;30:183–95.

Awad AG, Voruganti LNP, Heslegrave RJ. A conceptual model of quality of life in schizophrenia: description and preliminary clinical validation. Qual Life Res. 1997;6:21–36.

Bleuler E. Dementia praecox oder Gruppe der Schizophrenien. Leipzig/Wien: Franz Deuticke; 1911.

Bobes J, Gonzales MP. Quality of life in schizophrenia. In: Katschnig H, Freeman H, Sartorius N, editors. Quality of life in mental disorders. Chichester: Wiley & Sons; 1997. p. 165–78.

Bobes J, Garcia-Portilla P, Saiz PA, Bascaran T, Bousono M. Quality of life measures in schizophrenia. Eur Psychiatry. 2005;20:S313–7.

Bow-Thomas CC, Velligan DI, Miller AL, Olsen J. Predicting quality of life from symptomatology in schizophrenia at exacerbation and stabilization. Psychiatry Res. 1999;86:131–42.

Brooks R, Rabin R, De Charro F, editors. The measurement and valuation of health status using EQ-5D: a European perspective: evidence from the EuroQol BIOMED Research Programme. Springer Science & Business Media; Kluwer Academic Publishers - Dordrecht, Boston, London 2013.

Caron J, Mercier C, Diaz P, Martin A. Socio-demographic and clinical predictors of quality of life in patients with schizophrenia or schizo-affective disorder. Psychiatry Res. 2005;137:203–13.

Cramer J, Rosenheck R, Xu W, Henderson W, Thomas J, Charney D. Detecting improvement in quality of life and symptomatology in schizophrenia. Schizophr Bull. 2001;27:227–34.

Eack SM, Newhill CE. Psychiatric symptoms and quality of life in schizophrenia: a meta-analysis. Schizophr Bull. 2007;33:1225–37.

Eichler HG, Abadie E, Breckenridge A, Flamion B, Gustafsson LL, Leufkens H, Rowland M, Schneider CK, Bloechl-Daum B. Bridging the efficacy-effectiveness gap: a regulator's perspective on addressing variability of drug response. Nat Rev Drug Discov. 2011;10:495–506.

EMA. Reflection paper on the regulatory guidance for the use of health-related quality of life (HRQL) measures in the evaluation of medicinal products. 2005. http://www.ema.europa.eu/docs/en_GB/document_library/Scientific_guideline/2009/09/WC500003637.pdf. Accessed 28 Aug 2015.

Falissard B, Sapin C, Loze JY, Landsberg W, Hansen K. Defining the minimal clinically important difference (MCID) of the Heinrichs–Carpenter quality of life scale (QLS). Int J Methods Psychiatr Res. 2015. doi:10.1002/mpr.1483. Published online: 4 AUG 2015.

FDA. Guidance for industry on patient-reported outcome measures: use in medical product development to support labeling claims. 2009. http://www.fda.gov/downloads/Drugs/Guidances/UCM193282.pdf. Accessed 28 Aug 2015.

FDA. Guidance for industry and FDA staff: qualification process for drug development tools. 2014. http://www.fda.gov/downloads/drugs/guidancecomplianceregulatoryinformation/guidances/ucm230597.pdf. Accessed 28 Aug 2015.

Hasan A, Falkai P, Wobrock T, Lieberman J, Glenthoj B, Gattaz WF, Thibaut F, Möller HJ, WFSBP Task force on Treatment Guidelines for Schizophrenia. World Federation of Societies of Biological Psychiatry (WFSBP) guidelines for biological treatment of schizophrenia, part 2: update 2012 on the long-term treatment of schizophrenia and management of antipsychotic-induced side effects. World J Biol Psychiatry. 2013;14:2–44.

Hayhurst KP, Massie JA, Dunn G, Lewis SW, Drake RJ. Validity of subjective versus objective quality of life assessment in people with schizophrenia. BMC Psychiatry. 2014;14:365.

Hegarty JD, Baldessarini RJ, Tohen M, Waternaux C, Oepen G. One hundred years of schizophrenia: a meta-analysis of the outcome literature. Am J Psychiatry. 1994;151:1409–16.

Heinrichs DW, Hanlon TE, Carpenter WT. The Quality of Life Scale: an instrument for rating the schizophrenic deficit syndrome. Schizophr Bull. 1984;10:388–98.

Ibáñez E, Giner J, Cervera S, Baca E, Bobes J, Leal C. El Cuestionario Sevilla de Calidad de Vida: propiedades psicométricas. Actas Luso Esp Neurol Psiquiatr. 1997;25 Suppl 2:24–31.

Jääskeläinen E, Juola P, Hirvonen N, McGrath JJ, Saha S, Isohanni M, Veijola J, Miettunen J. A systematic review and meta-analysis of recovery in schizophrenia. Schizophr Bull. 2013;39:1296–306.

Jones PB, Barnes TRE, Davies L, Dunn G, Lloyd H, Hayhurts KP, Murray RM, Markwick A, Lewis SW. Randomized controlled trial of the effect on quality of life of second- vs. first-generation antipsychotic drugs in schizophrenia – cost utility of the latest antipsychotic drugs in schizophrenia study (CUtLASS 1). Arch Gen Psychiatry. 2006;63:1079–86.

Karow A, Wittmann L, Schöttle D, Schäfer I, Lambert M. The assessment of quality of life in clinical practice in patients with schizophrenia. Dialogues Clin Neurosci. 2014;16:185–95.

Kinon BJ, Chen L, Ascher-Svanum H, Stauffer VL, Kollack-Walker S, Zhou W, Kapur S, Kane JM, Naber D. Challenging the assumption that improvement in functional outcomes is delayed relative to improvement in symptoms in the treatment of schizophrenia. Schizophr Res. 2010;118:176–82.

Lehman AF, Ward NC, Linn LS. Chronic mental patients: the quality of life issue. Am J Psychiatry. 1982;10:1271–6.

Leucht S, Corves C, Arbter D, Engel RR, Li C, Davis JM. Second-generation versus first-generation antipsychotic drugs for schizophrenia: a meta-analysis. Lancet. 2009a;373:31–41.

Leucht S, Arbter D, Engel RR, Kissling W, Davis JM. How effective are second-generation antipsychotic drugs? A meta-analysis of placebo-controlled trials. Mol Psychiatry. 2009b;14:429–47.

Leucht S, Cipriani A, Spineli L, Mavridis D, Örey D, Richter F, Samara M, Barbui C, Engel RR, Geddes JR, Kissling W, Stapf MP, Lässig B, Salanti G, Davis JM. Comparative efficacy and tolerability of 15 antipsychotic drugs in schizophrenia: a multiple-treatments meta-analysis. Lancet. 2013;382:951–62.

Marquis P, Caron M, Emery MP, Scott JA, Arnould B, Acquadro C. The role of health-related quality of life data in the drug approval processes in the US and Europe. Pharm Med. 2011;25:147–60.

McLeod LD, Coon CD, Martin SA, Fehnel SE, Hays RD. Interpreting patient-reported outcome results: US FDA guidance and emerging methods. Expert Rev Pharmacoecon Outcomes Res. 2011;11:163–9.

Naber D. A self-rating to measure subjective effects of neuroleptic drugs, relationships to objective psychopathology, quality of life, compliance and other clinical variables. Int Clin Psychopharmacol. 1995;10 Suppl 3:133–8.

Naber D, Lambert M. The CATIE and CUtLASS studies in schizophrenia. CNS Drugs. 2009;23:649–59.

Nasrallah HA, Duchesne I, Mehnert A, Janagap C, Eerdekens M. Health-related quality of life in patients with schizophrenia during treatment with long-acting, injectable risperidone. J Clin Psychiatry. 2004;65:531–6.

Nilsson LL, Levander S. Quality of life and schizophrenia: no subjective differences among four living conditions. Nord J Psychiatry. 1998;52:277–83.

Oliver JPJ, Huxley PJ, Bridges K, Mohamad H. Quality of life and mental health services. London: Routledge; 1996.

Phillips GA, Van Brunt DL, Roychowdhury SM, Xu W, Naber D. The relationship between quality of life and clinical efficacy from a randomized trial comparing olanzapine and ziprasidone. J Clin Psychiatry. 2006;67:1397–403.

Pukrop R, Schlaak V, Möller-Leimkühler AM, Albus M, Czernik A, Klosterkötter J, Möller HJ. Reliability and validity of Quality of Life assessed by the Short-Form 36 and the Modular System for Quality of Life in patients with schizophrenia and patients with depression. Psychiatry Res. 2003;119:63–79.

Ritsner M, Modai I, Endicott J, Rivkin O, Nechamkin Y, Barak P, Goldin V, Ponizovsky A. Differences in quality of life domains and psychopathologic and psychosocial factors in psychiatric patients. J Clin Psychiatry. 2000;61:880–9.

Ritsner M, Ponizovsky A, Endicott J, Nechamkin Y, Rauchverger B, Silver H, Modai I. The impact of side-effects of antipsychotic agents on life satisfaction of schizophrenia patients: a naturalistic study. Eur Neuropsychopharmacol. 2002;12:31–8.

Ritsner MS, Lisker A, Arbitman M. Ten-year quality of life outcomes among patients with schizophrenia and schizoaffective disorders: I. Predictive value of disorder-related factors. Qual Life Res. 2012;21:837–47.

Schneider K. Klinische Psychopathologie. Fünfte, neu bearbeitete Auflage der Beiträge zur Psychopathologie. Stuttgart: Georg Thieme Verlag; 1959.

Schrank B, Bird V, Tylee A, Coggins T, Rashid T, Slade M. Conceptualising and measuring the well-being of people with psychosis: systematic review and narrative synthesis. Soc Sci Med. 2013;92:9–21.

Silverstein SM, Bellack AS. A scientific agenda for the concept of recovery as it applies to schizophrenia. Clin Psychol Rev. 2008;28:1108–24.

Siu CO, Harvey PD, Agid O, Waye M, Brambilla C, Wing-Kit C, Remington G. Insight and subjective measures of quality of life in chronic schizophrenia. Schizophr Res Cogn. 2.3 2015; 127–132. (In press). http://dx.doi.org/10.1016/j.scog.2015.05.002.

Speight J, Barendse SM. FDA guidance on patient reported outcomes. BMJ. 2010;340:c2921.

Swartz MS, Perkins DO, Stroup TS, Davis SM, Capuano G, Rosenheck RA, Reimherr F, McGee MF, Keefe RSE, McEvoy JP, Hsiao JK, Lieberman JA. Effects of antipsychotic medications on psychosocial functioning in patients with chronic schizophrenia: findings from the NIMH CATIE study. Am J Psychiatry. 2007;164:428–36.

The Whoqol Group. The World Health Organization quality of life assessment (WHOQOL): development and general psychometric properties. Soc Sci Med. 1998;46:1569–85.

Voruganti LNP, Awad AG. Personal evaluation of transitions in treatment (PETiT): a scale to measure subjective aspects of antipsychotic drug therapy in schizophrenia. Schizophr Res. 2002;56:37–46.

Ware JE, Sherbourne CD. The MOS 36-item short-form health survey (SF-36): I. Conceptual framework and item selection. Med Care. 1992;30:473–83.

Wehmeier PM, Kluge M, Schacht A, Helsberg K, Schreiber W. Correlation of physician and patient rated quality of life during antipsychotic treatment in outpatients with schizophrenia. Schizophr Res. 2007;91(1):178–86.

Wilkinson G, Hesdon B, Wild D, Cookson R, Farina C, Sharma V, Fitzpatrick R, Jenkinson C. Self-report quality of life measure for people with schizophrenia: the SQLS. Br J Psychiatry. 2000;177:42–6.

Wilson IB, Cleary PD. Linking clinical variables with health-related quality of life: a conceptual model of patient outcomes. JAMA. 1995;273:59–65.

Xiang YT, Chiu HF, Ungvari GS. Quality of life and mental health in Chinese culture. Curr Opin Psychiatry. 2010;23:43–7.

Xiang YT, Hou YZ, Yan F, Dixon LB, Ungvari GS, Dickerson F, Li WY, Li WX, Zhu YL, Chan SSM, Lee EHM, Chiu HFK, Chiu HF. Quality of life in community-dwelling patients with schizophrenia in China. J Nerv Ment Dis. 2012;200:584–7.

Zipursky RB, Agid O. Recovery, not progressive deterioration, should be the expectation in schizophrenia. World Psychiatry. 2015;14:94–6.

Chapter 12
Quality of Life and Health Costs: The Feasibility of Cost-Utility Analysis in Schizophrenia

A. George Awad and Lakshmi N.P. Voruganti

Schizophrenia is a disabling mental disorder that impacts on several domains of mental functioning as well as general behavior (see Chap. 1 by M. Seeman). It generally pursues a chronic course with acute psychotic exacerbations that may require frequent hospitalization. It affects about 1 % of the population, yet patients with schizophrenia were estimated to use 8 % of all hospital beds in Canada (Goeree et al. 1999). A similar report in the United States estimated that patients with schizophrenia occupy up to 25 % of all hospital beds (Davies and Drummond 1990). In Australia the number of persons with schizophrenia is estimated to be less than 10 % of the number of patients treated for myocardial infarction, yet the cost of treatment of schizophrenia is almost 75 % of those treated for myocardial infarction (Davies and Drummond 1990). In the United States, one report estimated the cost as high as over $62.7 billion in the year 2002, with $22.7 billion in direct healthcare, which included hospitalizations, outpatient and community care, and crisis interventions (Wu et al. 2005). In the United Kingdom, the care of patients with schizophrenia consumes over 5 % of NHS budget (Hargreaves 2003). In England alone the cost of schizophrenia was estimated to be around £6.7 billion in 2004/2005, with approximately two billion being spent on direct costs (Mangalore and Knapp 2007). In Canada, the economic burden of schizophrenia was estimated to be $2,035 billion for the year 2004 (Goeree et al. 2005). In essence, schizophrenia is a costly disorder particularly that it generally has an early onset in life and requires indefinite clinical, social, and economic support, not to mention the person and family

A.G. Awad (✉)
Department of Psychiatry, The Institute of Medical Science, University of Toronto,
Toronto, ON, Canada
e-mail: gawad@hrh.ca

Lakshmi N.P. Voruganti, MD, Msc, PhD
Department of Psychiatry, Oakville-Trafalgar Memorial Hospital,
3001 Hospital Gate, Oakville, ON L6M 0L8, Canada
e-mail: doctor@voruganti.net

© Springer International Publishing Switzerland 2016
A.G. Awad, L.N.P. Voruganti (eds.), *Beyond Assessment of Quality of Life in Schizophrenia*, DOI 10.1007/978-3-319-30061-0_12

sufferings, which are difficult to put a value on. Though estimates of costs vary among various studies, as well as among different countries, depending on methodology of computing costs, as well as the rigor of the survey itself, it is generally accepted that the cost is high. Over the past decade, in the face of continually escalating health costs, governments and health providers have put caps on health services, psychiatric and mental health services not excluded. Additionally, there has been increasing pressures to demonstrate cost-effectiveness of various approaches in management, with the objective, if not actual cost reduction, of at least attaining cost containment. Though antipsychotic medications, which evolved over the past 60 years as the cornerstone of clinical management in schizophrenia, cost less than 5 % of the direct costs (Knapp 1997), the recent introduction of the relatively expensive second wave of antipsychotics that started in the late 1990s has ignited a major pharmacoeconomics debate of whether the higher acquisition costs of the new antipsychotics translate to more improvement and less side effects which in the long run may reduce the overall direct costs. It is recognized that hospitalization is the most expensive component of direct costs, which means that slowing down hospitalization rates can cut direct costs considerably.

12.1 Antipsychotic Medications and Their Role in Clinical Management

The antipsychotic chlorpromazine is hailed as the first and effective antipsychotic, as it got introduced in the early 1950s. The introduction of chlorpromazine and subsequent development of similar antipsychotics have ushered in a new era in the management of psychotic conditions, including schizophrenia, and facilitated restructuring of psychiatric and mental health systems. It allowed for shifting of clinical care from hospital to the community, ushering in the deinstitutionalization movement. Many mental hospitals were closed or downsized, as the care shifted to the community that had not been prepared to receive many of the precipitously discharged patients. Families also frequently assumed care of their relatives, which added a significant burden on families and caregivers. Although the introduction of chlorpromazine and other antipsychotics has been in some way revolutionary, patients frequently paid a high price, in terms of side effects; some of them were more than inconvenience as they produced irreversible neurological symptoms. Additionally, antipsychotic medications, though proven effective in the management of positive symptoms such as agitation or delusions, were not effective in a broad range of other symptoms, including deficit and negative symptoms such as apathy, social withdrawal, as well as impairment of cognitive functioning (Awad et al. 1995). It was not until 40 years later that another generation of antipsychotics was developed and introduced for practice. The second generation of antipsychotics was marketed as superior and better tolerated by patients, yet similarly proved to be not effective against the broad range of other symptoms, such as negative symptoms and cognitive impairment. Though their side effects were generally better than the old medications, they contributed their own side effects, such as significant weight gain and impairment of neuroendocrine functions including higher rates of diabetes, which constituted a public health problem (Ohlsen et al. 2008). Yet, the cost of the new antipsychotics proved to be much higher, relative to the very low cost of the old antipsychotics, particularly that pharmacy budgets for schizophrenia were computed for a long time at the far cheaper cost of the old medications. That is where the debate still continues about whether the benefits of the new antipsychotics are worth the cost (Lieberman et al. 2005; Jones et al. 2006; Ohlsen et al. 2008; Geddes et al. 2000; Leucht et al. 2003).

12.2 Cost-Effectiveness of Antipsychotic Medications

In our publication in 1995, responding to the question about how to define the aim of antipsychotic medications, what are they and are they being achieved, we identified them as: efficacy without adverse effects, improved quality of life, cost-effectiveness, and positive long-term outcomes such as improved functional and social functioning (Awad et al. 1995). In essence, as we have argued over the years, the optimal outcome in the treatment of schizophrenia, in addition to symptom improvement, has to include improvement in quality of life as well as aspects of functioning, particularly social functioning (Awad and Voruganti 2004, 2013). This constitutes a significant conceptual shift from just symptom improvement to a broader aspect of improved functioning (Awad and Voruganti 2012, 2013). As it soon became clear in the early years after the introduction of the first antipsychotic, chlorpromazine, antipsychotic medications were not capable of improving functioning alone, but at best made it possible for patients to benefit from other psychosocial and vocational approaches that can influence functioning. In essence, raising the quality of life and the level of functioning for patients with schizophrenia requires different approaches in addition to medication, such as rehabilitation, living assistance, and socioeconomic support, all of which lead to higher costs, at least, in the initial stages (Awad and Voruganti 1999). It is clear that the higher level of quality of life attained by treatment has a more likelihood that persons with schizophrenia will become productive members of society, reasonably integrated into their communities. The alternative will be frequent relapses, expensive hospitalizations, and crisis intervention services, which will significantly increase the cost. In other words, the most cost-effective treatment is the one that brings about the highest level of quality of life. As health-related quality of life has become the ideal of modern medicine, improvement in quality of life can serve all the players in the healthcare system: patients and their families, clinicians, service providers, and, eventually, the society at large. Therefore, the most optimal approach in cost-effectiveness is a model that can combine assessment of quality of life as well as costs, such as the cost-utility analysis which represents an example of the usefulness of the construct of quality of life and its application in pharmacoeconomics studies.

12.3   Cost-Utility Analysis in Schizophrenia

Cost-utility analysis has been increasingly used in health economic evaluations as the approach is grounded on well-defined economics and theory of decision-making under uncertainty (von Neuman and Morgenstern 1944; Torrence 1986). It elicits individuals' preferences for a particular health status, based on their quality of life. In other words, utility measurement could be viewed as an alternative means of appraising the quality of life of individuals suffering from chronic illnesses such as schizophrenia. Utility measurement traditionally involves two steps: identifying the different health states experienced by individuals during the course of their illness and assigning them numerical values, which are known as utilities (Drummond et al. 1987; Drummond and Davies 1991). It is clear that the use of utility measures in clinical populations requires a good degree of cooperation and cognitive intactness, as it involves critical self-appraisal, comparative evaluation, abstract thinking, and making trade-offs, as well as assigning numerical values to health states. Cognitive demands imposed by these tasks may pose significant challenges for individuals with severe mental disorder which left clinicians being skeptical about the applicability of cost-utility analysis in mental disorders. On the other hand, such skepticism has not been shared by many other clinicians as well as health economists, who believed in the reliability and validity of such an approach in dealing with clinical and policy-relevant questions (Revicki et al. 1996). A number of researchers have managed to apply utility measurement approaches as a method of quantifying health status and quality of life (Chouinard and Albright 1997; Revicki et al. 1996). These attempts, though exploratory in nature, were innovative, leaving a scope for developing alternative methods for eliciting health utilities in schizophrenia.

12.4   Feasibility of Utility Approaches in Schizophrenia

In an effort to clarify such issues, we undertook a large feasibility study of assessing health utilities in schizophrenia (Voruganti et al. 2000; Awad and Voruganti 1999). Our study examined the feasibility and psychometric aspects of obtaining accurate health state descriptions and their utilities from symptomatic, but stable, patients with schizophrenia. The study used a cross-sectional case-controlled design that included 120 clinically stable patients with schizophrenia and a control group of 32 treated and recovered patients with major depression. The objectives of the study were to explore a number of questions: Can patients with schizophrenia recall and describe various health states experienced during the course of their illness, can patients with schizophrenia judge various health states and assign them reliable and valid values, does performance of patients with schizophrenia vary from that of other patients with major depression, can the severity of symptoms and the degree of insight affect the reliability and validity of the utility rating, how far do the patients' utility ratings concur with their clinicians' utility ratings, and, finally, how far do the ratings obtained from traditional quality of life measures correlate with the utility values derived from such new techniques?

Methodologically, we based the appraisal and assignment of utility values to health states, the choice of utility measurements, and the techniques used on four premises defined a priori. Firstly, all different health states associated with schizophrenia are considered to be chronic and better than death. Secondly, patients themselves are deemed to be the most suitable judges of their own health state. Our reason for such a choice is that it would be difficult for anyone without schizophrenia to approximate the experience of living with hallucinations and delusions, an experience which is hard for non-schizophrenia proxies to fully appreciate. Thirdly, global quality of life measures were used, since little is known about the key determinants of quality of life in schizophrenia. Fourthly, traditional measures of quality of life in schizophrenia were also used to cross-validate the utility values obtained.

Conventional methods of utility measures were chosen: magnitude estimation (ME), rating scale (RS), standard gamble (SG), time trade-off (TTO), and willingness to pay (WTP). These measures developed by health economists combine quality and quantity of life to drive quality-adjusted life-years (QALYs) (Von Neuman and Morgenstern 1947; Drummond et al. 1987; Froberg and Kane 1989a, b, c; Revicki et al. 1996, 1997).

Our results revealed that patients with schizophrenia, compared with control patients with depression, were able to distinguish and describe the specified health states with an equal degree of ease and accuracy (Table 12.1). Scores obtained from visual analogue ratings ranging between 1 and 10, about aspects of feasibility of

Table 12.1 Feasibility aspects of utility measurement

Criterion	ME	RS	SG	TTO	WTP
Clarity of test procedure					
Schizophrenia group	9.38	9.63	4.32	9.38	9.17
Depression group	10.0	9.96	6.57	9.96	9.95
Cognitive burden					
Schizophrenia group	6.47	8.61	3.47	7.56	7.38
Depression group	8.45	9.51	5.58	8.57	8.50
Self-rated accuracy					
Schizophrenia group	5.5.6	8.73	6.78	8.35	8.10
Depression group	5.98	9.93	7.89	9.92	9.90
Interviewers' global ratings					
Schizophrenia group	3.26	8.78	3.56	8.43	8.12
Depression group	4.58	9.93	4.78	9.92	9.90

Reprinted from reference: (Voruganti et al. 2000). Permission granted by Springer
Scores obtained from visual analogue ratings, ranging between 1 and 10, with 1 representing the most difficult and 10 representing the least
Values are means
ME magnitude estimation, *RS* rating scale, *SG* standard gamble, *TTO* time trade-off, *WTP* willingness to pay

utility measurements such as clarity of test procedure, showed patients with schizophrenia scores were comparable to those obtained from the control sample of depressed patients. Similarly, cognitive burden was rated between both groups as generally similar, though the group with schizophrenia experienced more difficulty on specific tasks, i.e., magnitude estimation and standard gamble; both were eventually dropped from the protocol. It is possible that both tasks were perceived as difficult and likely related to the well-recognized aversion of patients with schizophrenia to risk-taking. In essence, "rating scales," "time trade-off," and "willingness to pay" approaches emerged as the favored methods of utility evaluation in our sample of patients with schizophrenia. The test-retest reliability of utility ratings ($r = 0.87$–0.97; $p < 0.001$) was high (Table 12.2). Additionally, convergent validity of utility measures and standard measures of quality of life proved to be significant (Table 12.3). We also found that reliability and validity of patients' appraisals were unaffected by severity of symptoms or insight. Since we only included in our sample symptomatic but stable patients, the applicability of such an approach to acutely ill or chronically deteriorated subjects is not known. One interesting finding was that patients' and proxies' ratings of patients' health significantly concurred in situations when the proxy (in our study the nurse-clinician) was familiar with the patient. The implication of such observation is that the patients themselves are more accurate in judging and assigning utilities rather than using surrogates, which add to the meaning of real "preference-based evaluation."

Though our results may have dispelled the prevailing skepticism among some researchers, that patients with schizophrenia are generally unable to participate in preference-based evaluation, however, in reviewing the literature, so far there have been very few studies using or refining the utility analysis approach. We believe that utility evaluation involves a dynamic interaction between the rater and the subject and demands an active participation on behalf of the patients. In our feasibility

Table 12.2 Test-retest reliability coefficients for the study subjects with schizophrenia and control patients with treated depression

Health states	RS	TTO	WTP
Worst health state (H_w)			
Schizophrenia group	0.87*	0.97*	0.91*
Depression group	0.66*	0.89*	0.90*
Current health state (H_c)			
Schizophrenia group	0.89*	0.86*	0.93*
Depression group	0.88*	0.98*	0.97*
Most desired health status in future (H_f)			
Schizophrenia group	1.00	1.00	0.93*
Depression	1.00	1.00	0.94*

Reprinted from reference: (Voruganti et al. 2000). Permission granted by Springer
Values indicate Pearson's product-moment correlation coefficients
RS rating scale, *TTO* time trade-off, *WTP* willingness to pay
*$p < 0.001$

Table 12.3 Intercorrelations between quality of life and utility measures (for the current health state) [schizophrenia group]

	RS	TTO	WTP	SG	SIP	QLS	GAF	Gurin's
RS	1.00	0.67*	0.002	0.73*	0.29*	0.17	0.06	0.71*
RRO		1.00	0.09	0.74*	0.12	0.03	0.01	0.47*
WTP			1.00	0.09	0.26*	0.05	0.29*	0.01
SG				1.00	0.41*	0.64*	0.58*	0.41*
SIP					1.00	0.28*	0.34*	0.24*
QLS						1.00	0.76*	0.04
GAF							1.00	0.05
Gurin's								1.00

Reprinted from reference: (Voruganti et al. 2000). Permission granted by Springer
GAF Global Scale of Adaptive Functioning, *Gurin's* Gurin's quality of life scale, *QLS* Quality of Life Scale, *RS* rating scale, *SG* standard gamble, *SIP* Sickness Impact Profile, *TTO* time trade-off, *WTP* willingness to pay
*$p < 0.001$

study, patients felt empowered and appreciated that their opinions were included, which likely has contributed to improved motivation. On the other hand, utility measures demand time and certain expertise. Unfortunately, utility analysis does not provide a profile of quality of life, but instead establishes a numerical score to be used for comparisons. Such a numerical score may not prove very useful in planning treatment approaches, since clinicians need to know the profile of the individual's strengths and weaknesses, in order to develop corrective measures. On the other hand, it seems that the utility approach is more suited for health economic evaluations in the course of resource allocation (see Chap. 13 by Holloway and Carson). In our programmatic comparisons it is clear that utility analysis can be a difficult concept, particularly for clinicians as the results are often expressed in a language not familiar to clinicians, which can impede rather than facilitate communication. Challenges to using this approach lies in getting clinicians and health economists to understand each other's language and in being able to translate utility analysis results into meaningful information for clinical decision-making. Compared to assessment of individual quality of life, which relates to the particular individual, utility analysis seems likely more applicable to the assessment of health value, from a societal perspective. Nevertheless, we believe the utility approach is attractive and worth further exploration, and refinement, as it appears feasible at least among the group of stable patients with schizophrenia. It is one of the very few cost-effectiveness approaches that combines appraisal of quality of life and cost. It can provide a tool in outcomes studies as well as in clinical trials that involve patients with schizophrenia. On the other hand, we share a cautious note with Hansen et al. (2006): "…caution should be exercised when reviewing pharmacoeconomics data, as results indicate that serious discrepancies can occur between different methods of analysis." We support the authors' conclusion about the need for standardized pharmacoeconomics models.

12.5   Summary

This chapter reviews our feasibility studies of applying utility concepts to schizophrenia as an approach of combining quality of life and cost analysis. Based on our data, we argue that stable patients with schizophrenia are able to participate with a reasonable degree of ease in preference-based evaluations. The test-retest reliability of utility ratings was high, and also convergent validity of utility measures and standard measures of quality of life was shown to be significant. Unfortunately, utility measures do not provide a profile of quality of life and seem to be more suited to the assessment of health from a broad societal perspective. It requires close collaboration between clinicians and health economists in understanding each other's language as well as refining the concept, to enhance its use in clinical situations.

References

Awad AG, Voruganti LNP. Cost-utility analysis in schizophrenia. J Clin Psychiatry. 1999;60 Suppl 3:22–9.

Awad AG, Voruganti LNP. Impact of atypical antipsychotics on quality of life in patients with schizophrenia. CNS Drugs. 2004;18:877–93.

Awad AG, Voruganti LNP. Measuring quality of life in patients with schizophrenia – an update. Pharmacoeconomics. 2012;30:183–95.

Awad AG, Voruganti LNP. The impact of newer antipsychotics on patient-reported outcomes in schizophrenia. CNS Drugs. 2013;27:625–36.

Awad AG, Voruganti LNP, Heselgrave RJ. The aim of antipsychotic medications: what are they and are they being achieved? CNS Drugs. 1995;4:8–16.

Chouinard G, Albright P. Economic and health state utility determinations for schizophrenic patients treated with Risperidone or haloperidol. J Clin Psychopharmacol. 1997;17:298–307.

Davies LM, Drummond MF. The economic burden of schizophrenia. Psychiatr Bull. 1990;14:522–5.

Drummond MF, Davies L. Economic analysis alongside clinical trials, 1991. Int J Technol Assess Health Care. 1991;7:4561–73.

Drummond M, Stoddart G, Torrence G. Cost-utility analysis. In: Methods for the economic evaluation of health care programs. Oxford: Oxford Medical Publications; 1987. p. 113–38.

Froberg D, Kane R. Methodology for measuring health state preferences I measurement strategy. J Clin Epidemiol. 1989a;42:345–54.

Froberg D, Kane R. Methodology for measuring health state preferences II scaling methods. J Clin Epidemiol. 1989b;42:459–71.

Froberg D, Kane R. Methodology for measuring health state preferences III population and context effects. J Clin Epidemiol. 1989c;42:585–92.

Geddes J, Freemantle N, Harrison P, Bebbington P. Atypical antipsychotics in the treatment of schizophrenia: systemic overview and motor-regression analysis. BMJ. 2000;321:1371–6.

Goeree R, O'Brien BJ, Goering P, Blackhouse G, Agro K, Rhodes A, Watson J. The economic burden of schizophrenia in Canada. Can J Psychiatry. 1999;44:464–72.

Goeree R, Farahati F, Burke N, Blackhouse G, O-Reilly D, Pyne J, Tarride JE. The economic burden of schizophrenia in Canada 2004. Curr Med Res Opin. 2005;21:2017–28.

Hansen K, Toumi M, Francois C, Launois R. Pharmacoeconomic modelling in schizophrenia: trap or support for decision makers? Eur J Health Econ. 2006;7:19–29.

Hargreaves S. NICE guidelines address social aspects of schizophrenia. BMJ. 2003;29:326.

Jones PE, Barnes TR, Davies L, Dunn G, Lloyd H, Hayhurst K, Murray R, Markwick A, Lewis SW. Randomized controlled trial of the effect on quality of life of second- vs first generation drugs in schizophrenia: cost utility of the latest antipsychotic drugs in schizophrenia study (CUtLASS). Arch Gen Psychiatry. 2006;63:179–1087.

Knapp M. Costs of schizophrenia. Br J Psychiatry. 1997;171:509–18.

Leucht S, Wahelbeck K, Hamman J, Kissling W. New generation antipsychotics vs low-potency conventional antipsychotics: a systematic review and meta-analysis. Lancet. 2003;36:1581–9.

Lieberman JA, Stroup TS, McEvoy JP, Swartz MS, Rosenheck RA, Perkins DO, Keefe RS, Davis SM, Davis CE, Lebowitz DB, Severe J, Hsiao JK. Clinical antipsychotic trials of intervention effectiveness (CATIE) investigators effectiveness of antipsychotic drugs in patients with schizophrenia. N Engl J Med. 2005;22:1209–23.

Mangalore R, Knapp M. Cost of schizophrenia in England. J Ment Health Policy Econ. 2007;10:231–48.

Ohlsen R, Taylor D, Tandon K, Aitehison KJ. Returning to the issue of the cost-effectiveness of antipsychotics in the treatment of schizophrenia. Clin Neuropsychiatry. 2008;5:184–94.

Revicki D, Shakespeare A, Kind P. Preferences for schizophrenia-related health states: a comparison of patients, care givers and psychiatrists. Int Clin Psychopharmacol. 1996;11:101–8.

Revicki D, Brown RE, Keller M. Cost-effectiveness of new antidepressants compared with tricyclic antidepressants in managed care settings. J Clin Psychiatry. 1997;58:47–58.

Torrence GW. Measurement of health state utilities for economic appraisal. J Health Econ. 1986;5:1–30.

Von Neuman J, Morgenstern O. Theory of games and economic behaviour. Princeton: Princeton University Press; 1947.

Voruganti LNP, Awad AG, Oyewumi LK, Corfese L, Zirul S, Dhawan R. Assessing health utilities in schizophrenia – a feasibility study. Pharmacoeconomics. 2000;17:273–86.

Wu EQ, Brinbaum HG, Shi L, Ball DE, Kessler RC, Moulis M, Aggarwal J. The economic burden of schizophrenia in the United States 2002. J Clin Psychiatry. 2005;66:1122–9.

Chapter 13
Health-Related Quality of Life in Schizophrenia: Health Policy and Resource Allocation

Frank Holloway and Jerome Carson

13.1 Introduction

Imagine being a senior person within your Ministry of Health, responsible for recommending decisions about how scarce resources are allocated. You are aware of the zeitgeist that supports improving the quality of life and well-being of all citizens – what government does not publicly want the quality of life of its citizens to improve? This chapter attempts to review how the QoL construct may influence the decisions you recommend about spending on mental health care and more specifically treatment of people living with schizophrenia.

There are important contextual points. Mental health spending as a proportion of total health spending varies markedly between countries. It is both absolutely and proportionately much less in very poor countries and sharply increases as countries move into the 'high-income' category in terms of GDP (WHO 2015). In wealthy countries, mental health spending decreased following the economic downturn of 2008. The worldwide growth in the numbers of older people, with their inevitably increasing health and social care needs, presents enormous challenges to the health and social care infrastructure of all countries. Economic uncertainty and demographic change make the argument for investment in treatment for schizophrenia ever more difficult.

F. Holloway, FRCPsych (✉)
Emeritus Consultant Psychiatrist, South London and Maudsley NHS Foundation Trust, Beckenham, UK

Maudsley Hospital, Denmark Hill, London SE5 8AZ, UK
e-mail: f.holloway1@googlemail.com

J. Carson
Professor of Psychology, School of Education and Psychology, University of Bolton, Bolton BL3 5AB, UK
e-mail: j.carson@bolton.ac.uk

13.2   Understanding Quality of Life

Quality of life is a notoriously difficult concept. In a detailed assessment of two widely used measures of HRQoL, the EQ-5D (Brooks 1996) and the SF-36® (Ware and Sherbourne 1992), Brazier et al. (2014) identify no less than six overlapping approaches to the measurement of QoL.

1. *Objective indicators* relate to income, living conditions, access to resources and participation in occupational and social roles.
2. *Need satisfaction* is based on Maslow's hierarchy of needs, from the most basic human needs to higher-order needs such as 'self-actualisation'.
3. *Subjective well-being* can be either current hedonic state – 'happiness' – or reflect overall life satisfaction and satisfaction within particular life domains.
4. *Psychological well-being* includes constructs such as morale, self-esteem, self-efficacy and a sense of autonomy and control.
5. *Health-related QoL* (HRQoL) has been defined as 'A person's subjective perception of the impact of health status, including disease and treatment, on physical, psychological and social functioning and well-being' (Bowling 2002). The English National Institute for Health and Care Excellence (NICE) provides an alternative definition: 'A combination of a person's physical, mental and social well-being' (NICE 2013).
6. *Capability* is an approach developed by the welfare economist Amartya Sen. It focuses on what people are actually able to do in order to achieve outcomes that they value. In this model poverty, ignorance and oppression result in capability deprivation (Sen 1993).

Each approach has generated a large literature and has been subject to significant criticism (Brazier et al. 2014). All have had an impact on the discourse surrounding QoL and mental health policy and practice.

13.3   Quality of Life and Health Economics

Sen's capability approach is a reaction to traditional ways that economists assess value in order to inform public policy. The currently dominant paradigm is that of 'utility', which is a measure of the strength of the preferences an individual would have about a particular outcome and the test of this utility against the cost of an intervention or activity. The concept of utility underlies a cost-benefit analysis (CBA)[1] or cost-effectiveness analysis (CEA)[2] that might be undertaken to justify a particular course of policy action.

[1] Cost-benefit analysis may be defined as a systematic process for calculating and comparing benefits and costs of a project, decision or government policy.
[2] Cost-effectiveness analysis is a form of economic analysis that compares the relative costs and outcomes of two or more courses of action.

Within health care, the measure of utility recommended by many agencies is the QUALY (quality-adjusted life year). This is calculated by multiplying survival in life years with the 'utility' associated with a particular health state. Full health rates as 1 and death rates at 0. Given appropriate outcome and cost data, the health benefit of an intervention (e.g. a hip replacement or coronary bypass operation) in terms of QUALYs and the costs of the intervention per QUALY gained can be calculated. In principle, one could choose to do 'x' instead of 'y' because 'x' provided more QUALYs per unit cost within an overall ambition to use scarce resources to maximise health gain.

This allows comparison between chalk and cheese: 'x' might be psychological therapy for mild depression and 'y' might be surgical treatment for varicose veins. In England, the cost per QUALY is used as a limiting factor in decisions by the NICE as to whether to recommend a particular health-care intervention for general use within the NHS. Acceptable cost per QUALY is currently £30,000 (NICE 2013) – at the time of writing roughly US$45,000.

The EQ-5D and the SF-36® are 'preference-based' measures of QoL designed to be generally applicable to health status. They elicit patient responses to a set of questions about health status, including mental health and functioning. Changes in health status as a result of an intervention can be assessed. Then, using research data on the preferences of a panel of respondents, a particular QUALY rating can be allocated to a score on the change in the HRQoL measure. Change scores can be used to calculate the costs per QUALY gained by any intervention that is evaluated using one of these 'preference-based' measures. The EQ-5D is the measure preferred by NICE to generate QUALYs for the purpose of the cost-effectiveness analysis of a health technology (NICE 2013).

13.4   Quality of Life in Mental Health Care

One of the major aims of deinstitutionalization was to improve the quality of life of people living with severe mental illness (Marcheschi et al. 2015). We have previously argued that in the context of mental health services QoL is best understood in terms of two dimensions (Holloway and Carson 2002). The first is objective life conditions, such as income, housing, family support and employment (**1** in the Brazier typology). The second is subjective assessment of QoL both overall (Global Subjective Quality of Life) and within particular life domains that include those readily measured 'objectively' and the person's perspective on their physical and mental health (**3** in the Brazier typology). Subjective QoL is now widely used as an outcome measure in studies of specific treatments and service structures in mental health (Marcheschi et al. 2015). All those using the construct of subjective QoL as applied to severe mental illness are following in the footsteps of Lehman's (1988) groundbreaking work. There is a well-recognised and troubling problem that people with schizophrenia report rather better subjective QoL than would be expected given their objective life conditions. It is also abundantly evident that subjective QoL is strongly influenced by mood state (Saarni et al. 2010).

The application of HRQoL (**5** in the Brazier typology) as applied to schizophrenia is explored in detail elsewhere in this book (see Chap. 2 Voruganti and Awad; Chap. 3 Awad and Voruganti; Chap. 4 Voruganti and Awad; Chap. 11 Karow). There is very significant concern that the available generic 'preference-based' HRQoL measures, such as the EQ-5D and the SF-36®, do not well reflect the health outcomes of people with a mental illness, particularly severe mental illnesses such as schizophrenia (Brazier 2010; Saarni et al. 2010). In principle, this may disadvantage mental health problems in decisions on the allocation of resources for health care.

13.5 The Impact of Schizophrenia

Schizophrenia has very significant effects on the sufferer, their family and society at large. These go far beyond the experience of the particular symptoms (positive and negative psychotic symptoms, thought disorder, mood disorder) that tend to be the focus of interest of psychiatrists. Long-term impairment in functioning is common. Physical health is often poor and mortality rates are substantially increased. People with a diagnosis of schizophrenia experience marked impacts on their social networks (which are smaller and nonreciprocal), intimate relationships, employment, finances and housing. Unemployment and homelessness are much commoner than in the general population. Unemployment results in poverty. These are all 'objective' indicators of QoL. People with a diagnosis of schizophrenia are much more likely to become victims of crime and exploitation and somewhat more likely to be perpetrators, particularly of violence. Carers experience significant impacts on their lives both emotionally and practically.

The extensive societal costs associated with schizophrenia (and indeed all other mental disorders) can be presented in a variety of ways. Health economists have calculated the very substantial monetary costs associated with the illness. These include not only the direct costs of health and social care, social security payments and the costs of informal care but also broader impacts on society in terms of lost productivity and excess mortality (Knapp et al. 2004: Andrews et al. 2012).

An alternative approach in measuring health impacts is the DALY (disability-adjusted life year), which can be defined as 'The sum of years of potential life lost due to premature mortality and the years of productive life lost due to disability'. DALYs have been used by the World Health Organization to calculate the global burden of disease (WHO 2008). Neurological, mental and substance misuse disorders (NMS) contribute a third of the global burden in both high-income and low- and middle-income countries, with schizophrenia worldwide being the third most significant NMS disorder after unipolar depression and alcohol use disorders. Because of Europe's ageing population, schizophrenia contributes proportionately less to the burden of disease in terms of DALYs and falls lower down the ranking of NMS disorders (Wittchen et al. 2010). The global burden data provides a powerful argument for the investment of resources into the treatment of NMS conditions and research into more effective treatments (Collins et al. 2011). Mental health care loses out both in terms of allocated health budget and, even more so, research funding, compared with other contributors to the global burden of disease.

13.6 Measuring Economic Performance and Social Progress

The traditional measure of the health of an economy is the gross domestic product (GDP) – 'the monetary value of all the finished goods and services produced within a country's borders in a specific time period'. GDP figures make headlines and preoccupy politicians. There is growing belief that GDP on its own is inadequate. A report by the Commission on the Measurement of Economic Performance and Social Progress (CMEPSP), which was co-authored by Joseph Stiglitz and Amartya Sen, concluded that '… conventional, market-based measures of income, wealth and consumption are insufficient to assess human well-being' (Stiglitz et al. 2009 pg 144).

This has resulted in increasing interest in the use of measures of quality of life and well-being as an alternative or complement to GDP (Grasso and Canova 2007; Stiglitz et al. 2009; Bache 2013; O'Donnell et al. 2014). The English Department of Health (2014c) offered a number of arguments for giving priority to well-being in policy formulation. Subjective well-being has not changed in the UK over the past 40 years despite marked economic growth. GDP does not measure everything that is important in measuring social progress and indeed includes things that actually decrease well-being (such as the costs of commuting or cleaning up an oil spill!). It is also clear from international comparators there are diminishing returns to well-being from growth in GDP.

In the UK, the Office for National Statistics (ONS) now measures national well-being (ONS 2015). This is a complex task that is fraught with conceptual and methodological difficulty. ONS includes 43 indicators that assess ten dimensions of well-being: personal well-being, our relationships, health, what we do, where we live, personal finance, the economy, education and skills, governance (essentially participation in the democratic process) and the natural environment. The ONS assessment includes both objective and subjective indicators. For example, the 'health' domain includes both life expectancy and satisfaction with one's health. Personal well-being, rated in four ways, is entirely dependent on the ratings of subjective response to questions or questionnaires – including ratings of quality of life and life satisfaction. Subjective well-being is assessed by the answers to four questions that were initially proposed by researchers at the London School of Economics (Dolan and Metcalfe 2012): (1). *Overall, how satisfied are you with your life nowadays?* (2). *Overall, to what extent do you feel the things you do in your life are worthwhile?* (3). *Overall, how happy did you feel yesterday?* (4). *Overall, how anxious did you feel yesterday?*

The ten ONS dimensions of national well-being are strikingly similar to those adopted by CMEPSP (Stiglitz et al. 2009, pp 14–15) and the 'social indicators' approach (Grasso and Canova 2007). However, the 'social indicators' approach, which provides a single index of QoL by country using national statistics, focuses explicitly on the 'objective' externals (what is available to people in society) rather than subjective evaluations of well-being and happiness per se. In the EU, the QoL index for member states correlates quite well with both GDP and subjective well-being (Grasso and Canova 2007).

13.7 Well-Being and Public Policy

A recent publication from ONS stated that 'The measurement of wellbeing is central to public policy... [for] 1) monitoring progress; 2) informing policy design; and 3) policy appraisal' (Dolan et al. 2011). The argument for using well-being to move beyond GDP as the metric of societal success and the monetized CBA framework for policy choice was well made in a recent report on *Well-being and Public Policy* (O'Donnell et al. 2014). The report was endorsed by, amongst others, the Managing Director of the IMF and the Secretary-General of the OECD. It was also praised by Martin Seligman, who is the leading proponent of Positive Psychology, itself one of the intellectual underpinnings of the well-being movement. The report makes a number of intriguing policy recommendations that include access to effective treatment for 'mental ill-health', addressing the developmental needs of children, improving communities, empowering citizens and fostering employment opportunities and improving well-being at work (O'Donnell et al. 2014 Ch 5).

In practice in the UK, well-being plays at best a small part in government decisions surrounding policies, programmes and projects. HM Treasury guidance (The Green Book), which is binding on government departments and agencies, requires an appraisal process that takes into account both the 'market' and 'non-market' impacts of a proposal that attach monetary values to the impacts of possible options (HM Treasury 2011). 'Non-market' impacts include health benefits, preferably measured in terms of QUALYs and costs per QUALY. Although it is acknowledged that in principle 'subjective well-being' or 'life satisfaction' could contribute to decision-making, the document expresses scepticism about incorporating well-being into the required economic analyses (HM Treasury 2011 pp 57–58).

13.8 Public Health and Public Mental Health: The English Experience

Well-being and quality of life have had an impact on public health policy in England, which emphasises the importance of promoting health and well-being (Department of Health 2010). The Public Mental Health agenda involve preventing disease, which crucially includes intervening early when problems first arise, and promoting mental health (Joint Commissioning Panel for Mental Health 2013). One of the five themes of the NHS Outcomes Framework is 'Enhancing quality of life for people with long-term conditions' (Department of Health 2014b). However, the King's Fund (2015), which is the leading health-care think-tank in the UK, concluded that 'there has been little sign that the government has taken into account the impact of its wider NHS reforms and fiscal programme on public health, despite an initial focus to give well-being an equal status with maximising economic growth'.

Well-being has had its most significant impact in the field of mental health policy. Lord Layard (one of the authors of *Well-being and Public Policy*) has been a powerful advocate of the importance to policy of promoting 'happiness' amongst citizens (see Layard 2005). He and the psychologist David Clark have been instrumental in persuading government to invest massively in a national system for Improving Access to Psychological Therapy (IAPT), which offers rapid access for people experiencing anxiety and depression to cognitive behavioural therapy (Layard and Clark 2014). IAPT offers little or no benefit to people living with schizophrenia.

13.9 The Salience of HRQoL to Health Policy

Social policy does not arise in a vacuum. It is influenced by multiple factors that include technological developments, demographic changes, the local and global financial context, political cultures and the specific ideologies espoused by politicians in power. Contingent events, such as high-profile tragedies that appear in the media, are an important policy driver. One element that is often not recognised is the body of professional opinion within a specific policy field, such as mental health care. Professionals are undoubtedly influenced by the research literature, which now includes a fair amount of evidence about the effects of specific treatments and service configurations on the QoL of patients/service users (see Chap 11, Karow).

HRQoL has its most obvious and direct impact on health policy in two spheres. The first is as an outcome measure used by regulators to inform the process of approval of treatments, particularly pharmacological treatments and in the arguments pharmaceutical companies use in seeking to market their wares. Pharmacoeconomics as applied to schizophrenia is discussed in detail elsewhere in this book as a discipline in itself and from the perspective of the pharmaceutical industry and regulators (see Chap. 15 Revicki; Chap. 12 Buller; and Chap. 13 Broich et al.).

The second and linked impact of HRQoL lies in the analytic methodologies employed to formulate clinical guidelines and appraisals of health technologies, including novel medications. We have already noted the methodology employed by NICE, which develops clinical guidelines and appraises health technologies. NICE makes explicit use of HRQoL data in formulating its recommendations (NICE 2013).

There are across the world numerous clinical guidelines relating to the treatment of schizophrenia, all of which are variations on a theme. Guidelines are guidelines and do not necessarily represent government policy, actual investment in treatments and services or clinical practice. The most recent iteration of the NICE guideline for schizophrenia (NCCMH 2014), to which service providers in England and Wales are expected to adhere, repeatedly mentions QoL, either in broad terms or in the context of HRQoL as an outcome measure. However, the guideline almost as often alludes to the promotion of 'recovery' and 'recovery-oriented services'. ('Recovery' is a complex and indeed contested term. Roberts and Wolfson (2004) provide an accessible introduction.)

13.10   Mental Health Policy and Practice

The World Health Organization recommends the development of mental health policies and plans (WHO 2009). Most countries now have a policy that is regularly updated. In Western Europe, there tend to be additional specific policies supporting the implementation of community care (Medeiros et al. 2008). In order to identify the importance of QoL for mental health policy, we reviewed policy documents from six Anglophone countries: Australia, Canada, England, Ireland, New Zealand and the USA. The status of these documents is very variable on a spectrum from the merely advisory (USA, Ireland, Canada) towards the formulation of specific government policies (England, New Zealand and Australia). What is striking about these documents is that although 'QoL', broadly defined, receives mention, the rhetoric of 'recovery' is far more prominent (see Table 13.1).

It is easy to produce a policy document. Influencing practice is another matter altogether, particularly in countries that have a federal structure, such as the USA, Canada and Australia. In the USA, health care is highly fragmented with multiple funding streams, including monies from the Federal and State Governments and payments from health insurers, and a wide array of for-profit and not-for-profit service providers. In this environment, transformation of the mental health-care system

Table 13.1 Mental health policy documents: references to 'quality of life' versus 'recovery'

	Quality of life	Recovery	Ratio
Australia[a]	1	58	1:58
Canada[b]	14	102	1:7.3
England[c]	2	15	1:7.5
Ireland[d]	18	116	1:6.4
New Zealand[e]	3	26	1:8.7
USA[f]	4	70	1:17.5

[a]Commonwealth of Australia (2009)
[b]Mental Health Commission of Canada (2012)
[c]Department of Health (2014b)
[d]Department of Health and Children (2006)
[e]Ministry of Health (2012)
[f]New Freedom Commission (2003)

is extraordinarily complex (Hogan 2008). In England, where almost all funding comes directly from the state, the Department of Health was able to use its powers of resource allocation to transform mental health services during the first decade of the twenty-first century (Appleby 2007).

Until 2012 the English Department of Health collected very detailed information on mental health spending. A series of annual reports dating back 11 years document investment in assertive outreach, crisis resolution and early onset psychosis teams and IAPT (Mental Health Strategies 2013).[3] Mental health promotion accounted for 0.05 % of total mental health spending. Investment in specialist accommodation has been substantial whilst spending on supporting people to live in their own homes was much more modest. A significant though steadily declining amount of money went to services offering activities and employment opportunities, which we know are crucial to subjective QoL.

Despite investment in specific community services, secure hospital care is the single largest item of expenditure and is increasing, as a result of factors that have nothing to do with QoL, wellness or 'recovery'.

13.11   Conclusions

Deinstitutionalisation was driven in part by concern about the quality of life of long-stay mental hospital residents. More recently, measurement of HRQoL has become a key component of decision-making by authors of clinical guidelines and medicine regulators. Well-being, one of many approaches to understanding QoL, has been promoted as an alternative to GDP in the measurement of the health of society. Health policy freely uses the rhetoric of well-being although its practical impact is far from clear. QoL appears in many national mental health policy documents but is now clearly losing out, at least in terms of rhetoric, to a newer paradigm – 'recovery'.

References

Andrews A, Knapp M, McCrone P, Parsonage M, Trachtenberg M. Effective interventions in schizophrenia the economic case: a report prepared for the Schizophrenia Commission. London: Rethink Mental Illness; 2012.
Appleby L. Mental health ten years on: progress on mental health care reform. London: Department of Health; 2007.
Bache I. Measuring quality of life for public policy: an idea whose time has come? Agenda-setting dynamics in the European Union. J Eur Public Policy. 2013;20(1):21–38.
Bowling A. Measuring health: a review of quality of life and measurement scales. Milton Keynes: Oxford University Press; 2002.

---

[3] The series ended in 2012 just as it became clear that mental health spending was decreasing in real terms.

Brazier J. Is the EQ-5D fit for purpose in mental health? Br J Psychiatry. 2010;197:348–9. doi:10.1192/bjp.bp.110.082453.

Brazier J, Connell J, Papaioannou D, Mukuria C, Mulhern B, Peasgood T, et al. A systematic review, psychometric analysis and qualitative assessment of generic preference-based measures of health in mental health populations and the estimation of mapping functions from widely used specific measures. Health Technol Assess. 2014;18(34):vii–viii, xiii–xxv, 1–188.

Brooks R. EuroQol: the current state of play. Health Policy. 1996;37(1):53–72.

Collins PY, Patel V, Joestl SS, March D, Insel TR, Daar A; on behalf of the Grand Challenges in Global Mental Health Scientific Advisory Board and Executive Committee. Grand challenges in global mental health. Nature. 2011;474(7354):27–30. PMID 21734685.

Commonwealth of Australia. Fourth national mental health plan. An agenda for collaborative government action in mental health 2009-2014. Canberra: Commonwealth of Australia; 2009.

Department of Health. Healthy lives, healthy people: our strategy for public health in England. London: Department of Health; 2010.

Department of Health. Closing the gap: priorities for essential change in mental health. London: Department of Health; 2014a.

Department of Health. The NHS outcomes framework 2015/16. London: Department of Health; 2014b.

Department of Health. Wellbeing. Why it matters to health policy. 2014c. https://www.gov.uk/government/uploads/system/uploads/attachment_data/file/277566/Narrative__January_2014_.pdf). Accessed 28 July 2015.

Department of Health and Children. A Vision for change. Report of the Expert Working group on mental health policy. Dublin: Department of Health and Children; 2006.

Dolan P, Metcalfe R. Measuring subjective wellbeing: recommendations on measures for use by national governments. J Soc Policy. 2012;41(02):409–27. doi:10.1017/S0047279411000833.

Dolan P, Layard R, Metcalfe R. Measuring subjective well-being for public policy. Newport: Office for National Statistics; 2011.

Grasso M, Canova L. An assessment of the quality of life in the European Union based on the social indicators approach. Soc Indic Res. 2007. doi:10.1007/s11205-007-9158-7.

HM Treasury. The green book. Appraisal and evaluation in central government. London: The Stationery Office; 2011. www.gov.uk/government/uploads/system/uploads/attachment_data/file/220541/green_book_complete.pdf. Accessed 14 Nov 2015.

Hogan M. Transforming mental health care: realities, priorities and prospects. Psychiatr Clin N Am. 2008;31:1–9.

Holloway F, Carson J. Quality of life in severe mental illness. Int Rev Psychiatry. 2002;14:175e184.

Joint Commissioning Panel for Mental Health. Guidance for commissioning public mental health services. 2013. http://www.jcpmh.info/wp-content/uploads/jcpmh-publicmentalhealth-guide.pdf. Accessed 14 Nov 2015

Knapp M, Mangalore R, Simon J. The global costs of schizophrenia. Schizophr Bull. 2004;30:279–93.

Layard R. Happiness. Lessons from a new science. London: Allen Lane; 2005.

Layard R, Clark DM. Thrive: the power of evidence-based psychological therapies. London: Penguin; 2014.

Lehman AF. A quality of life interview for the chronically mentally ill. Eval Program Plann. 1988;11(1):51e62.

Marcheschi E, Laike T, Brunt D, Hansson L, Johansson M. Quality of life and place attachment among people with severe mental illness. J Environ Psychol. 2015;41:145–54.

Medeiros H, McDaid D, Knapp M (2008) Shifting care from hospital to the community in Europe: economic challenges and opportunities. MHEEN II policy briefing 4. http://eprints.lse.ac.uk/4275/1/MHEEN_policy_briefs_4_Balanceofcare%28LSERO%29. pdf Accessed 3/03/16.

Mental Health Commission of Canada. Changing directions, changing lives: the mental health strategy for Canada. Calgary: Mental Health Commission of Canada; 2012.

Mental Health Strategies (2013) 2011/12 National Survey of Investment in Adult Mental Health Services. https://www.gov.uk/government/publications/investment-in-mental-health-in-2011-to-2012-working-age-adults-and-older-adults.

Ministry of Health. The mental health and addictions service development plan 2012-2017. Wellington: Ministry of Health; 2012.

National Collaborating Centre for Mental Health. Psychosis and schizophrenia in adults. The NICE guideline on treatment management. Leicester: British Psychological Association; 2014. http://www.nice.org.uk/guidance/cg178/evidence/cg178-psychosis-and-schizophrenia-in-adults-full-guideline3. Accessed 8 Aug 2015.

National Institute for Health and Care Excellence. Guide to the methods of technology appraisal. 2013. http://publications.nice.org.uk/pmg9. Accessed 28 July 2015.

New Freedom Commission on Mental Health. Achieving the promise: transforming mental health care in America. Final report. Rockville: Department of Health and Human Services; 2003. DHHS pub no SMA-03-3832.

O'Donnell G, Deaton A, Gurand M, Halpern D, Layard R. Wellbeing and policy. London: Legatum Institute; 2014.

Office for National Statistics. Measuring national wellbeing. 2015. http://www.ons.gov.uk/ons/guide-method/user-guidance/well-being/index.html. Accessed 28 July 2015.

Roberts G, Wolfson P. The rediscovery of recovery: open to all? Adv Psychiatr Treat. 2004;10:37–49.

Saarni SI, Viertio S, Perala J, Koskinen S, Lonnqvist J, Suvisaari J. Quality of life of people with schizophrenia, bipolar disorder and other psychotic disorders. Br J Psychiatry. 2010;197:386–94.

Sen AK. Capability and wellbeing. In: Nussbaum MC, Sen AK, editors. The quality of life. New York: Oxford Clarendon Press; 1993. p. 30–53.

Stiglitz JE, Sen A, Fitoussii J-P. Report by the commission on the measurement of economic performance and social progress. 2009. http://www.insee.fr/fr/publications-et-services/dossiers_web/stiglitz/doc-commission/RAPPORT_anglais.pdf. Accessed 14 Nov 2015.

The Kings Fund. Has the government delivered a new era for public health? The Kings Fund verdict. 2015. Posted April 15 2015. http://www.kingsfund.org.uk/projects/verdict. Accessed 31 July 2015.

Ware JE, Sherbourne CD. The MOS 36-item short-form health survey (SF-36): I. Conceptual framework and item selection. Med Care. 1992;30:473–83.

Wittchen HU, Jacobi F, Rehm J, et al. The size and burden of mental disorders and other disorders of the brain in Europe 2010. Eur Neuropsychopharmacol. 2010;21:655–79.

World Health Organization. The global burden of disease: 2004. Geneva: Update World Health Organisation; 2008.

World Health Organization. Improving health systems and services for mental health. Geneva: World Health Organization; 2009.

World Health Organization. Mental health atlas 2014. Geneva: World Health Organization; 2015.

Chapter 14
Beyond Assessment of Quality of Life in Schizophrenia: Cultural, Clinical, and Research Perspectives from India, a Case Study

Santosh K. Chaturvedi, M. Krishna Prasad, and Abhishek Pathak

14.1 Introduction

Schizophrenia is a complex, severe, and debilitating disorder having multifactorial causation. Quality of life (QOL) is often considered equivalent to standard of living in Indian society including the health sector. The concept of QOL is relatively recent and has become an important part of mental health care only recently, though not as popular in clinical practice as in many developed parts of the world. As sociocultural factors play a significant contribution in this concept, Indian region-related factors are bound to have an influence. Many definitions are popular among health professionals including the comprehensive definition proposed by the World Health Organization (WHO). The WHO definition includes not only a person's physical health, psychological state, level of independence, social relationships, personal beliefs, and environment, all of which are shaped by culture and value systems. Culture in this context refers to the unique behavior patterns and lifestyle shared by a group of people, which distinguish it from others (Tseng 2003a). For years, there was not enough attention on quality of life in the care of persons with schizophrenia in India. Clinical drug trials on psychotropics did not include measures of QOL and assessed only symptom remissions and reliefs. Gradually, the concept of QOL was introduced, and now, it constitutes a relevant factor in assessing the outcome of schizophrenia.

S.K. Chaturvedi, MD, FRCPsych (✉)
Department of Mental Health Education, National Institute of Mental Health & Neuro Sciences, Bangalore 560029, India

Department of Psychiatry, National Institute of Mental Health & Neuro Sciences, Bangalore 560029, India
e-mail: skchatur@gmail.com

M.K. Prasad, MD • A. Pathak, MD
Department of Psychiatry, National Institute of Mental Health & Neuro Sciences, Bangalore 560029, India

© Springer International Publishing Switzerland 2016
A.G. Awad, L.N.P. Voruganti (eds.), *Beyond Assessment of Quality of Life in Schizophrenia*, DOI 10.1007/978-3-319-30061-0_14

This chapter aims to review the perspective of the QOL of schizophrenia in India, explore the role of cultural factors on QOL and how it compares with the rest of the world and the role of clinical variables and how they influence QOL, and explore evidence-based research from India on QOL. Global burden of illness resulting from schizophrenia is monumental, yet it is greatly underrepresented in conventional government statistics in India (Solanki et al. 2010). The prevalence rate for Schizophrenia in India has been estimated to vary from 1.8 to 3.3/1000 (ICMR 1987; Reddy and Chandrashekar 1998; Ganguli 2000). Current treatment guidelines focus not only on symptomatic recovery but also on improving the functioning and quality of life of an individual.

14.2 Cultural Perspective from India

India as a nation is conglomerate of multiethnic, multicultural, and multireligious societies which exemplify unity in diversity. The anthropological survey of India had initially listed 6748 communities in India and later on went to identify and study 4635 communities in the People of India project at the field level (www.ansi.gov.in/people_india.htm). On a cultural level, however, these communities were found to have many similarities. The people of India have many religious beliefs and follow several sects, sometimes cults. More recently in the last few decades in contrast to earlier times, large-scale sociocultural change has been taking place rapidly around the globe, and these trends follow in India as well (Khandelwal et al. 2004). Culture is expected to have a patho-plastic, patho-elaborative, patho-facilitative, or patho-reactive effect on the course and development of schizophrenia. International research indicates that the symptomatology, help-seeking behavior, and course of schizophrenia are strongly influenced by cultural interpretations (Sartorius et al. 1987).

14.3 Culture and Schizophrenia in India

Cultural factors in schizophrenia have been studied in the Indian setting. The follow-up study of patients diagnosed with schizophrenia in the International Pilot Study of Schizophrenia (IPSS) showed that, in spite of clinical similarity, there were remarkable variations in course and outcome within and across different cultures and those in developing countries including Agra (India) had a better outcome than those in developed countries (Leff et al. 1992). Other studies, Determinants of Outcome of Severe Mental Disorders (DOSMeD), Madras Longitudinal study, and Study of Factors Associated with the Course and Outcome of Schizophrenia (SOFACOS), also observed the outcome to be more favorable in India (Craig et al. 1997; Thara et al. 2004; Verghese et al. 1989). QOL was not a key outcome variable measured in these, though.

The IPSS found that four symptoms, auditory hallucinations, delusions, social withdrawal, and flat affect, were common to all cultures (Leff et al. 1992). The DOSMeD study found that the symptom profile of patients was quite similar in developing and developed centers, apart from visual hallucinations being more frequent in the former and affective symptoms (mainly depression) in the latter (Craig et al. 1997). Persecutory, grandiose, and fantastic or bizarre delusions have been reported to be more common among Africans, Asians, and other non-Western people (Vishwanath and Chaturvedi 2012). Paranoid and religious contents are extremely common in non-Western cultures and are, perhaps, related to the common acceptance of magico-religious beliefs in these countries (Vishwanath and Chaturvedi 2012). Religious delusions are common in Christian societies, whereas these are rarer in Hindu, Muslim, or Buddhist societies (Chandrasena 1987). Magico-religious delusions have also been found to be greater in rural societies, especially in women >30 years of age (Vishwanath and Chaturvedi 2012). Indian studies have found first-rank symptoms (FRS) to be generally culture-free. However, there is a lower occurrence of FRS in non-Western countries (Vishwanath and Chaturvedi 2012). Chandrasena (1987) proposed that the low rates are related to the high prevalence of subcultural beliefs and delusions in non-Western cultures and their overlap with FRS. The WHO multicentric studies found that acute schizophrenic episodes and catatonic schizophrenia were the commonest subtypes in developing centers and paranoid schizophrenia in the developed ones (Leff et al. 1992; Craig et al. 1997). There are differences in the frequency of types of negative symptoms between patients in India and the United States (Chaturvedi 1986). Symptoms in schizophrenia such as not eating, not sleeping, and negative symptoms were reported to be more distressing in Indian patients, compared to aggression and positive symptoms among those from the United Kingdom (UK) (Gopinath and Chaturvedi 1992).

The QOL of Indian and Swedish patients with schizophrenia in majority of the domains was essentially the same despite the differences in culture and general standard of living. The Indian patients were not more dissatisfied than their Swedish counterparts with housing and environment including community services (Gupta et al. 1998). The Swedish patients were more dissatisfied with contacts than their Indian counterparts suggesting that the joint family system and close social ties that are prevalent in India do help to maintain contacts.

From a clinical standpoint, there is evidence to suggest that positive, negative, and cognitive deficits as well as depressive symptoms influence QOL (George et al. 1996; Dan et al. 2011; Patra and Mishra 2012; Chugh et al. 2013). In another study from eastern India (Patra and Mishra 2012), being male, unmarried, and with a higher education predicted a poorer QOL in the acute phase of schizophrenia. This study also found depression and anxiety to be strongest predictors of QOL in schizophrenia in this population. In schizophrenia patients under remission at Ranchi (Kujur et al. 2010), males had better QOL on all domains of World Health Organization Quality of Life-BREF (WHOQOL-BREF) (WHO 1996; Saxena et al. 1998), while females had higher scores on disability.

Comparison within India is highlighted by a multicentered investigation (Verghese et al. 1989) on factors associated with the course and outcome of schizophrenia. The three centers which differed in sociocultural factors – Lucknow (rural background from North India), Madras (urban patients from South India), and Vellore (semi-urban patients from South India) – had similar rates of outcome. The best clinical outcome was seen in about 45 % of patients at the 2-year follow-up. About 40 % showed good occupational adjustment and 34 % good social interaction. About 66 % of patients showed a good overall outcome. At 2-year follow-up, the course and outcome were similar in the three centers, except Madras, where it was slightly worse, maybe due to being more urban than other centers.

There have been many explanations about the reasons for the differences in symptomatology, favorable outcome, and QOL. It has been proposed that a low level of linguistic competence, as in cultures such as in India, leaves anxiety unbound in the initial stages of schizophrenia, causing catatonic symptoms and less elaborate delusions (Kulhara and Chakrabarti 2001). The exact nature of social, cultural, or environmental factors contributing to the better outcome in developing countries has been the subject of much debate. Effects of industrialization, differences in physical environment or family atmosphere, have all been considered as responsible factors. The support available from extended families in India perhaps protect from the deleterious effects of schizophrenia (Kulhara and Chakrabarti 2001). However, the effects of sociocultural changes in the last few decades, like urbanization, industrialization, and globalization, may become apparent and may have narrowed the differences then by changing social frameworks (families becoming nuclear and losing the protection offered by joint and extended families) and by altering environmental factors (because of improved perinatal care, those with insults in utero may survive, i.e., those who are going to have the worst outcomes).

Factors such as existence of joint families, sharing of income within these families, lack of emphasis on education, and low priority to leisure have been offered to explain the differences in QOL of patients with schizophrenia in India when compared to developed countries (Gupta et al. 1998; Lobana et al. 2001). In India, a significant degree of social support is offered by extended family such as parents, brothers, sisters, and their families sometimes across generations. The family is also more aware of the patient's problems than in Western cultures (Lobana et al. 2001). Another factor that may contribute to the differences in QOL when compared to the developed world is the consideration of marriage as a sacred union in India and societal norms expecting the spouse, more commonly the wife, to take care of the sick partner at significant personal cost and suffering (Lobana et al. 2001).

14.4   Stigma and Quality of Life in India

Schizophrenia has been associated with poor QOL and negative self-concept when there is high perceived stigma (Rai et al. 2014). Stigma is reported to be related to the cultural features of illness-related experience and behavior in people suffering from schizophrenia in Bangalore, India (Loganathan and Murthy 2008). Both men and women experience stigma in India; the subjective experiences and the social roles through which it is experienced differ by gender and sociocultural context (Loganathan and Murthy 2011). This difference in emphasis is expected, considering the customary gender roles and life trajectories in India. Men experience stigma in relation to their work roles and occupational functioning, while women experience stigma more in their marital life and functioning, during pregnancy and childbirth. Men with schizophrenia reported not disclosing their illness to others, staying unmarried, experiencing shame and ridicule, and worrying about what others thought of them (Loganathan and Murthy 2011). On the other hand, in traditional rural and religious places, persons with mental illnesses are considered special and chosen one by God and provided alms and food, especially in the temples, dargahs, and religious places.

14.5 Drug-Related Issues and Quality of Life

The impact on QOL of atypical antipsychotics has had an amusing trajectory. The first few years of introduction of olanzapine saw thin emaciated patients put on weight, much to the surprise and relief of their relatives. This was viewed as a factor leading to a good quality of life; however, as years went by, people realized the ill effects of obesity and metabolic syndromes. Atypical antipsychotics have demonstrated a broader efficacy profile and better tolerability pattern than conventional ones but results concerning their greater benefits in improving the quality of life of schizophrenic patients are controversial at present (Bobes et al. 2007). The impact of extrapyramidal symptoms on the quality of life of schizophrenic patients remains unclear. Other side effects, such as weight gain and sexual dysfunction, have been shown to be negatively associated with quality of life (Bobes et al. 2007). There were no significant differences between antipsychotics (77 % were on atypical antipsychotics) when quality of life was an outcome measure in one study (Shrivastava et al. 2012). In another study, electroconvulsive therapy (ECT) led to not only symptomatic improvement but also significant improvement of QOL (Garg et al. 2011). One reason why ECT is still a popular method of treatment in India and is acceptable to patients and families is the rapid improvement in mental health, recovery, and regaining their quality of life.

Ethnic differences in pharmacokinetics and pharmacodynamics are well documented. It is now well recognized that differences in the distribution of polymorphic variants of cytochromes P450 (CYP) enzymes exist between different ethnic groups (Tseng 2003b). These differences will influence both effects and side effects caused by antipsychotic drugs, therefore impacting the QOL differentially across ethnicities. Cultural beliefs may also influence the general attitude to taking drugs, labeling, and reporting of both therapeutic and adverse effects. They thus have a significant influence on compliance and may influence quality of life. "English" (allopathic) medicines may be viewed as being more potent than traditional Ayurvedic ones; therefore, "English" medicines are often used by laymen only to a limited extent with the very young and the very old, who are considered too weak to tolerate the potent "English" medicines (Tseng 2003b). In many societies, including India, it is generally viewed that injectable agents, in contrast to oral, are more potent and have more immediate effects (Tseng 2003b). Clearly, there are distinct differences among people of different ethnic and/or racial backgrounds, but such diversity has superimposed on it interindividual diversity.

14.6 Factors Influencing Quality of Life in Schizophrenia in India

Psychopathology and severity of symptoms – Many studies have reported inverse correlation between severity of symptoms and quality of life (Chaturvedi et al. 1995; Awad et al. 1995; George et al. 1996; Gupta et al. 1998; Hansson et al. 1999; Browne et al. 2000; Solanki et al. 2008, 2010; Patra and Mishra 2012). Several authors have reported that negative QOL/subjective well-being correlates more strongly with depression and anxiety than with psychotic symptoms (Awad et al. 1995; Ritsner et al. 2003). Patra and Mishra (2012) observed that more severe positive as well as negative symptoms predicted a poorer quality of life as positive symptoms show statistically significant negative correlation with QOL in psychological domains. Poorer QOL was also reported to be related to negative symptoms (Solanki et al. 2008; Gupta et al. 1998). Another Indian study observed that cognitive deficits were more in those with predominant negative symptoms and the cognitive deficits were found to add to the poor quality of life of persons with schizophrenia (George et al. 1996). Persons without employment and of rural background had significantly greater cognitive deficits. The authors concluded that if a patient in spite of the chronic illness has cognitive abilities well preserved, the patient may have a better quality of life and social functioning. Helping the patients to overcome or improve their cognitive functions may help in elevating the quality of life and better day-to-day functioning (George et al. 1996).

Insight – The presence of insight in schizophrenia was associated with lower QOL scores in the physical, psychological, and environmental domain, but higher scores on the social domain (Radhakrishnan et al. 2012).

Psychosocial and demographic factors – Many psychosocial and demographic factors influence QOL of an individual. No significant sex differences were reported in studies from developing countries (Aleman et al. 2003). However, it was observed that the clinical remission and recovery was higher in females as compared to males (Carpiniello et al. 2012). In a study done by Patra and Mishra 2012, male gender, unmarried status, and more than 10 years of schooling showed poorer QOL in physical and psychological domains of World Health Organization Quality of Life (WHOQOL) (The WHOQOL Group 1994, 1995). Female gender, married status, and lower educational attainment were associated with better QOL with only environmental domain of WHOQOL being adversely affected.

People with schizophrenia in low- and middle-income countries are more likely to be employed than their Western counterparts. An annual rate of employment was found to be 63–73 % in the first 10 years of follow-up of schizophrenia (Srinivasan and Thara 1997). Moreover, among untreated Indian people with schizophrenia, almost one-third were employed (Padmavathi et al. 1998). Generally, high employment rates (up to 75 %) have been found in India (Thara et al. 2004). Solanki et al. (2008) reported about 30 % of patients with schizophrenia to be unemployed. QOL was better in those who were educated and employed (Murali et al. 1995). Solanki et al. 2008 observed that occupation had negative correlation with social relationship domain of QOL. This observation can be attributed to strong family ties and social support system in developing countries, and employed individuals have aspirations for decent housing and social relationship.

Most studies from the West have reported low rates of marriage for people with schizophrenia (Nanko and Moridaria 1993; Harrison et al. 2001). In contrast, a 10-year follow-up study (Thara and Eaton 1996) from India found a high marital rate (70 %). Married individuals have better outcome and quality of life (Thara et al. 2003).

Duration of untreated psychosis – Duration of untreated psychosis (DUP) is associated with poorer outcome, with the relationship being strongest in the initial months of psychosis (Drake et al. 2000). Large numbers of patients come late for treatment in developing countries owing to lack of awareness, a strong belief in magico-religious causes, poor accessibility to health-care systems, and lack of community care (Isaac et al. 1981; Padmavathi et al. 1998). There is also evidence that in low- and middle-income (LAMI) countries, a substantial proportion of patients with psychosis seek treatment from traditional healers and use indigenous methods based on their non-biomedical beliefs or pathways to care. In clinical practice, we do encounter patients who have had previous episodes of psychosis which remitted spontaneously or by indigenous methods (Chaturvedi 2009). A substantial portion of patients with schizophrenia remain untreated in India due to poor mental health resources and awareness. Consequently, many patients become homeless and end up living on streets as vagabonds, beggars, or as sadhus (hermits). Increasingly, many families are no longer willing to take care of mentally ill relatives so they end up on the streets. This has more to do with the transition in the Indian society as the strong family and social networks that used to provide support to people with mental illness are breaking down.

Side effects due to medications – Antipsychotic agents have a wide range of adverse effects and can cause lots of emotional distress in a patient. Extrapyramidal symptoms (EPS) are especially seen with conventional antipsychotic agents, and in the acute phase, EPS, in particular akathisia and Parkinsonism, and, in chronic phase, tardive dyskinesia have been associated with deteriorating QOL/subjective well-being (Chaturvedi et al. 1995; Solanki et al. 2008; Patra and Mishra 2012). Besides EPS, adverse effects such as weight gain, sedation, and sexual dysfunction are also associated with poor QOL/subjective well-being (Hofer et al. 2002 & Allison et al. 2003). The cultural aspects of such side effects have been discussed above.

Religion, spirituality, and quality of life in schizophrenia – Both religion and spirituality play an important role in the lives of Indians including persons with mental illness. Many Indians use religion and spirituality to cope up with mental illnesses. Religion and spirituality encourages healthy lifestyle and also provides various avenues for social support. Religion and spirituality also determine the outcome

Table 14.1 Sociodemographic and clinical correlates of QOL

1.	Female gender, married status, being educated/employed are associated with better QOL
2.	Inverse correlation between severity of symptoms and quality of life
3.	Cognitive deficits/negative symptoms contribute toward poor QOL
4.	Side effects like weight gain, EPS, sedation, and sexual dysfunction are associated with poor quality of life
5.	Religious/spiritual practices improve QOL
6.	Indigenous methods of treatment complement modern medicine ["Dawa (medication) and/ or Dua (blessing)"]

and quality of life in schizophrenia (Grover et al. 2014). Religion and spirituality are associated with better clinical outcome and reduction in relapse rate (Huguelet et al. 1997; Mohr et al. 2011). Positive religious coping has also been associated with higher quality of life in the domain of psychological health (Shah et al. 2011; Nolan et al. 2012). The WHO considers spirituality, religion, and personal beliefs as an important area in the evaluation of the quality of life (Grover et al. 2014). Shah et al. (2011) reiterated that apart from pharmacological and non-pharmacological interventions, psychiatrists should also assess spiritual and religious domains and encourage their patients to follow their religious practices and spiritual beliefs. Spiritual QOL is another important dimension, which needs to be considered, both for the persons with schizophrenia and their caregivers.

An Indian study documented that many patients access the services of faith healers in order to cure their mental illness (Kulhara et al. 2000). Another study from South India found out that 58 % of the patients afflicted with psychosis seek the services of faith healers before accessing psychiatric services (Campion and Bhugra 1997). Traditional healing methods are known to complement modern medicine in treatment of psychiatric disorders (Saravanan et al. 2008). Religious and spiritual domains have largely been ignored in psychiatric assessment. Psychiatrists need to be empathetic toward the religious and spiritual needs of the patients as unfulfilled spiritual needs of the patient adversely affect the outcome and in turn quality of life of these patients (Clark et al. 2003).

The important sociodemographic and clinical factors associated with QOL of schizophrenia in India are summarized in Table 14.1.

14.7 Measurement of QOL in a Cultural Context: Examples from India

In a country where concept of QOL had a late entry in mental health care, measurement of QOL was an even more distant issue. Initially, Western instruments were employed, with or without linguistic and cultural adaptations. Clinicians and researchers noted items in the Western scales were not easily understandable and inappropriate. One of the major challenges lies with the international and cross-cultural development and use of quality-of-life measures, especially in mental health. During the process of cross-cultural instrument development, the concept of differential item functioning (DIF) is important for understanding the implications of minimizing or enhancing cross-cultural DIF (Bullinger et al. 2007). To address the issue of cross-cultural QOL instrument development, two methods have been employed – culture-free instruments (by identifying and eliminating culture-specific responses to items) and culture-sensitive instruments (by explicitly attending to and sometimes enhancing culture-specific responses). Both methods are useful but for different purposes. WHOQOL, long, and BREF versions have been cross-culturally validated (15 countries including India) instruments that have also been translated into Hindi with crosslinguistic equivalence, but there have been conceptual and scalar concerns (Saxena et al. 2005). Majority of the Indian studies on QOL in schizophrenia have used WHOQOL-BREF. Quality of Life Interview (QOLI) (Lehman 1998) (modified as per the Indian cultural background) has demonstrated convergent validity with a disease-specific instrument Quality of Life Scale (QLS) as well as a generic instrument, WHOQOL-BREF (Lobana et al. 2002). Generic scales such as Quality of Life Enjoyment and Life Satisfaction Questionnaire (QOLES) (Endicott et al. 1993) and schizophrenia-specific scales such as Quality of Life Self-Report 100 (QLS100) (Skantze et al. 1992) and Quality of Life Scale (QLS) (Heinrichs et al. 1984) have also been used in Indian researches (George et al. 1996; Gupta et al. 1998) (Table 14.2).

Interestingly, a study documented that in an Indian setting subjective and objective assessments of QOL can be substituted for each other (Lobana et al. 2001). This may not be true for individual domains of activity such as finances, social relations, and daily activities. There is a greater degree of agreement between the patient and the caregiver about QOL suggesting that relatives may be used to provide proxy ratings for QOL in an Indian context (Lobana et al. 2001).

In a multicentric study conducted across India, needs as reported by patients with severe mental illness including schizophrenia were those of money, welfare benefits, transport, information about the illness and treatment, relief of psychological distress, company, household skills, and intimate relationships (Grover et al. 2015). Patients with chronic mental illnesses, including schizophrenia, from rural areas did not avail any disability benefits other than the disability pension disbursed by the state (Kashyap et al. 2012). Schizophrenia accounted for highest number of certifications for disability. Majority of the patients who seek disability benefits are males though levels of disability are comparable in males and females. Work-related disability is relatively higher among males; and females continue to be financially dependent on the family members (Balhara et al. 2013). The impact of these disability benefits on QOL has not been reported.

Poor subjective well-being was reported by patients with schizophrenia in another study from India (Kumar et al. 2013). Indian caregivers perceived difficulties in several areas such as finance, family relationship, well-being, and health, but they still perceived burden to be lesser compared to Malaysian counterparts (Talwar and Matheiken 2010). The extent of burden among families of schizophrenic patients was found to be more than those of bipolar disorder in Hyderabad, southern India (Narasipuram and Kasimahanti 2012). The spouses of patients with schizophrenia

Table 14.2 Indian studies on quality of life in patients

Authors	Description	Results	Cultural factors
Radhakrishnan et al. (2012)	Compared QOL in 50 patients each with systemic lupus erythematosus (SLE) and schizophrenia using the WHOQOL-BREF scale	QOLs in schizophrenia and SLE were comparable on all domains except the social domain; the factors that mediate QOL in both these illnesses were different	Insight associated with poorer QOL in physical, psychological, and environmental domain, but higher scores on the social domain
Patra and Mishra (2012)	Psychopathology and quality of life were assessed in patients attending outpatient department. WHOQOL-BREF scale, the positive and negative syndrome scale (PANSS) (Kay et al. 1987) were used	Male gender, unmarried status, and higher educational status predicted a poorer quality of life	Marriages considered a sacred union. This might explain better QOL among married
Dan et al. (2011)	Sixty patients with schizophrenia were divided into two groups (with and without depression) and were assessed on Lehman Quality of Life Interview (QOLI) – Brief Version for QOL	General psychopathology had significant effect, whereas depression had no significant effect on QOL in patients with schizophrenia	Social support attributed to strong family bonding and social support system in Indian culture
Solanki et al. (2010)	Fifty obsessive-compulsive disorder (OCD) and 47 schizophrenia subjects were evaluated on the WHOQOL-BREF, the global assessment of functioning scale, and the Indian disability evaluation assessment scale	No difference between the two groups on QOL domains. OCD patients had lower disability	Perception of quality of life among Indian patients might differ from that of persons living in developed countries
Solanki et al. (2008)	Fifty patients diagnosed with schizophrenia were evaluated on the WHOQOL-BREF and PANSS	Poor QOL in patients with schizophrenia despite improvement in symptoms	Only 30 % patients were found to be unemployed
Lobana et al. (2001)	Subjective and objective QOL assessed in 38 patients with schizophrenia using the Quality of Life Interview – Brief Version and WHOQOL-BREF. Family members were also interviewed	Both objective and subjective QOL scores correlated well with total QOL scores. Similar degree of correlation was found between patients and their relatives	In Indian setting, Subjective QOL (SQOL) and Objective QOL (OQOL) can be substituted for each other

(continued)

Study	Methods	Findings	Comments
Gupta et al. (1998)	Quality of life (QOL) was assessed in three groups of patients, consisting of 30 schizophrenic patients with duration of illness <2 years, 30 schizophrenic patients with duration of illness more than 2 years, and 30 dysthymic patients using Quality of Life Enjoyment and Life Satisfaction Questionnaire (QOLES), brief psychiatric rating scale (BPRS), scale for the assessment of positive symptoms (SAPS), scale for the assessment of the negative symptoms (SANS), Hamilton depression rating scale (HDRS)	Poor QOL in schizophrenia and dysthymia despite significant improvement with pharmacological treatment. Dysthymic patients were significantly less satisfied than schizophrenic patients with duration of illness <2 years in the domain of physical health	Schizophrenia patients had greater satisfaction with regard to knowledge, education, and finance. Can be attributed to cultural factors as shared family environment, income, and the lack of emphasis on education
George et al. (1996)	120 chronic schizophrenic patients were included to assess their cognitive functions and quality of life, using mini-mental status examination, Quality of Life Scale, scale for assessment of positive symptoms, and scale for assessment of negative symptoms	Cognitive deficits greater in those without employment, those from the rural background, and those with predominant negative symptoms. Cognitive deficits added to the poor QOL of schizophrenia patients	Studied rural–urban differences in India
Chaturvedi et al. (1995)	120 patients of chronic schizophrenia assessed on mini-mental status examination, Quality of Life Scale, SANS, SAPS, and scale for assessment of family distress	QOL better in paranoid schizophrenia and those with low family distress. QOL poorer in those with negative symptoms	Low family distress explained by joint family system and strong familial bonds in India

were found to spend numerous care hours in a study at a tertiary center at Delhi (Kaushik and Bhatia 2013). Longer care hours significantly contribute to higher care burden and poor quality of life in caregivers.

Measurement of quality of life is important not only for patient care but also for allocation of mental health resources and formulating policies (Awad et al. 1997). Multiple scales measuring quality of life in patients with schizophrenia have been published and used for clinical as well as research purpose. Some of the measures available for assessment of QOL in the Indian setting are as follows (Chaturvedi et al. 2000):

1. PGI well-being scale (Hindi adaptation) (Verma et al. 1983)
2. Subjective well-being inventory (SUBI) (Sell and Nagpal 1992)
3. WHOQOL-100 and WHOQOL-BREF (WHOQOL Group 1994 & 1995; Saxena et al. 1998)
4. Quality of Life Scale for schizophrenia (Heinrichs et al. 1984)
5. EuroQol (EQ-5D) (The EuroQOL Group 1990)

For review of current Quality of Life Scales in use, please see Chapter 5, by Bobes and Bobes-Bascaran, as well as the reviews by Awad et al. 1997, Awad and Voruganti 2012.

Indian studies on persons with schizophrenia and their caregivers are summarized in Tables 14.2 and 14.3, including cultural factors identified in these studies.

14.8 Challenges in Measuring QOL in India

It is not an easy task to assess QOL in schizophrenia in the Indian setting. There is no absolute equivalent phrase for "quality of life" in Indian languages. The commonly used phrase *jeevan ki gunvatta* translates to properties of life or standard of living. No wonder there are numerous challenges in measuring QOL in mental health in India (Table 14.4) and in developing countries (Table 14.5). Some of these are:

Table 14.3 Indian studies on quality of life in caregivers

Authors	Description	Results	Cultural factors
Panigrahi et al. (2014)	QOL of 50 caregivers of schizophrenia patients evaluated using Quality of Life Enjoyment and Satisfaction Questionnaire, short form Q-LES-Q-SF	Parents had the poorest QOL compared to other caregivers. QOL moderately low in caregivers	Parents look after their offsprings with schizophrenia
Kate et al. (2014)	One hundred primary caregivers of patients with schizophrenia were assessed on WHOQOL-BREF, WHOQOL Spirituality, Religiousness, and Personal Beliefs (WHOQOL-SRPB scales) (WHOQOL-SRPB Group 2006) and family burden interview schedule and coping checklist	Those who use coercion frequently had poor QOL in the spiritual strength facet of WHOQOL-SRPB scale	QOL of caregivers influenced by spiritual factors

Table 14.4 Challenges in measuring QOL

1.	Limited psychometric properties
2.	Most of the tools available are too lengthy to use in clinical trials
3.	QOL is difficult to assess in children, depressed individuals, patients with comorbid intellectual disability, cognitive deficits, illiterate patients
4.	Spiritual and religious domains are largely neglected
5.	Measurement tools are not culturally congruent

Table 14.5 Challenges for QOL research in developing countries

1.	Most of the studies conducted in developing countries are of cross-sectional design
2.	Lower in hierarchy in terms of evidence-based research
3.	Almost all the studies are conducted in hospital settings
4.	Lack of universal consensus on definitions and domains of QOL
5.	Neglecting role of cultural, racial, and ethnic factors on QOL
6.	Subjective perception of QOL in developing countries is different

(i) The current QOL measures are often too lengthy for use in clinical trials, need to be completed by experts rather than the patient, are insensitive to clinical changes, or are limited in terms of psychometric properties (Wilkinson et al. 2000).

(ii) Some groups in which it is difficult to assess QOL are children, where subjective assessment is difficult due to inadequate cognitive development, elderly with cognitive deficits, and the illiterate (Chaturvedi et al. 2000).

(iii) An important but neglected dimension of quality of life is the spiritual dimension. A part of the difficulty also arises from the complexities in understanding or defining spiritual quality of life (Chaturvedi et al. 2000). As such, spirituality aspect is not probed in schizophrenia.

(iv) The instruments described above have been developed in Western countries, and many domains in these instruments may not be culturally congruent (Burns and Patrick 2007). Cultural factors play an important role in functional outcome of an individual. However, these factors have been largely ignored in these instruments.

(v) Moreover, self-reporting measures are vulnerable to biases, and there is growing discrepancy between subjective and objective dichotomies (Awad and Voruganti 2012). One of the important aspects of cross-cultural adaptation is to ensure semantic equivalence between the original tool and the adapted versions (Chandra 2000).

14.9 Critical Appraisal of Indian Research on QOL in Schizophrenia

The concept of "quality of life" has gained prime importance in psychiatry following deinstitutionalization and increased focus on recovery-oriented services. The concept of QOL is perhaps more important in psychiatric disorders as they have a chronic and debilitating course despite pharmacological management (Gupta et al. 1998). Most studies of QOL have been conducted in Western countries, and there is dearth of literature on quality of life in schizophrenia in developing countries. Cultural factors play an important role in influencing outcome of schizophrenia and hence quality of life (Kulhara 1994). Perception of quality of life is different in developing countries like India and Western countries. Indians give more importance to satisfaction, including peace of mind and spiritual aspects, unlike Europeans who give more emphasis on their physical and physiological needs, and functional aspects (Chaturvedi 1991). Measuring QOL solely on the basis of subjective reports has its own limitations because chronic mental illnesses can alter the perception of quality of life (Sainfort et al. 1996). QOL research faces many challenges like lack of universal consensus on definitions and domains of QOL, lack of psychometrically validated instruments, and neglecting role of cultural, racial, and ethnic factors on QOL (Gupta et al. 1998). In the past two decades, some Indian studies on QOL have been published. However, almost all of them had cross-sectional designs. Some studies had small sample sizes and were undertaken during the acute phase of the illness. Almost all the studies were conducted in hospital-based settings, and hence, findings are difficult to generalize in community settings (Patra and Mishra 2012). In some, WHOQOL-BREF was used which is a generic instrument and has not been designed specifically for schizophrenic patients (Solanki et al. 2010).

14.10   Improving Quality of Life of Patients with Schizophrenia and Caregivers in India

In the last decade, interest in quality of life has been generated due to two main reasons, firstly as part of the larger drive toward "health for all" and the promotion of physical, mental, and social well-being. Secondly, a fundamental rethinking of the goal of rehabilitation as an indicator of good QOL has been perceived by the patients and their relatives (Chaturvedi et al. 2000). In order to maintain a good QOL, the priorities and goals of an individual must be taken into consideration (Chaturvedi et al. 2000). To improve QOL, it is necessary to narrow down the gap between aspirations and current reality. Patients should be taught to bring down their expectations into tune with the current reality and encouraged to explore new areas of interest which are realistic and achievable (Vasudevan 2000). Clinically, it is observed that assessing quality of life systematically actually improves the patients' and families' satisfaction with care and their QOL.

The purpose of rehabilitation and recovery-oriented approach is to narrow this gap between expectations and achievements, by enhancing their potentials. The main objective of a psychiatric rehabilitation service is to contribute to the recovery by enhancing functioning in a role valued by society and selected by the individual (Anthony et al. 2002). Psychiatric rehabilitation comprises a wide range of interventions that target functional outcomes rather than control of illnesses and thereby helps in improving the quality of life. Rehabilitation starts right from the first time the patient has come into contact with a psychiatrist. A clinician should not wait for the patient to become asymptomatic (Chandrashekar et al. 2010). One study in India found out that 90 % of patients with schizophrenia desired rehabilitation in one form or another and most exhibited multiple needs (Nagaswami et al. 1985). However, in a developing country like India, psychiatric rehabilitation services are scarce and confined only to a few apex institutions. Early attempts at rehabilitation can improve the functioning and QOL of the patients as well as their caregiver in the long term (Channabasavanna 1987).

It is acknowledged that integrating mental health services with primary health services will go a long way in implementation of mental health services at grass root level. Focus should shift from mental hospitals to general hospital psychiatric units, private clinics, and community care at primary health-care level. These strategies will improve the accessibility to mental health services and therefore improve quality of life (Wig 1997). In India, besides the distressing symptoms in the mentally ill, a majority of mentally ill patients experience financial, domestic, social, and occupational difficulties. It also must be acknowledged that often the cost of treatment could possibly have a greater negative effect on the quality of subsequent life than any positive effect of the offered treatment. Essential antipsychotic drugs should be made easily available at all health-care levels.

14.11 Conclusions

Assessing and improving QOL of person with schizophrenia should be central goal of mental health care, and local traditional and sociocultural factors must be given due importance. To introduce QOL into routine mental health care, it is necessary to be explicit about its relevance to needs of health personnel, its usefulness for health-care industries and pharmaceuticals, its political value, and its progress in saving life and maintaining it. Preferably, local measures must be developed, to address local sociocultural aspects. The caregivers should not be neglected, and a good QOL of caregivers is important to maintain a good QOL of their patient. The staff stress and QOL of the mental health professionals does not get addressed often. QOL should become a routine clinical and research theme in the care of persons with schizophrenia in India also, as in many parts of the world.

References

Aleman A, Kahn RS, Selten JP. Sex differences in the risk of schizophrenia: evidence from meta-analysis. Arch Gen Psychiatry. 2003;60:565–71.
Allison DB, Mackem JA, McDonnel DD. The impact of weight gain on quality of life among persons with schizophrenia. Psychiatr Serv. 2003;54:565–7.
Anthony WA, Cohen MR, Farkas M, Gagne C. Psychiatric rehabilitation. 2nd ed. Boston: Boston University, Center for Psychiatric Rehabilitation; 2002.

Awad AG, Voruganti LN. Measuring quality of life in patients with schizophrenia. An update. Pharmacoeconomics. 2012;30:183–95.

Awad AG, Hogan TP, Voruganti LN, et al. Patients' subjective experiences on antipsychotic medications: implications for outcome and quality of life. Int Clin Psychopharmacol. 1995;10 Suppl 3:l23–32.

Awad AG, Voruganti LNP, Heslegrave RJ. Measuring quality of life in patients with schizophrenia. Pharmacoeconomics. 1997;11(1):32–47.

Balhara YP, Verma R, Deshpande SN. A study of profile of disability certificate seeking patients with schizophrenia over a 5 year period. Indian J Psychol Med. 2013;35:127–34.

Bobes J, Garcia-Portilla MP, Bascaran MT, et al. Quality of life in schizophrenic patients. Dialogues Clin Neurosci. 2007;9(2):215–26.

Browne S, Clarke M, Gervin M, et al. Determinants of quality of life at first presentation with schizophrenia. Br J Psychiatry. 2000;I76:I7.V6.

Bullinger M, Schmidt S, Naber D. Cross cultural quality of life research in mental health. In: Ritsner MS, Awad AG, editors. Quality of life impairment in schizophrenia, mood and anxiety disorders. 1st ed. Dordrecht: Springer; 2007. p. 67–98.

Burns T, Patrick D. Social functioning as an outcome measure in schizophrenia studies. Acta Psychiatr Scand. 2007;116:403–18.

Campion J, Bhugra D. Experiences of religious healing in psychiatric patients in south India. Soc Psychiatry Psychiatr Epidemiol. 1997;32(4):215–21.

Carpiniello B, Pinna F, Tusconi M, Zaccheddu E, Fatteri F. Gender differences in remission and recovery of schizophrenic and schizoaffective patients: preliminary results of prospective cohort study. Schizophr Res Treatment. 2012;2012:576369.

Chandra PS. Measurement in quality of life. In: Chaturvedi SK, Chandra PS, editors. Quality of life in health & disease. Bangalore: Malalur printers; 2000. p. 27–36.

Chandrasena R. Schneider's first-rank symptoms: an international and interethnic comparative study. Acta Psychiatr Scand. 1987;76:574–8.

Chandrashekar H, Prashanth NR, Kasthuri P, Madhusudhan S. Psychiatric rehabilitation. Indian J Psychiatry. 2010;52:S278–80.

Channabasavanna SM. Rehabilitation in psychiatry. Indian J Psychiatry. 1987;29:1.

Chaturvedi SK. Negative symptoms in schizophrenia: cross-cultural differences. Indian J Psychiatry. 1986;2:59–65.

Chaturvedi SK. What's important for QOL to Indians in relation to cancer. Soc Sci Med. 1991;33:92–4.

Chaturvedi SK. Duration of untreated psychosis in LAMI countries. Br J Psychiatry. 2009;194:188.

Chaturvedi SK, Murali T, Gopinath PS. Quality of life of chronic schizophrenics-II. In: Kalyansundaram S, Varghese M, editors. Innovations in psychiatric rehabilitation. Bangalore: The Richmond fellowship society (India); 1995. p. 233–6.

Chaturvedi SK, Savithasri EV, Rajashekhar K. Quality of life general concepts and research in India. In: Chaturvedi SK, Chandra PS, editors. Quality of life in health & disease. Bangalore: Malalur printers; 2000. p. 1–11.

Chugh PK, Rehan HS, Unni KE, Sah RK. Predictive value of symptoms for quality of life in first-episode schizophrenia. Nord J Psychiatry. 2013;67(3):153–8.

Clark PA, Drain M, Malone MP. Addressing patients' emotional and spiritual needs. Jt Comm J Qual Saf. 2003;29:659–70.

Craig TJ, Siegel K, Hopper S, et al. Outcome in schizophrenia and related disorders compared between developing and developed countries. A recursive partitioning re-analysis of the DOSMeD data. Br J Psychiatry. 1997;170:229–33.

Dan A, Kumar S, Avasthi A, Grover S. A comparative study on quality of life of patients of schizophrenia with and without depression. Psychiatry Res. 2011;189(2):185–9.

Drake RJ, Haley CJ, Akhtar S. Causes and consequences of duration of untreated psychosis in schizophrenia. Br J Psychiatry. 2000;177:511–5.

Endicott J, Nee J, Harrison W, Blumenthal R. Quality of life enjoyment and satisfaction questionnaire: a new measure. Psychopharmacol Bull. 1993;29:321–6.

Ganguli HC. Epidemiological finding on prevalence of mental disorders in India. Indian J Psychiatry. 2000;42:14–20.

Garg R, Chavan BS, Arun P. Quality of life after electroconvulsive therapy in persons with treatment resistant schizophrenia. Indian J Med Res. 2011;133:641–4.

George MR, Chaturvedi SK, Murali T, Gopinath PS, Rao S. Cognitive deficits in relation to quality of life in chronic schizophrenics. NIMHANS J. 1996;14:1–5.

Gopinath PS, Chaturvedi SK. Distressing behaviour of schizophrenics at home. Acta Psychiatr Scand. 1992;86:185–8.

Grover S, Davuluri T, Chakrabarti S. Religion, spirituality, and schizophrenia: a review. Indian J Psychol Med. 2014;36(2):119–24. doi:10.4103/0253-7176.130962.

Grover S, Avasthi A, Shah S, et al. Indian psychiatric society multicentric study on assessment of health-care needs of patients with severe mental illnesses. Indian J Psychiatry. 2015;57:43–50.

Gupta S, Kulhara P, Verma SK. Quality of life in schizophrenia and dysthymia. Acta Psychiatr Scand. 1998;97:290–6.

Hansson L, Middelboe T, Merinder L, et al. Predictors of subjective quality of life in schizophrenic patients living in the community. A Nordic multicentre study. Int J Soc Psychiatry. 1999;45:247–58.

Harrison G, Hopper K, Craig T. Recovery from psychotic illness: a 15- and 25-year international follow-up study. Br J Psychiatry. 2001;178:506–17.

Heinrichs DW, Hanlon TE, Carpenter WT Jr. The Quality of Life Scale: an instrument for rating the schizophrenic deficit syndrome. Schizophr Bull. 1984;10(3):388–98.

Hofer A, Kemmler G, Eder U, et al. Attitudes toward antipsychotics among outpatient clinic attendees with schizophrenia. J Clin Psychiatry. 2002;63:49–53.

http://www.ansi.gov.in/people_india.htm.

Huguelet P, Binyet-Vogel S, Gonzalez C, Favre S, McQuillan A. Follow-up study of 67 first episode schizophrenic patients and their involvement in religious activities. Eur Psychiatry. 1997;12(6):279–83.

ICMR. Collaborative study on severe mental morbidity report. New Delhi: Indian Council of Medical Research and Department of Science and Technology; 1987.

Isaac M, Kapur RL, Chandrasekhar CR. Management of schizophrenia patients in the community. An experimental report. Indian J Psychol Med. 1981;4:23–7.

Kashyap K, Thunga R, Rao AK, Balamurali NP. Trends of utilization of government disability benefits among chronic mentally ill. Indian J Psychiatry. 2012;54:54–8.

Kate N, Grover S, Kulhara P, Nehra R. Relationship of quality of life with coping and burden in primary caregivers of patients with schizophrenia. Int J Soc Psychiatry. 2014;60(2):107–16.

Kaushik P, Bhatia MS. Burden and quality of life in spouses of patients with schizophrenia and bipolar disorder. Delhi Psychiatry J. 2013;16(1):83–9.

Kay SR, Flszbein A, Opfer LA. The positive and negative syndrome scale (PANSS) for schizophrenia. Schizophr Bull. 1987;13:261–76.

Khandelwal SK, Jhingan HP, Ramesh S, Gupta RK, Srivastava VK. India mental health country profile. Int Rev Psychiatry. 2004;16(1–2):126–41.

Kujur NS, Kumar R, Verma AN. Differences in levels of disability and quality of life between genders in schizophrenia remission. Ind Psychiatry J. 2010;19:50–4.

Kulhara P. Course and outcome of schizophrenia: some transcultural observations with particular reference to developing countries. Eur Arch Psychiatry Clin Neurosci. 1994;244:227–35.

Kulhara P, Chakrabarti S. Culture and schizophrenia and other psychotic disorders. Psychiatr Clin North Am. 2001;24:449–64.

Kulhara P, Avasthi A, Sharma A. Magico-religious beliefs in schizophrenia: a study from north India. Psychopathology. 2000;33(2):62–8.

Kumar P, Nehra DK, Verma AN. Subjective well-being and coping among people with schizophrenia and epilepsy. Dysphrenia. 2013;4(1):25–30.

Leff J, Sartorius N, Jablensky A, Korten A, Ernberg G. The international pilot study of schizophrenia: five-year follow-up findings. Psychol Med. 1992;22(1):131–45.

Lehman AF. A Quality of Life Interview for the chronically mentally ill (QOLI). Eval Prog Planning. 1988;11:51–62.

Lobana A, Mattoo SK, Basu D, Gupta N. Quality of life in schizophrenia in India: comparison of three approaches. Acta Psychiatr Scand. 2001;104:51–5.

Lobana A, Mattoo SK, Basu D, Gupta N. Convergent validity of Quality of Life Interview (Qoli) in an Indian setting: preliminary findings. Indian J Psychiatry. 2002;44(2):118–24.

Loganathan S, Murthy SR. Experiences of stigma and discrimination endured by people suffering from schizophrenia. Indian J Psychiatry. 2008;50(1):39–46.

Loganathan S, Murthy RS. Living with schizophrenia in India: gender perspectives. Transcult Psychiatry. 2011;48(5):569–84.

Mohr S, Perroud N, Gillieron C, Brandt PY, Rieben I, Borras L, Huguelet P. Spirituality and religiousness as predictive factors of outcome in schizophrenia and schizo-affective disorders. Psychiatry Res. 2011;186(2–3):177–82.

Murali T, Chaturvedi SK, Gopinath PS. Quality of life of chronic schizophrenics-I. In: Kalyansundaram S, Varghese M, editors. Innovations in psychiatric rehabilitation. Bangalore: The Richmond fellowship society (India); 1995.

Nagaswami V, Valecha V, Thara R, Rajkumar S, Menon SM. Rehabilitation needs of schizophrenic patients. Indian J Psychiatry. 1985;27:213–20.

Nanko S, Moridaria J. Reproductive rates in schizophrenic outpatients. Acta Psychiatr Scand. 1993;87:400–4.

Narasipuram S, Kasimahanti S. Quality of life and perception of burden among caregivers of persons with mental illness. AP J Psychol Med. 2012;13(2):99–103.

Nolan JA, McEvoy JP, Koenig HG, Hooten EG, Whetten K, Pieper CF. Religious coping and quality of life among individuals living with schizophrenia. Psychiatr Serv. 2012;63(10):1051–4.

Padmavathi R, Rajkumar S, Srinivasan TN. Schizophrenic patients who were never treated a study in an Indian urban community. Psychol Med. 1998;28:1113–7.

Panigrahi S, Acharya RK, Patel MK, Chandrani KV. Quality of life in caregivers of patients with schizophrenia and its correlation with severity of illness. Int J Eng Science. 2014;3(6):55–60.

Patra S, Mishra A. Association of psychopathology with quality of life in acute phase of schizophrenia; an experience from east India. Ind Psychiatry J. 2012;21(2):104–8.

Radhakrishnan R, Menon J, Kanigere M, Ashok M, Shobha V, Galgali RB. Domains and determinants of quality of life in schizophrenia and systemic lupus erythematosus. Indian J Psychol Med. 2012;34:49–55.

Rai A, Khess CR, Bhattacharjee D, et al. Self-concept, stigma and quality of life in chronic schizophrenia and chronic skin disorders: a comparative study. Delhi Psychiatry J. 2014;17(1):65–73.

Reddy MV, Chandrashekar CR. Prevalence of mental and behavioral disorders in India: a meta-analysis. Indian J Psychiatry. 1998;40:149–57.

Ritsner M, Kurs R, Gibel A, et al. Predictors of quality of life in major psychoses: a naturalistic follow-up study. J Clin Psychiatry. 2003;64:308–15.

Sainfort F, Becker M, Diamond R. Judgments of quality of life of individuals with severe mental disorders: patient self-report versus provider perspectives. Am J Psychiatry. 1996;153:497–502.

Saravanan B, Jacob KS, Deepak MG, Prince M, David AS, Bhugra D. Perceptions about psychosis and psychiatric services: a qualitative study from Vellore, India. Soc Psychiatry Psychiatr Epidemiol. 2008;43(3):231–8.

Sartorius N, Jablensky A, Ernberg G, et al. Course of schizophrenia in different cultures: some results of a WHO international 5 year follow up study. In: Hafner H, Gattaz WF, Janzarik W, editors. Search for the cause of schizophrenia. Berlin: Springer; 1987. p. 107–13.

Saxena S, Chandiramani A, Bhargava R. WHOQOL-Hindi: a questionnaire for assessing quality of life in health care settings in India. Natl Med J India. 1998;11:160–6.

Saxena S, Quinn K, Sharan P, Naresh B, Yuantao H, Power M. Cross-linguistic equivalence of WHOQOL-100: a study from north India. Qual Life Res. 2005;14(3):891–7.

Sell H, Nagpal R. Assessment of subjective well being. New Delhi: World Health Organisation; 1992.

Shah R, Kulhara P, Grover S, Kumar S, Malhotra R, Tyagi S. Contribution of spirituality to quality of life in patients with residual schizophrenia. Psychiatry Res. 2011;190(2–3):200–5.

Shrivastava A, Johnston M, Terpstra K, et al. Atypical antipsychotics usage in long-term follow-up of first episode schizophrenia. Indian J Psychiatry. 2012;54:248–52.

Skantze K, Malm U, Dencker SJ, et al. Comparison of quality of life with standard of living in schizophrenia out-patients. Br J Psychiatry. 1992;161:797–801.

Solanki RK, Singh P, Midha A, Chugh K. Schizophrenia: impact on quality of life. Indian J Psychiatry. 2008;50:181–6.

Solanki RK, Singh P, Midha A, Chugh K, Swami MK. Disability and quality of life in schizophrenia and obsessive compulsive disorder: a cross sectional comparative study. East Asian Arch Psychiatry. 2010;20:7–13.

Srinivasan TN, Thara R. How do men with schizophrenia fare at work? A follow up study from India. Schizophr Res. 1997;25:149–54.

Talwar P, Matheiken ST. Caregivers in schizophrenia: a cross cultural perspective. Indian J Psychol Med. 2010;32(1):29–33.

Thara R, et al. Twenty-year course of schizophrenia: the Madras Longitudinal Study. Can J Psychiatry. 2004;49(8):564–9.

Thara R, Eaton WW. Outcome of schizophrenia: the Madras longitudinal study. Aust N Z J Psychiatry. 1996;30:516–22.

Thara R, Kamath S, Kumar S. Women with schizophrenia and broken marriages – doubly disadvantaged? I. Patient perspective. Int J Soc Psychiatry. 2003;49:225–32.

The EuroQol Group. EuroQol – a new facility for the measurement of health related quality of life. Health Policy. 1990;16:199–208.

The WHOQOL Group. Development of the WHOQOL: rationale and current status. Int J Ment Health. 1994;23:24–8.

The WHOQOL Group. The World Health Organization Quality of Life assessment (WHOQOL): position paper from the World Health Organization. Soc Sci Med. 1995;10:1403–9.

Tseng WS. Culture, behavior and pathology. In: Tseng WS, editor. Clinician's guide to cultural psychiatry. 1st ed. California: Academic; 2003a. p. 1–53.

Tseng WS. Ethnicity, culture and drug therapy. In: Tseng WS, editor. Clinician's guide to cultural psychiatry. 1st ed. California: Academic; 2003b. p. 343–52.

Vasudevan S. Quality of life in health and disease: a spiritual perspective. In: Chaturvedi SK, Chandra PS, editors. Quality of life in health & disease. Bangalore: Malalur printers; 2000. p. 12–7.

Verghese A, John JK, Rajkumar S, et al. Factors associated with the course and outcome of schizophrenia in India. Results of a two-year multicentre follow-up study. Br J Psychiatry. 1989;154:499–503.

Verma SK, Dubey BL, Gupta D. PGI general well being scale: some correlates. Indian J Clin Psychol. 1983;10:299–304.

Vishwanath B, Chaturvedi SK. Cultural aspects of major mental disorders: a critical review from an Indian perspective. Indian J Psychol Med. 2012;34(4):306–12.

WHOQOL SRPB Group. A cross-cultural study of spirituality, religion, and personal beliefs as components of quality of life. Soc Sci Med. 2006;62:1486–97.

Wig NN. Keynote address. In: Kulhara P, Avasthi A, Verma S, editors. Schizophrenia-Indian scene. Mumbai: Searle (India); 1997.

Wilkinson G, Hesdon B, Wild D, et al. Self-report quality of life measure for people with schizophrenia: the SQLS. Br J Psychiatry. 2000;177:42–6.

World Health Organization. WHOQOL-BREF: introduction, administration, scoring and generic version of the assessment, field trial version. Geneva: World Health Organization; 1996.

Part IV
Reinventing Quality of Life in Schizophrenia

Chapter 15
Reinventing Quality of Life: Refining the Concept and Going Beyond Assessments

A. George Awad

In spite of the broad popularity of the concept of quality of life in medicine and generally in its broad societal usage, why then is the interest in measuring quality of life in schizophrenia has been somewhat eroded in recent years? Obviously, there is no single answer to such a challenging question, but it seems to relate to a number of issues specific to the schizophrenia disorder itself and its impact on a wide range of mental deficits, as well as the impact of its treatment, i.e., the various and significant side effects of antipsychotic medications. Equally significant is the lack of research interest to go beyond assessments of quality of life into the broader applications that can impact clinical management and other important health outcomes. The excellent contributions to this book by the various internationally known experts in the field, coming from a broad range of theoretical and scientific background, all attest that the concept of quality of life in schizophrenia is alive and continues to be of great interest, but requires to be invigorated. New conceptual thinking, refinement of methodology, and going beyond measurement, into researching models for integration in clinical care as well as in pharmaco- and health economics, are all needed.

15.1 Refining the Concept of Quality of Life in Schizophrenia and Improving Measurements

Schizophrenia is widely recognized to impact on a number of important mental domains and behavior and also on several aspects of functioning. Its management, including the benefits and limitations such as the broad range of side effects of

A.G. Awad
Department of Psychiatry, The Institute of Medical Science, University of Toronto,
Toronto, ON, Canada
e-mail: gawad@hrh.ca

© Springer International Publishing Switzerland 2016
A.G. Awad, L.N.P. Voruganti (eds.), *Beyond Assessment of Quality of Life in Schizophrenia*, DOI 10.1007/978-3-319-30061-0_15

219

medicines, as well as the frequent inadequacy of psychosocial and vocational support, is at play, effecting the eventual outcome. In other words, the multidimensionality of the schizophrenia disorder and its treatment requires integrative multidimensional conceptual approaches, both theoretical and clinical. As is clear in this book and from the literature at large, there is a noticeable deficit in formulating conceptual models that can clarify the underpinnings of the concept itself and also informs the development of better scales based on well-tested models. The few models that have been proposed so far, unfortunately, did not get adequate attention nor have been vigorously tested.

15.2   Quality of Life in Schizophrenia as a Biopsychosocial Construct

Historically, the concept of quality of life has been conceived as a psychosocial phenomenon. Appraisal of quality of life in general requires accurate judgment by the patients of their inner feelings as well as their state of well-being and level of satisfaction, all requiring a degree of cognitive and affective intactness. Such a requirement is not only important for reliability of the assessments but also to enable the person to interact effectively with their environment. Significant alterations of such brain functions can impact negatively on patients' appraisal of their level of satisfaction. Additionally, antipsychotic medications can frequently lead to affective blunting in addition to an altered mood state, such as subjective dysphoric reactions. Recently, in a neuroimaging experimental design, we clarified the role of dopamine in the genesis of neuroleptic-induced dysphoric and affective states in schizophrenia (Voruganti and Awad 2006, Voruganti et al. 2001). It is now widely accepted that the neurobiological basis for the schizophrenia disorder itself continues to be related to dopamine, in large part. It is well known that dopamine has also been implicated in the mediation of pleasurable responses, as well as in reward and reinforcement behavior (Voruganti and Awad 2007). It is accepted that the meso-limbic and mesocortical dopamine systems in the brain are the neurobiological substrate associated with varied subjective responses to drugs. Alteration in these systems, either by disease such as schizophrenia or drugs, can lead to negative subjective responses that include altered mood states. With the evolving data about the negative impact of depression and altered mood states on assessment of quality of life (see Chap. 9 by Karow et al.), one cannot escape the need for broadening the concept of quality of life to include a neurobiological component. Another line of research is to explore the impact of cognitive impairment on quality of life. Unfortunately, the data continues to be conflictual, likely as a result of methodological issues and how the concept of quality of life is either measured subjectively or objectively. Using "objective" measures, cognitive functioning seems to correlate with quality of life, while such a relationship seems to be absent when subjective approaches for assessment of quality of life are used.

Recently, a study seems to suggest that some of the new-generation antipsychotics seem to correlate quality of life with symptomatic improvement, meaning that some antipsychotics may have a direct neurobiological impact on quality of life beyond their impact through symptomatic improvement (Philips et al. 2006). Obviously, association cannot be interpreted as causation, and one study cannot be construed as proof, particularly that the study in question was part of a pharmaceutical clinical trial for a new antipsychotic. We believe that the issue raised is important and of worth for future explorations, but it requires a more rigorous and purpose-built design.

15.3   Models for Integration of Quality of Life in Clinical Care Plans

One of the major reasons that contributed to the decline in interest in quality of life measurement in schizophrenia is the lack of models that integrate quality of life assessment in clinical care. As presented in Chap. 10 by Giacco and Priebe, it is possible to develop protocols which can do that. One of the early conceptual models proposed by Calman (Calman 1984) lends itself easily to integrate quality of life in care plans. As quality of life is identified according to that model as the gap between expectations and actual accomplishment, this provides an excellent framework in which expectations in clinical care are identified a priori by the patient, their family, and the clinicians. Obviously, expectations have to be reasonable, practical, and achievable. The advantage of such a model is that it involves the patients in their own care and also puts some responsibility on the patient to share with clinicians in the achievement of their own recovery: Clinical improvement is then judged relative to the predefined expectations. This is just an example of one model. Schizophrenia as a multidimensional disorder can provide several opportunities for development of a broad range of conceptual formulations. Without demonstrating that quality of life can impact clinical care, the concept will remain remote and perceived as not practical.

15.4   Quality of Life: Pharmaco- and Health Economics

Quality of life in schizophrenia is not only a desirable outcome but also can be a mediator of other important outcomes such as satisfaction and adherence to therapeutic regimens, including antipsychotic medications. On the other hand, very few clinical trials of new antipsychotics included any serious assessment of quality of life and, if any, frequently were included as an afterthought. The pharmaceutical industry has been reluctant to include such assessments, particularly that it has not been required by regulatory agencies. There has also been the prevailing skepticism about the reliability of patients' self-reports, as well as adequacy of measurement tools. Recently, regulatory bodies indicated their willingness to consider accepting quality of life data in the process of approving applications for new antipsychotics, provided the reliability of methodology is assured. Indeed, the FDA in the last few years has issued guidance documents for such submissions, in the context of patient-reported outcomes (see Chap. 11 by Buller and Sapin). That not only opens the door but also invites researchers to refine and improve methodological issues in the assessment and interpretation of quality of life data.

Similarly, quality of life needs to play a significant role in health policy and pharmacoeconomics. The rising cost of health care is evolving as a societal concern, and one way for cost containment is to prove the value of various interventions. Cost-effectiveness analysis, unfortunately, has not been broadly applied in psychiatric disorders and much less so in schizophrenia. Cost-utility analysis is one of the many economic approaches that has the advantage of combining cost and quality of life. We believe there is enough evidence to demonstrate the feasibility of cost-utility approaches in schizophrenia, though we admit that it can benefit from further refinement, which can come from further research as well as the close collaboration of clinicians and health economists. There is also a need for a standardized approach toward data analysis, in order to make comparison of data more reliable and predictable (see Chap. 12 by Awad and Voruganti). Using quality of life for health resource allocation makes a good deal of sense and serves the interest of the individual and the society, yet it requires a good deal of advanced and standardized methodological approaches, as well as political will and leadership (see Chap. 13 by Holloway and Carson).

15.5   Quality of Life and Economic and Cultural Differences Across Societies

It is recognized that there exists wide cultural and economic differences among various societies which can significantly impact on the expectations of quality of life. Well-developed societies with their ability to provide better health care, as well as reasonable rehabilitation programs, housing, and economic support, make it possible to require a higher level of quality of life. In less developed economic societies, with their limited health care and economic systems, the content and meaning of "quality of life" can be different, at least in terms of health attributes and standards of living. This inevitably may introduce the notion of the "relativity" of the construct of quality of life. Though the expectations of quality of life will continue to be the same everywhere else, the psychosocial determinants may look different or may include unique components such as spirituality and cultural and religious beliefs, as illustrated by the comprehensive case study from India (see Chap. 14 by Chaturvedi et al.). This makes the most important point that any transcultural assessment of quality of life has to include the "individual self-assessment" in addition to other standards of living determinants.

15.6   Use of New Electronic Technologies for Improving Outcome Assessments and New Scale Development

The rapid development and introduction of new electronic technology provide an opportunity in experience sampling methods, which allow having patients' experiences in real time, which can supplement traditional retrospective assessments (see Chap. 8 by de Wit et al.). It can provide a reliable longitudinal self-report. It can save time and cost of conducting clinical trials and also can standardize the time of sampling among participants. Obviously, the disadvantage is that it eliminates face-to-face contact between the research subject and the investigator. On the other hand, it makes it possible to have multiple measurements that can help in establishing patterns. We believe that the new advances in electronic technology need to be embraced rather than feared, as the net benefits are expected to outweigh any disadvantages.

Development of new measurement scales using new modern information theories, computer adaptive technology, and item banks can enhance the reliability of measurement tools (see Chap. 7 by Bjorner and Bech). It can make the process of measurement more predictable and also can provide standardized common metrics that can enhance comparative effectiveness.

15.7   Clarification of Terminology

It is obvious that the field needs clarification of many terms that are frequently in use to avoid misconceptions, such as what is meant by "objective measure." What is needed is the development of an agreed-upon "Glossary of Terms" in quality of life in schizophrenia that researchers and journal editors adhere to.

In conclusion, we are grateful for all the contributors of this book, for their unique insights and expertise which, hopefully, can be the beginning of a serious conversation about reinvigorating the concept of quality of life in schizophrenia and other psychiatric disorders and make it an important contributor to quality care and also a tool for making rational health policy decisions and appropriate resource utilization.

References

Calman KC. Quality of life in cancer patients – an hypothesis. J Med Ethics. 1984;10:124–7.

Philips GA, Van Brunt DL, Roychowdhury SM, Xu W, Naber D. The relationship between quality of life and clinical efficacy from a randomized trial comparing olanzapine and ziprasidone. J Clin Psychiatry. 2006;67:1937–403.

Voruganti LNP, Awad AG. Subjective and behavioural consequences of striatal dopamine depletion in schizophrenia - Findings from an in vivo SPECT study. Schizophre Res. 2006;88:178–86.

Voruganti LNP, Awad AG. Role of dopamine in pleasure, reward and subjective responses to drugs – the neuropsychopharmacology of quality of life in schizophrenia. In: Ritsner M, Awad AG, editors. Quality of life impairment in schizophrenia, mood and anxiety disorder. Dordrecht: Springer; 2007. p. 21–31.

Voruganti LNP, Slomka P, Zabel P, Costa G, So A, Mattar A, Awad AG. Subjective effects of AMPT - induced dopamine depletion in schizophrenia: Correlation between dysphoric responses and striatal D2 binding ratios on SPECT imaging. Neuro Psychopharmacology. 2001;25:642–50.

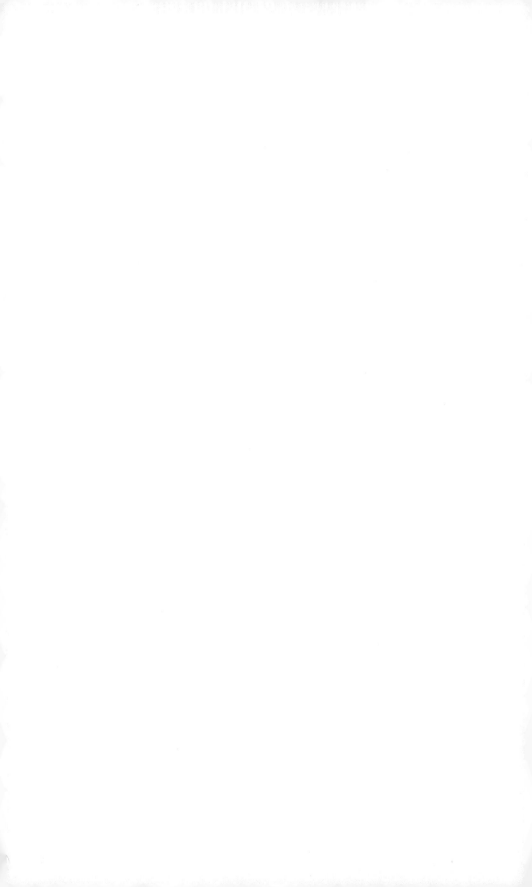

Printed in the United States
By Bookmasters